T0369648

Advance Praise Page

"This is a careful, detailed look at the Chinese response to COVID-19 that sheds much light on what happened. It also uncovers many lessons not only for China but for every country—and we can only hope the world learns them."—John Barry, author of *The Great Influenza*

"In *Wuhan*, Dali Yang provides a riveting and comprehensive account of how SARS-CoV-2 emerged and evolved into a global pandemic. By focusing on the dynamics that led to the initial outbreak spiraling out of control, the book highlights the bureaucratic-pathological tendencies in China's policy process. *Wuhan* will undoubtedly capture the interest of students of public health, public policy, and Chinese politics, while also holding relevance for anyone deeply concerned about the future of our planet."—Yanzhong Huang, Council on Foreign Relations

"In this remarkable book, Dali Yang offers a gripping account of the outbreak of COVID-19 in China: day by day, and even hour by hour. It will be the definitive account of the outbreak and the Chinese government's mishandling of it."—Bruce Dickson, George Washington University

"Dali Yang has been one of very top scholars of Chinese bureaucratic politics over the past 30 years. Now, he offers a comprehensive, straightforward, and accessible analysis of the recent era's most spectacular breakdown of Chinese bureaucracy during the early days of Covid . Looking at the granular unravelling of information gathering, inconsistency in messaging and ideological framing, and the shifting dynamics of central-local relations, he provides a compelling account of how China's most tragic governance failure in 40 years allowed the worst pandemic in a century to spiral out of control."—William Hurst, University of Cambridge

"Dali Yang has made a career of thinking dispassionately and insightfully about the Chinese Communist Party and the governance of China. This deeply informed and meticulous analysis of the vexed question of what happened in Wuhan in 2019–2020 is a priceless contribution to a heated debate."—Paul Monk, former head of the China desk in Australia's Defence Intelligence Organisation

"Dali Yang has given us the most detailed look yet at the early stages of the COVID outbreak in China. It is a book that only he could write, drawing on extensive primary evidence and decades of expertise on the politics of public health. This is one of the most important books on Chinese politics ever written."—Rory Truex, Princeton University

"Dali Yang has produced an urgent, compelling, readable account of how the COVID-19 crisis unfolded in China, and beyond. He pulls from a wide range of sources, including official communiques, lab reports, revealing social media threads that outran Chinese censors, and from first-hand accounts by many players close to the action. Yang's account of the crisis in China offers universal lessons and warnings on how people and governments process and use information during crises. In all, it makes for a kind of forensic/policy thriller that is also a tour de force of scholarship and reporting."—Ted C. Fishman, bestselling author of *China, Inc.*

"Thorough and thoughtful, *Wuhan* details the conflicts over information and between institutions that ultimately spiraled into the global COVID-19 pandemic. Dali Yang's deeply researched volume sheds new light on the early actions of the doctors, bureaucrats, officials, and politicians facing the novel coronavirus over these crucial weeks, deepening our understanding of its origins and politics in the country where it originated."—Jeremy Wallace, Cornell University

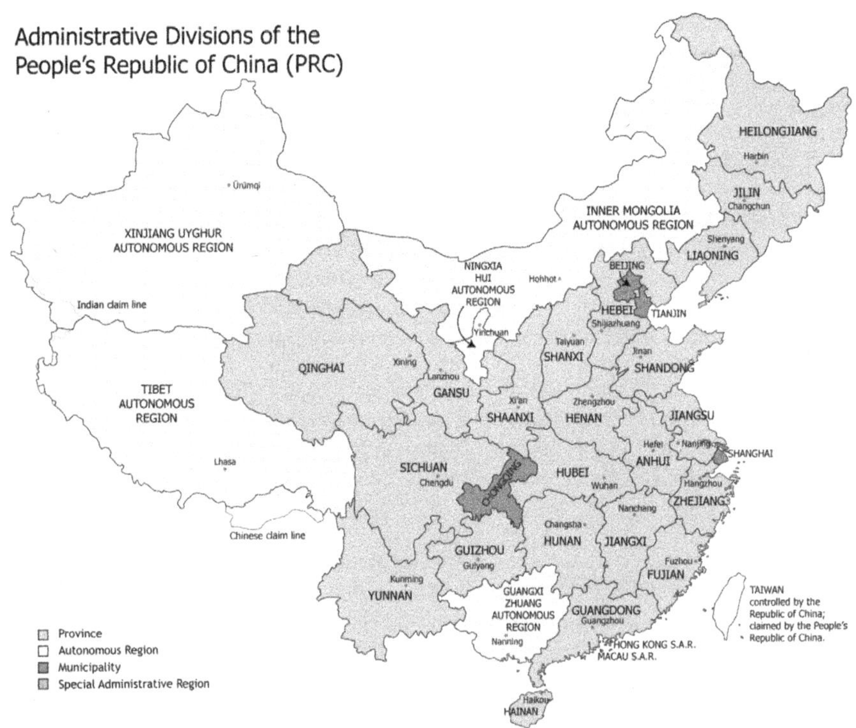
Administrative Divisions of the People's Republic of China (PRC)
HEILONGJIANG
Harbin
JILIN
Changchun
Ürümqi
INNER MONGOLIA AUTONOMOUS REGION
Shenyang
LIAONING
XINJIANG UYGHUR AUTONOMOUS REGION
NINGXIA HUI AUTONOMOUS REGION
Hohhot
BEIJING
Indian claim line
HEBEI
TIANJIN
Shijiazhuang
Yinchuan
Taiyuan
Jinan
QINGHAI
Xining
SHANXI
SHANDONG
Lanzhou
GANSU
TIBET AUTONOMOUS REGION
Xi'an
Zhengzhou
SHAANXI
HENAN
JIANGSU
Hefei
Nanjing
SHANGHAI
Lhasa
SICHUAN
Chengdu
CHONGQING
HUBEI
ANHUI
Wuhan
Hangzhou
Nanchang
ZHEJIANG
Chinese claim line
Changsha
HUNAN
JIANGXI
GUIZHOU
Guiyang
Fuzhou
FUJIAN
Kunming
YUNNAN
GUANGXI ZHUANG AUTONOMOUS REGION
Nanning
GUANGDONG
Guangzhou
TAIWAN controlled by the Republic of China; claimed by the People's Republic of China.
HONG KONG S.A.R.
MACAU S.A.R.
Haikou
HAINAN
Province
Autonomous Region
Municipality
Special Administrative Region

Wuhan

How the COVID-19 Outbreak in China Spiraled Out of Control

Dali L. Yang

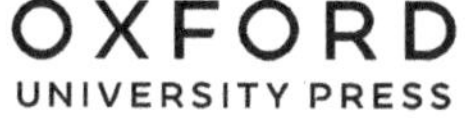
OXFORD
UNIVERSITY PRESS

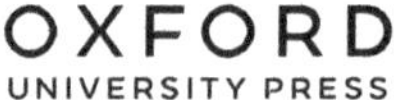

Oxford University Press is a department of the University of Oxford. It furthers the University's objective of excellence in research, scholarship, and education by publishing worldwide. Oxford is a registered trade mark of Oxford University Press in the UK and certain other countries.

Published in the United States of America by Oxford University Press
198 Madison Avenue, New York, NY 10016, United States of America.

Library of Congress Control Number: 2023033993

ISBN 978-0-19-775626-3

DOI: 10.1093/oso/9780197756263.001.0001

Printed and bound by CPI Group (UK) Ltd, Croydon, CR0 4YY

In Memoriam

Deng Xiuyun (1921–2019)
Huang Mingxia (1937–2020)

Contents

Figures and Tables

Acknowledgments

My father passed away when I was just a toddler. I only discovered in my college years that he succumbed to an infectious disease, which caused devastation in a remote corner of China where he had relocated our family before the Cultural Revolution. His passing prompted my mother's return to our hometown, with a toddler (i.e., me) in tow. This tragic trajectory, marked by trials and tribulations, inadvertently paved the way for my college admission in Beijing in 1979 and, subsequently, my pursuit of graduate education in the United States.

The profound impact of an infectious disease on my family ignited a fascination within me about the intersection of public health and politics. In the decade leading up to the COVID-19 pandemic, I engaged in a number of research projects on health politics in China, from the spread of HIV/AIDS in Henan to the politics of the severe acute respiratory syndrome (SARS) outbreak in 2003. In a twist of fate, I was undertaking field research in Beijing during the SARS crisis in the spring of 2003.

When news of the novel coronavirus outbreak in Wuhan emerged, I promptly integrated the ongoing crisis into my teaching and research, unaware then that documenting the unfolding epidemic would become a multi-year mission. The inception of this book is owed to Jessica Chen Weiss of Cornell University. Jessica took a liking to a Twitter thread I wrote on the handling of the outbreak in Wuhan and invited me to write for the *Washington Post Monkey Cage*, which she co-edited at the time. Space constraints necessitated cutting a significant section on China's central government response, an omission that gnawed at me and compelled me to delve deeper and present the full picture.

Ted Fishman, renowned author of *China Inc.*, and Charles Myers, then with the University of Chicago Press, offered unwavering support as I began to conceptualize this book project. As the city of Chicago went under a shelter-in-place order amid the spread of COVID-19, Ted, a fellow Hyde Park resident, and I bonded in our walks through the park, discussing our respective endeavors. Ted's patience, inquisitiveness, and insightful questions provided much-needed encouragement and served as a critical sounding board. Enid Rieser, my longtime neighbor, was an exemplar of living a resilient life during the pandemic. As my favorite local historian, she offered invaluable context to the pandemic when she related her family's experience with the great influenza of 1918–1919.

I am deeply indebted to the numerous individuals in China who generously granted me their time for interviews. Although they shall regrettably stay nameless, my gratitude toward them is no less profound. They entrusted me with their experiences and observations concerning government decision-making processes; operational procedures of organizations including local Centers for Disease Control and Prevention (CDCs), hospitals, and research organizations; as well as local community responses to the outbreak and subsequent lockdown. I gained invaluable insights from specialists associated with health commissions and CDCs at the national level, in Hubei and several other provinces, and in the cities of Wuhan, Beijing, Shenzhen, and Shanghai. Discussions with several eminent experts in Chinese law and regulation, based in Wuhan, Beijing, Shanghai, and Hong Kong, were tremendously enlightening.

Except for a few instances noted, I have used these interviews as deep background briefings. With the advantage of time, I have referenced materials and information that are formally published or accessible online in open sources. However, the interviews frequently guided me toward avenues of exploration that I might not have ventured into independently. I also drew inspiration from interviewees in China who expressed admiration for this project and urged me to bring it to fruition in order that China and the global community might benefit from the project's findings.

Given the restrictive environment in China regarding outbreak reporting, researching, and publishing, I want to express my sincere admiration and gratitude toward the brave journalists in China who covered the epidemic in Wuhan. These individuals faced not only the viral threat but also numerous other hurdles to report on the escalating crisis, shedding light on the inner operations of medical and health organizations and, more generally, on the outbreak and subsequent "war against the novel coronavirus." My profound gratitude also extends to the individuals who committed their time and energy and risked the wrath of the state to archive and preserve online Chinese publications and memories that were repeatedly made to disappear from websites in China.

My discussions with and the probing questions from numerous journalists writing in English and other languages, including, but not limited to, Chris Buckley, Jane Cai, Chao Deng, Jiayang Fan, Anna Fifield, Nectar Gan, Tom Hancock, Dake Kang, Ananth Krishnan, Lily Kuo, Jane Li, Jun Mai, Amy Qin, Austin Ramzy, Christian Shepherd, Gerry Shih, Helen-Ann Smith, Alice Su,

Jing Xuan Teng, Yew Lun Tian, Lingling Wei, and Sophia Yan, have enriched my understanding greatly.

I am incredibly fortunate to have benefited from the skilled editorial leadership of David McBride at Oxford University Press. Niko Pfund, the Press's president and academic publisher, took a distinct interest in this project and helped with the final iteration of the title. Phoebe Aldridge-Turner, the project manager, has been an absolute delight to collaborate with. Lavanya Nithya efficiently guided the project through production. Andrew Pachuta copy-edited the manuscript, offering varios suggestions for improvement.

The manuscript reviewers for Oxford University Press provided comprehensive and thoughtful critiques on the near-final version of the manuscript. Their challenging questions, engaging discussion on some of the most complex aspects of studying pandemic origins, and constructive recommendations served as essential scaffolding for the manuscript's revision.

Sara Doskow offered valuable feedback on an early draft of the manuscript. Ted Fishman, Michael Worobey, and William Parish made insightful comments on several draft chapters. Not only have I learned from Yanzhong Huang's significant writings on health governance in China, but our conversations on the COVID-19 pandemic have also been enriching. Joshua Lustig, the editor of *Current History*, extended an invitation to write about the zero-COVID regime, a task that was intellectually invigorating and allowed me to improve my perspective on the initial outbreak response.

Sections from this project were shared at the annual meetings of the American Political Science Association and the Association of Asian Studies and at workshops or seminars at Georgetown, Princeton, and Rutgers Universities. I am grateful to Thomas Banchoff, Xian Huang, Lizhi Liu, Ning Leng, Rory Truex, and the seminar participants for their invaluable comments and feedback.

The successful completion of this project owes a great deal to the intellectually stimulating environment provided by the University of Chicago. The foundation for much of my research was established during my tenure as the faculty director of the University of Chicago Center in Beijing. I owe a considerable debt of gratitude to the visionary leadership of the late president and chancellor Robert J. Zimmer. I'm profoundly grateful to David A. Greene and Provosts Thomas Rosenbaum, Eric Isaacs, Daniel Diermeier, and Ka Yee Lee for their encouragement and consistent support. My heartfelt appreciation extends to John Mark Hansen and Amanda Woodward, former and current deans of the Social Sciences Division, for their backing and to William Howell, chair of the Political Science Department, for his enlightened leadership.

Being a part of such a vibrant and resilient community, both offline and online, has been a privilege. Discussions with colleagues from diverse fields across campus, particularly the biological, physical, and social sciences, enriched my understanding of various aspects of the COVID-19 pandemic. I am particularly grateful to the following distinguished individuals in the medical field for their inspiration and invaluable assistance over the course of many years: Andrew Davis, Anne Hong, Michael Millis, Olufunmilayo Olopade, Kenneth S. Polonsky, Renslow Sherer, and Shu-Yuan Xiao. The opportunity to explore broad themes related to China and the COVID-19 pandemic with students in my courses on Chinese politics and public policy has been incredibly rewarding, and I am grateful for the engaging discussions and challenging questions that arose and the sense of community during pandemic times.

Over the summers of 2020–2023, I was fortunate to have two or three University of Chicago undergraduate students join me each year as Metcalf interns, including Evelyn Li, Catherine G. Lyons, Cynthia Ma, Jinhao Pan, Rachel Wang, Flannery Xu. They joined me to diligently track pandemic policies and responses and investigate special topics of interest. The 2022 cohort also offered valuable feedback on the draft chapters of the initial manuscript. Symonne Liu went beyond the call of duty to assist with proofreading. This Metcalf internship program has been supported by the University of Chicago's Office of Career Advancement, under the capacious leadership of Meredith Daw. I extend my special thanks to Chiara Montanari, Eugene Chan, and Katie Fassbinder for their effective program support.

My family has played a significantly more hands-on role in this project than in my previous works, providing a constant stream of love and inspiration. My wife, Ling, and I engaged in countless discussions about the pandemic responses during our strolls through the stunning natural landscapes of Jackson Park, a gem within the Chicago Park District. She often shared with me her discoveries about China's pandemic response and her observations on local developments in the Chicago area. Our children, Ethel, Claudia, and Edward, provided varied forms of support and were always eager to inquire about the book's progress and anticipated completion. They patiently listened to my passionate discourse on my findings and offered valuable feedback, each contributing insights from their unique perspectives.

This book is dedicated to the cherished memory of my mother-in-law and my mother, both of whom we sadly lost within months of each other in late 2019 and early 2020. My mother-in-law was a dedicated teacher who earned the respect of her many students and everyone fortunate enough to have known her. Born in 1921 and denied formal education, my mother weathered the most turbulent decades of China's long twentieth century. To her, I was a miracle child. There is not a day that goes by without my thoughts turning to her kindness, her insightful observations, and, above all, her magnanimous spirit.

My mother and mother-in-law would have been overjoyed to learn that, as I was concluding this book, Ethel and Jamie were uniting in matrimony, while my youngest child, Edward, followed in his sisters' footsteps and successfully graduated from college. As their generation steps into the future, I'm filled with hope and optimism. The wisdom and transformations ignited by the challenges of the COVID-19 pandemic have equipped them with valuable insights and resilience. My wish is that their generation will continue to make strides in shaping a world that is less burdened by war and infectious diseases.

Abbreviations

ARDS	acute respiratory distress syndrome
BAL	bronchoalveolar lavage
BMHC	Beijing Municipal Health Commission
CAMS	Chinese Academy of Medical Sciences
CCP	Chinese Communist Party (also CPC)
China CDC	Chinese Centers for Disease Control and Prevention (also CCDC)
CPLAC	Central Political and Legal Affairs Commission
CT	computed tomographic
ECMO	extracorporeal membrane oxygenation
fangkong	pinyin transliteration of the Chinese original short form for "prevention and control"
GDP	gross domestic product
GISAID	Global Initiative on Sharing All Influenza Data
HFMD	hand, foot, and mouth disease
HPHC	Hubei Provincial Health Commission
HUST	Huazhong University of Science and Technology (Wuhan)
ICDC	Institute for Communicable Disease Control and Prevention
ICU	intensive care unit
IVDC	Institute for Viral Disease Control and Prevention
JPCM	Joint Prevention and Control Mechanism (of the State Council)
MERS	Middle East respiratory syndrome
MOH	Ministry of Health
NHC	National Health Commission
NNDSS	National Notifiable Disease Surveillance System
PBSC	Politburo Standing Committee
PCCM	Pulmonary and Critical Care Medicine
PCR	polymerase chain reaction
PHEIC	public health emergency of international concern
PPC	Provincial People's Congress
PRC	People's Republic of China
PUE	pneumonia of uncertain etiology or pneumonia of uncertain cause
Q&A	question- and- answer
SARS	severe acute respiratory syndrome
SCEM	State Council Executive Meeting
SPHCC	Shanghai Public Health Clinical Center

TCM	traditional Chinese medicine
WCH	Wuhan Central Hospital
WHO	World Health Organization
WIV	Wuhan Institute of Virology (of the Chinese Academy of Sciences)
WMHC	Wuhan Municipal Health Commission
VPUE	viral pneumonia of uncertain etiology

Note on Names, Dates, Online Sources, and Translations

Chinese names are presented in the Chinese format, with the surname preceding the given name. For instance, in the name Zhong Nanshan, Zhong is the surname, not Nanshan. Exceptions exist for Chinese authors who publish in English and present their names in accordance with English-language conventions. Translations are by the author, unless otherwise indicated. Pinyin serves as the method for the transliteration of Chinese names and terms.

It should be noted that the nomenclature for the COVID-19 disease underwent multiple revisions during the Wuhan outbreak and lockdown. Generally, I refer to the terminology in use at that particular time. On February 7, 2020, the National Health Commission (NHC) of China named the disease 新型冠状病毒肺炎, or "novel coronavirus pneumonia" in English. However, on February 11, 2020, the World Health Organization referred to the disease as "coronavirus disease 2019 (COVID 19)." Subsequently, on February 22, 2020, the NHC announced that the English name would change to COVID-19, but the Chinese name would remain the same.

Due to censorship and technical issues, links to Chinese sources on numerous websites are often unreliable. In this book, the links to Chinese sources in the notes were checked and available as of September 1, 2023, unless otherwise noted. Readers outside of the People's Republic of China (PRC) can usually access the items no longer available at the original links by searching for the title, which will often lead to alternative sites with the same items.

Dates in the endnotes adhere to the ISO 8601 format, adopted by the International Organization for Standardization in 1988. Dates are written with the year first, followed by the month, and finally the day. For example, the first day of January 2020 is written as 2020-01-01.

1
Thinking about China's Response to the COVID-19 Outbreak

> A healthy society should not have only one voice.
>
> —**Dr. Li Wenliang**[1]

Dr. Zhong Nanshan was a national hero during the SARS (severe acute respiratory syndrome) epidemic in 2003. Based in Guangzhou, he correctly diagnosed that mysterious pneumonia disease as viral despite pressure from Beijing. He also spoke up about the severity of that outbreak when national officials sought to downplay it in early April 2003.

On January 20, 2020, the 83-year-old Dr. Zhong took on the awesome burden of breaking the bad news about the outbreak in Wuhan. For several days, Dr. Zhong had been on a multi-city emergency itinerary that included a high-profile expert visit to Wuhan and a whole day of meetings in Beijing on January 20. At 9:44 PM, the visibly exhausted Dr. Zhong appeared on the *News 1+1* program of China Central Television. Contrary to the obfuscations from Wuhan, he informed the audience bluntly that the novel coronavirus found in Wuhan, later named "SARS-coronavirus 2" (SARS-CoV-2), "is certainly transmissible from human to human." Health workers in Wuhan were among the infected, he noted. Confirming rumors that began to circulate in December 2019, Dr. Zhong observed that the patients' symptoms were like those for the much-dreaded SARS. He warned the public to put on facemasks and to not go to Wuhan.[2]

Seventeen years after the SARS crisis of 2002–2004, the *News 1+1* interview with Dr. Zhong became the first Chinese official communication of yet another novel coronavirus epidemic. It also marked the beginning of national mobilization in China.[3] In the morning of January 23, 2020, the Wuhan leadership, on the order of General Secretary and President Xi Jinping, sealed off Wuhan, a city of about 11 million people, from the rest of the country. The Wuhan lockdown would last 76 days.

By imposing the cordon sanitaire on Wuhan, China persuaded the World Health Organization (WHO) to refrain from immediately declaring the emergence of the novel coronavirus (2019-nCoV) a public health emergency of international concern (PHEIC). The PHEIC declaration happened on January 30, 2020. On February 11, 2020, the International Committee on Taxonomy of Viruses named the novel coronavirus first identified in Wuhan as "SARS-CoV-2" and thus a genetic sibling to the virus responsible for the SARS epidemic of 2003.[4] On the same day, the WHO named the disease caused by SARS-CoV-2 "coronavirus disease COVID-19," or COVID-19.

The WHO declared the COVID-19 outbreak a global pandemic exactly a month later. When Wuhan reopened on April 8, 2020, the COVID-19 pandemic was still in its infancy for the rest of the world. According to a WHO study, in its first 2 years (2020–2021) alone, the estimated worldwide death toll associated directly or indirectly with the COVID-19 pandemic was about 14.9 million (ranging from 13.3 to 16.6 million).[5] The COVID-19 pandemic had become the worst plague of the twenty-first century.[6]

*****

I was in Beijing for research on China's governance during the SARS crisis of 2003.[7] Like many others who had experienced the ups and downs of the SARS crisis, I was immediately hooked when the first pieces of information about an outbreak of SARS-like pneumonia cases in Wuhan began to circulate on Chinese social media on December 30, 2019.

The SARS crisis was the first pandemic of the twenty-first century.[8] It started in Guangdong, China at the end of 2002, and the coronavirus that caused SARS was believed to have jumped from wildlife such as civet cats to humans.[9] Before SARS was contained, the SARS-coronavirus (SARS-CoV-1) reached 29 countries and territories, spreading fear and destruction along the way. In Beijing, authorities concealed the outbreak from the public for weeks, at one point putting some patients in ambulances roaming around the city when a WHO expert mission made hospital visits.[10] In late April 2003, China's newly installed leaders Hu Jintao and Wen Jiabao sacked Health Minister Zhang Wenkang and Beijing mayor Meng Xuenong and unleashed a massive public campaign against SARS. As part of the campaign, the city of Beijing built the Xiaotangshan SARS Hospital, then the largest field hospital for the quarantine and treatment of infected patients, in about a week. By hard work and luck, the SARS crisis was over by summer 2003.

The SARS crisis left painful memories for China's leaders, healthcare professionals, and many members of the public.[11] It also helped catalyze important governance reforms in China, especially in public health.[12] Massive investments were made to enhance disease prevention and control capabilities, and the Chinese Centers for Disease Control and Prevention (China CDC) quickly built a nationwide online disease reporting and surveillance network system. Such capacity-building also helped to instill growing confidence in China's health emergency preparedness.

When information about an outbreak of SARS-like pneumonia cases in Wuhan began to circulate at the end of 2019, it was inevitable for people who had experienced SARS to draw on that experience to make sense of the new and unusual pneumonia cases. In fact, the clinicians credited with identifying the initial cases in Wuhan drew on their SARS experiences. Even though the Wuhan Municipal Health Commission (WMHC) quickly denied that the unusual pneumonia cases were SARS, there was high hope and a significant amount of trust among the Chinese public that Chinese health authorities had learned the lessons from the SARS crisis and would be better at handling the outbreak in Wuhan.

As I eagerly searched for what I could find about the outbreak in Wuhan on December 30, 2019, the SARS crisis loomed large in the back of my mind. Unlike in 2003, when information traveled much more slowly in China, a good amount of information from Wuhan quickly circulated on social media in real time. Some of the online postings included portions of lab reports that pointed to a SARS-like coronavirus.

Two red letter–headed WMHC emergency notices also circulated in WeChat groups. They made no mention of a SARS or SARS-like coronavirus but referred to cases of pneumonia of uncertain etiology (PUE) or cause associated with a certain Huanan Seafood Market in Wuhan. These notices directed hospitals to submit information on PUE cases to the WMHC and to mobilize resources for patient treatment. "If there's a SARS outbreak as in 2003, we'd expect the official response to escalate soon," I tweeted hopefully early that evening.[13]

In contrast with 2003, the national party-state media in China was heavily engaged with the outbreak in Wuhan as soon as it became public. By late in the evening (around noon Beijing time on December 31, 2019), I noted that "The Wuhan health authorities have spoken to strongly suggest it's not exactly SARS (of the 2003 kind)."[14] There were also reports from China that experts organized by the National Health Commission (NHC) and the China CDC had reached Wuhan to conduct investigations. The *People's Daily* post on Weibo, China's Twitter-like service, appeared at 11:56 AM (Beijing time, December 31, 2019):

> According to multiple hospital sources in Wuhan, the cause of [these viral pneumonia cases] is not yet clear; it cannot be concluded that it is the SARS virus

> rumored online but it is more likely some other severe pneumonia. Even if it is the SARS virus, there is a mature prevention and control treatment system in place, so the public need not panic.[15]

The *People's Daily* Weibo post allowed moderated comments. The first comment that users could see was also widely shared. It offered an enormously assuring message: "Wuhan has the world's top virology research institute, there's nothing to worry about, don't panic."[16]

As I digested these releases in Chinese official media, I couldn't help but notice the contrast between the diagnostic information of patients I could read from Chinese social media postings and the reassuring tone in the official releases.[17] This contrast gave me a premonition that all might not go as well as projected in the official media. At 10:42 PM, I wrote that "I was in Beijing in 2003 during the SARS outbreak and remember well how the authorities kept lying for weeks until they couldn't hide it anymore."[18] Though China learned strong lessons from the SARS crisis and made major investments to strengthen public health institutions and capabilities, my previous research also reminded me that China's multi-level party-state hierarchy often followed its own political-institutional logic, not that of the virus, and that leaders made decisions under the influence of various forms of cognitive bias.[19]

When there is very limited information, my research background in Chinese politics and governance and contacts in China have proven handy for making sense of what was going on in Wuhan and how the Hubei/Wuhan authorities interacted with central authorities.[20] Like millions of others, I was angered but not surprised by the crackdown on Dr. Li Wenliang and other medical professionals for sharing information about the SARS-like coronavirus. I was also frustrated by official obfuscations on the identity and infectivity of the pathogen and of outbreak severity in January 2020 but again not surprised because "being intense internally but relaxed externally" was well known as the operating motto in Chinese health emergency response.

Still, I was shocked to learn that the much-vaunted national disease reporting system was not utilized for reporting the initial cases to the China CDC in December 2019 until the NHC and the China CDC had sent emergency response teams to Wuhan, and even then it was put into disuse until after Wuhan was in lockdown.[21] This naturally begged questions of what happened, why, and what might have been. The questions kept growing as it became known that NHC and China CDC experts and senior officials went to Wuhan on December 31, 2019; maintained their presence in Wuhan in the ensuing days and weeks; and yet did not publicly disclose human-to-human transmission of the novel coronavirus until January 20, 2020. Still more questions arose for me when Wuhan was sealed off from the rest of China and I joined in efforts to provide much-needed personal protection equipment to Wuhan and later to Chicago. After the Wuhan lockdown was lifted, China's tenacious pursuit of zero COVID until late 2022, including putting Shanghai, China's most populous and wealthiest city, under an extended siege in spring 2022, raised a different set of questions about the Chinese body politic.[22]

Pivotal historical events are important in themselves as well as transformative of existing structures.[23] Having already claimed millions of lives and disrupted the entire world in generation-defining terms, the COVID-19 pandemic is such a pivotal event. To understand how a small outbreak in Wuhan exploded into one of the most devastating pandemics in human history, it is essential to learn more about the choices and decisions of authorities in China in the initial handling of the Wuhan outbreak and the subsequent efforts to contain the epidemic and prevent its resurgence in China. This study thus contributes to the burgeoning literature on the COVID-19 pandemic by examining Chinese decision-making during the Wuhan outbreak and the ensuing lockdown. It is a study on how the Wuhan outbreak spiraled out of control despite China's experiences with SARS and other respiratory infectious diseases such as the H7N9 influenza. Since the Chinese health emergency response regime is part of a complex multi-level governance system dominated by the Communist Party, this is by necessity a study of the politics of health emergency response. The findings of this project should not only help us recognize the strengths and limitations of existing systems but also provide valuable knowledge and lessons for efforts to better prepare for future epidemics.

Organizations, Leadership, and Epidemic Information

In spring 2019, China CDC director general Gao Fu, known as George F. Gao in English, assured the public that "SARS-like events will not occur again."[24] In making that oft-recalled remark, Gao showed a technocrat's faith in the health emergency response system that had been enhanced in the post-SARS years to strengthen infectious disease prevention and control. Inadvertently, he also inserted himself in a long-standing debate about organizations, leadership, and disasters. More specifically, he represented a school of thinking known as "high reliability theory," which holds that it is possible and indeed necessary to build high reliability organizations and systems to deliver safety, reliability, and effectiveness in medicine and other domains.[25]

In contrast to high reliability theory, social scientists led by Charles Perrow, Scott Sagan, and Diane Vaughan, among others, have argued that "accidents" or disasters are unavoidable in systems of great complexity even if efforts could be made to reduce the probability of their occurrence.[26] According to Perrow's "normal accidents" theory, systems that exhibit both high complexity and tight coupling—strong interdependence among units—tend to be prone to system-wide risks. Moreover, efforts to layer on additional safety devices or measures also increase the complexity of the system and may instead produce unanticipated failures. The space shuttle disasters at NASA and the Chernobyl nuclear disaster are among the most striking examples of such phenomena. Vaughan argued that the *Challenger* space shuttle accident occurred in an organizational culture characterized by the "normalization of deviance."[27] In such an organizational culture, unacceptable practices or standards became acceptable. Tragically, efforts to change the organizational culture in NASA following the *Challenger* disaster were not effective, and the *Columbia* accident followed.[28]

The debate between normal accident theory versus high reliability theory has become the starting point for more open approaches to the study of disasters and disaster response.[29] It also offers valuable theoretical lenses and historical perspectives for examining China's handling of the initial outbreak in Wuhan and subsequent responses to the COVID-19 pandemic over time.

Both official discourse and academic studies from China have highlighted how China's leadership led by General Secretary Xi Jinping took prompt and decisive decisions to lock down Wuhan and contain the COVID-19 pandemic within China in the first half of 2020.[30] China's formidable determination and capability to implement the lockdown of more than 10 million people through to conclusion and then to pursue a zero-COVID policy for years are a constant reminder of the capacities of the Chinese party-state and the sacrifices that Chinese society could be made to endure for party-defined commonweal.

With the casualties and costs of the COVID-19 pandemic continuing to pile up in China and the rest of the world, the growing capacities for disease surveillance and testing in China and elsewhere point to the potential for saving lives and mitigating losses if infectious disease outbreaks could be prevented from spiraling out of control with enhanced pandemic preparedness.[31] None other than Xi Jinping lamented in early February 2020 that there had been "shortcomings in public health" as well as "formalism and bureaucratism in epidemic prevention and control work."[32] However, during the Wuhan lockdown, the Chinese party-state also imposed strict restrictions on research and publication of COVID-19-related research.[33] In consequence, official as well as academic publications from China have highlighted the effectiveness of non-pharmaceutical interventions centered on the lockdown but have elided the weaknesses and deficiencies in China's early epidemic response.[34]

It has long been known that non-democratic regimes tend to suffer from problems of information.[35] In Wuhan, the crackdown on medical professionals such as Dr. Li Wenliang, whose poignant words grace the beginning of this chapter as an epigraph, epitomized the politics of information suppression in the initial outbreak response.[36] Proponents of authoritarian advantage in dealing with epidemics are hard pressed to explain the juxtaposition between China's formidable disease surveillance and health emergency response capabilities and the extended delay in announcing human-to-human transmission of the novel coronavirus in January 2020.

Organizational Cultures, Information Flows, and Disasters

In researching for this project, I have engaged in an ethnography of decision-making in China's epidemic response. The more I have delved into the many interviews and reports about China's handling of the outbreak, the more I have felt compelled to reach back to the literature on disasters and disaster response because of its emphasis on the interaction of humans and organizations in complex systems.[37]

Decades of research on disasters, safety management, and organizational cultures have shown the vital importance of obtaining, sharing, and properly making use of information, especially anomalous information, based on the criteria of relevance, timeliness, and clarity.[38] The measure of an organization or system is how it processes and uses information and what information it ignores. In the literature on disasters, a disaster is not defined in purely physical terms but "as a significant *disruption or collapse of the existing cultural beliefs or norms* about hazards, and for dealing with them and their impacts."[39] The incidence of disaster is a process that includes an incubation period, errors and communication difficulties, and an element of surprise—cognitively, materially, as well as politically—for those who thought they were in control.

Organizational cultures are the shared assumptions or expectations invented or developed by a given group in processes of internal integration and external adaptation.[40] James Reason describes the ideal organizational culture for safety management as one in which individuals are willing and ready to report their errors and near-misses and share essential safety-related information, and, as a result, the leaders and managers of the system have access to current knowledge about the factors that affect system safety.[41] Real-world organizational practices rarely match Reason's ideal. One can nonetheless invert Reason's description of the good organizational culture for safety to approximate the organizational environment that is prone to safety lapses and even disasters. Incorporating style of information processing as a key marker, Ron Westrum has developed a spectrum of three types of organizational cultures—bureaucratic, generative, and pathological—for assessing the quality of organizational cultures for safety.[42] The generative type of organizational culture is performance- or mission-oriented and akin to Reason's ideal safety culture. It can "get the needed information to the right person in the right form and in the right time frame."[43] It scores high on measures of trust and cooperation, treatment of bearers of bad news and whistleblowers, and respect for the needs of the information recipient. It empowers rather than muzzles voices. By fostering a level playing field, it encourages the discovery and sharing of information horizontally and vertically. Decision makers in a generative organizational culture tend to receive relevant safety-related information timely and clearly and are thus equipped to make appropriate decisions to forestall disasters or respond to them.

At the other end of the Westrum spectrum is the pathological type of organizational culture wherein information is a political commodity prone to distortion and hoarding. This is an organizational environment centered on personal power and glory and filled with fear and threat. In a climate low on trust and cooperation, people watch their words carefully and keep quiet. Messengers of bad news are punished. Because of the suppression of safety-related information amid collective silence, "latent pathogens" tend to build up, creating the potential for disasters to occur.[44] Suppression of critical safety-related information, shirking of responsibility, and scapegoating tend to go together.

In between the generative and the pathological is the bureaucratic, which is characteristic of most organizations. The bureaucratic organization emphasizes rules and positions and is a potent structure for mobilizing resources in pursuit of various objectives. It also has well-known weaknesses when business as usual is no longer adequate. "Turfs" and hierarchies may hinder cooperation. Important safety-related information may become encapsulated and neglected. Table 1.1 is a summary of the three types of organizational culture and how they differ in information flows.

When we employ the organizational culture concept to facilitate analysis, we need to keep in mind that different organizations in the same organizational ecosystem may possess very different cultures. Moreover, subordinate organizations in a large and complex system may also have different types of

Table 1.1 Organizational Culture Types and Information Flows

Type of organizational culture	Orientation	Characteristics
Bureaucratic	Rules and regulations	Focus is on following rules and procedures. Communication is formal and often slow. Critical thinking and questions are not encouraged. Decisions are made based on rules in hierarchies, not necessarily what is most appropriate for the challenges at hand. This type of organizational culture falls between the generative and the pathological.
Generative	Mission and performance	Focus is on mission and performance. The discovery of information and the sharing of information horizontally and vertically are both encouraged. Critical thinking is encouraged. Decision-making is distributed and collaborative, characterized by trust and cooperation. Decision makers make appropriate decisions with relevant safety-related information. There is willingness to learn from failure.
Pathological	Power and control	Focus is on power and control. Information is hoarded and siloed. Abnormal information tends to be ignored. Communication is one way and limited. Messengers of bad news are not welcome. Decision-making is centralized and arbitrary. Degree of trust and cooperation is low. This type of organization tends to let safety lapses accumulate. Shirking of responsibility and scapegoating go hand in hand.

organizational cultures. Furthermore, organizational culture continues to evolve because of interactions with the environment and of the internal dynamics of agency–structure interactions.[45] Leaders of organizations are not simply passive processors of information but are decision makers with self-interest and varying degrees of discretion. Their leadership and decision-making styles can make a significant difference, shaping the cultures of organizations in terms of organizational openness, transparency, and more generally how organizations manage information.

The information processing and interpretive capacities of organizations that are nested in still larger organizations or systems are in turn affected by the imperatives of the larger organizations or systems. Generalizing from cases they had examined, Martin and Turner argued that the propensity for a system to amplify errors and misinformation and produce serious consequences such as disasters is related to how the system pursues order.[46] Systems that are preoccupied with the maintenance of order and stability may paradoxically be carriers of the pathological type of organizational culture and breeding grounds for instability. "The more extensive a negentropic order-seeking system becomes, the greater is the potential which it also develops for the orderly dissemination of unintended consequences."[47]

The typology of organizational cultures and the broader understanding of the dynamics of organizational leadership offer a useful analytical framework as we review how individuals and organizations in China obtained, processed, and responded to information of the emerging outbreak in Wuhan in December 2019 and after. On the one hand, all the key individuals and organizations involved in the health emergency response operated in a complex political-administrative landscape dominated by the party-state. To help with the understanding of the incentives and pathologies of China's party-state system, I shall lay out, in Chapter 2, the key features of China's neo-Communist Party-state system, including its preoccupation with stability maintenance and growing emphasis on party leadership. The health emergency response regime is part of this party-state and must contend with the needs for vertical and horizontal cooperation in a complex political-administrative hierarchy as well as societal involvement.

On the other hand, information tends to be scarce and fragmentary in the early phases of an outbreak. It should be obvious as well as important to note that specialists such as clinicians, epidemiologists, and virologists as well as the leaders of health organizations and administrations that participate in handling an initial outbreak must work with incomplete information and make decisions under uncertainty.

Cognitive Biases, Incentives, and Decision-Making in a Hierarchy

Within and across organizations, the roles of leaders and of leadership are important but are also hard to quantify and generalize.[48] Besides variations in personality, there can be many factors to consider about the roles of and incentives for leaders that shape their behavior, and I want to highlight two of them here. First, contemporary societies have increasingly turned to the quantification of performance using various metrics to evaluate the performance of organizations and of their leaders. In consequence, organizational leaders such as party secretaries, mayors, and hospital presidents are themselves responsive to the incentives facing them and their organizations. In the larger organizational setting of the Chinese party-state, these incentives have become increasingly rule-governed and metric-driven even while they fall under the leadership of the Communist Party elite.[49] In such a setting, considerations of power, rules, and performance are oftentimes in tension and thus mediated by the judgment of organizational leaders as decision makers. Metrics of evaluation intended to promote good governance may instead prompt officials seeking to look good to their superiors and other evaluators to engage in deliberate manipulations and distortions.[50] As I shall note, municipal leaders in major cities like Wuhan are acutely sensitive about maintaining their city's image and rankings, frequently going to great lengths, and even adopting measures that might seem unreasonable to outsiders, in order to achieve this goal.

Second, it is well acknowledged that individuals rely on heuristics and are susceptible to cognitive biases when making decisions under uncertainty.[51] Turner was among the first to recognize how decision makers' use of cognitive heuristics or simplifying assumptions could limit the range of considered scenarios and impact the precautions taken.[52] When these practices result in the neglect of certain information, anomalies, or considerations, allowing "unnoticed, mis-perceived, and mis-understood events" to accumulate, disruptions and even disasters may ensue.[53] In healthcare, particularly when responding to infectious disease outbreaks with long incubation periods and causative pathogens not easily visible to the human eye, cognitive biases tend to lead decision makers to "prioritize the readily imaginable over the statistical, the present over the future, and the direct over the indirect."[54] Even the most highly trained experts may still succumb to such biases and other psychological influences, such as motivated reasoning.[55]

Questions about the Chinese Body Politic and the Handling of the Coronavirus Outbreak in Wuhan

The general insights on organizations, decision makers, and hierarchies from the literature on crises and disasters are useful scaffolding when we seek to understand what took place in Wuhan in late 2019 and early 2020, in the context of the Chinese party-state and health emergency response regime. The official Chinese narrative on the initial outbreak response depicted near perfection, emphasizing openness, promptness, transparency, and responsibility.[56] However, any field epidemiologist, especially one experienced in epidemic outbreak studies, would instinctively question such lofty political rhetoric, given that many governments worldwide struggled with their initial COVID-19 responses.[57] Fortunately, a wealth of information from the early months of the Wuhan crisis became available, despite attempts to promote a unified narrative, conceal misjudgments and missteps, and enforce strict heavy-handed censorship on reporting, research, and publishing.

Throughout this book, I excavate from the rich veins of evidence from Wuhan and other parts of China, supplemented by in-depth background interviews with individuals who had access to the health emergency decision-making processes. I explore how clinicians, epidemiologists, scientists, hospital administrators, local and national health leaders, and patients infected with the novel coronavirus (later known as SARS-CoV-2) made crucial choices within China's multi-layered political-administrative system beginning in December 2019. These early decisions significantly influenced the scale and scope of the outbreak in Wuhan and beyond.

Following the imposition of cordon sanitaire, Wuhan reopened on April 8, 2020, and declared itself COVID-free in June 2020. In retrospect, Dr. Zhong's announcement of human-to-human transmission on January 20, 2020 and the imposition of cordon sanitaire in Wuhan on January 23, 2020, commonly known as the "Wuhan lockdown," were pivotal moments in China's COVID-19 response.[58] In this study, I differentiate between the pre-Wuhan lockdown period and the post-lockdown period. The 4 weeks or so prior to the Wuhan lockdown were among the most important weeks in the history of pandemics.

In epidemic outbreak responses, information about the causative pathogen is the currency of the realm, and the fate of the response hinges on decision makers' ability to collect, interpret, and act upon key pieces of epidemic information. As I detail in the book, the front-line respiratory medicine doctors who reported early cases in late December 2019 and early January 2020 suspected contagion and took appropriate precautions. Some also had access to diagnostic results identifying a SARS-like coronavirus in late December 2019. Despite the involvement of numerous experts, organizations, and political-administrative authorities in the initial health emergency response and considerable information about initial case clusters and the novel coronavirus, it took the Chinese health system and leadership over 3 weeks to publicly announce the human-to-human transmission of the novel coronavirus.

This project primarily examines the handling of emerging epidemic information during the outbreak in Wuhan, followed by a portrayal of the massive efforts to rescue Wuhan and contain the epidemic during the lockdown period: Who knew what about the earliest cases and about the causative pathogen, later named SARS-CoV-2? When and how did the information surface? How did the individuals and organizations with access to early outbreak information react? How did health and political authorities use available information and other resources to respond to the outbreak and specifically to interrupt viral transmission chains?

The answers to these questions will help address the following: What were the misjudgments, missteps, and deficiencies in collecting, accessing, and using epidemic information? Why did leading national experts like Xu Jianguo and health policymakers believe the outbreak was under control in mid-January 2020 while Wuhan became, in Guan Yi's words, an "unguarded city"? What did China CDC leaders mean when they referred to "limited human-to-human transmission"? What caused the delay in publicizing the novel coronavirus's contagious nature and human-to-human transmission? In other words, what made China's health emergency response system falter in Wuhan during the first 3 weeks of January 2020?

Once China's leaders recognized the necessity to contain the novel coronavirus, they sealed off Wuhan and the rest of Hubei from the rest of the country, mobilizing and unleashing the full power of the Chinese party-state to combat the coronavirus in Wuhan and nationwide. The campaign in Wuhan and the rest of Hubei successfully brought the epidemic under control within China. However, since SARS-CoV-2 had already spread in the weeks preceding the imposition of cordon sanitaire in Wuhan, China could not afford to relax its efforts after concluding its campaign to save Wuhan and the rest of Hubei. As the COVID-19 pandemic continued to devastate the rest of the world, China shifted to a persistent zero-COVID strategy to safeguard the accomplishments of the Wuhan lockdown. The pursuit of zero COVID became synonymous with heightened societal control and lasted until late 2022.[59] Consequently, China was the first to implement sustained lockdowns and the last to exit, leading to significant repercussions for Chinese society, the economy, and its relationships with the rest of the world.

The Chinese Communist Party-State and the Political-Institutional Context for Health Emergency Response

Possessing Leninist organizational discipline, Maoist mobilizational capabilities, and twenty-first-century digital technologies, the Chinese party-state stands unrivaled in its command of organizational and material resources and its dominance over society. Our examination of how the Chinese body politic has responded to SARS-CoV-2 begins with an overview of the Chinese party-state and its intricate multi-level governing hierarchy (Chapter 2). The Chinese public health emergency response system is an integral component of this elaborate system.

At the most basic level, there are five levels of government administration (central, provincial, municipal, district, street/town/township), each with its own administrative and parallel Communist Party leadership. All but the lowest government administrative level (street/town/township) possess their own health commissions or bureaus. The subnational CDCs in the provinces, municipalities, and districts (counties) follow technical guidance from the China CDC but are embedded in the health commissions (bureaus) of the respective territorial jurisdictions. Public hospitals physically located in the same city district may still belong to various levels of health commissions (bureaus).

This brief enumeration of the multiple layers of health administrations and variegated landscape of health-related organizations is suggestive of the complex institutional terrain for managing an infectious disease outbreak that spans organizational boundaries. As is generally known and as I'll elaborate in Chapter 2, much of this system, together with laws and regulations for infectious disease prevention and control and for health emergency response, was reconstituted and reinforced during and in the aftermath of the 2003 SARS crisis.[60] The online National Notifiable Disease Reporting System, the world's most extensive, was put into operation in 2004 to serve as the cornerstone for dealing with infectious disease outbreaks. This system, often referred to with considerable pride, had acquired mythical status in the minds of China's health leaders and the Chinese public prior to the Wuhan outbreak.

Known for its pursuit of the twin objectives of economic growth and sociopolitical stability, the contemporary Chinese party-state is an example of Turner's "negentropic order-seeking system."[61] When there are real or perceived threats such as labor demands, not-in-my-backyard protests, and local emergencies, local authorities through the party leadership impose or maintain order using the stability maintenance regime, an institutionalized multi-departmental mechanism that includes the police and the courts. They can enlist the propaganda system and the police to silence critics and manage the aggrieved.[62] This is a body politic that is primed to react strongly to any real or perceived threat. Yet, the obsession with order-seeking, as Turner contended, may also create the potential for the dissemination of unintended consequences and cause disasters to occur.[63] Meanwhile, as I elaborate in Chapter 2, the Chinese party-state is plagued by tendencies toward fragmentation and disjointedness in policymaking and implementation that can also hamper epidemic information flows, decision-making, and coordination during an outbreak.

The Order-Seeking Polity and the "Preventable and Controllable" Outbreak

Within the broader governance context for health emergencies, I delve into and explain how individuals and organizations responded to the outbreak in Wuhan and several other cities in China. Chapter 3 recounts the initial encounters by clinicians, independent clinical laboratories, and health administrators with the PUE cases that presented SARS-like symptoms. While the official story credits Dr. Zhang Jixian as the first doctor to report the PUE cases that were later identified as COVID-19 cases, this chapter reveals the involvement and persistence of clinicians in various hospitals as well as the contributions of commercial diagnostic laboratories that alerted clinicians and health leaders to the dangers of a SARS-like novel coronavirus early on. I also present, for the first time, the investigation conducted by a provincial–municipal–district joint team, highlighting what the team report focused on and overlooked.

From an emergency response perspective, Chinese public health experts and health leaders held a remarkably strong hand of cards in terms of information about the early cases on December 31, 2019. They possessed not only crucial information about the so-called PUE cases but also diagnostic results identifying a SARS-like novel coronavirus as the pathogen (Chapters 3 and 4). That evening, health officials and experts, including those from the NHC and China CDC, reviewed the outbreak situation in Wuhan. They recommended and secured approval for the closure of the Huanan Seafood Market as the presumed source of infections. They also formulated an anti-epidemic action program.

However, despite having highly significant information about the SARS-like pneumonia cases and China's vivid memories of the SARS crisis, it took more than 3 weeks for the national health leadership to finally inform the public, through Dr. Zhong Nanshan, that the novel coronavirus was transmissible from human to human. Despite the dedication and hard work of clinicians, epidemiologists, and scientists who cared for and observed patients, conducted contact tracing, and carried out genomic research in challenging circumstances, the crux of the matter is that the novel coronavirus spread in Wuhan and beyond unimpeded for much of January 2020 before the lockdown. In retrospect, the failure to implement *public* health measures to contain the virus during that period was monumental, especially because clinicians and virologists warned of the dangers in late December 2019 and early January 2020.

Chapters 5–10 outline the multiple and parallel bureaucratic and political processes that were activated in Wuhan and nationally to manage and control the availability and flow of epidemic information. These processes, complicated by principal–agent problems (Chapters 8 and 9), hindered the sharing and use of quality epidemic information that had become available, led to the disregard of valuable information about the contagiousness of the novel coronavirus, and failed to prompt the public to take protective action. The intricate fault lines of fragmented authoritarianism presented a substantial obstacle to cohesion between the National Health Authority, inclusive of the China CDC, and the health authorities of Hubei and Wuhan, which encompass their respective CDCs. They contributed to and were further exacerbated by a cognitive framework rooted in the belief that the virus had jumped from wildlife to humans in the Huanan Seafood Market and would therefore be of limited transmissibility at the time (Chapters 7 and 8).

All these weaknesses and deficiencies could have been alleviated, if not fully eliminated, had the larger system been more transparent, more open to new information and the consideration of alternative views, and more straightforward in communicating risk with the public. As John Barry underscored in his magisterial study of the great influenza pandemic of 1918–1919, authorities need to communicate openly with the public and to maintain public trust: "The way to do that is to distort nothing, to put the best face on nothing, to try to manipulate no one."[64]

However, the health emergency response in Wuhan diverged drastically from the tenets of transparency and open communication. To the contrary, the authorities managing the responses to the Wuhan outbreak focused on dominance and control, which stemmed from the Chinese party-state's order-and-stability complex and were reinforced by an increasingly complex array of evaluation metrics for individuals, hospitals, and local governments. The preoccupation with order and stability led in multiple ways to the suppression, distortion, and neglect of important pieces of disease information and, more generally, to an atmosphere of organized silence that strongly discouraged views deviating from the official stance and discourse (Chapters 5, 6, 8, and 9). The punishment of Dr. Ai Fen, Dr. Li Wenliang, and others for sharing disease information with fellow professionals resulted in the silencing of clinicians more broadly (Chapter 5). Despite the scientific culture of priority, scientists at multiple research laboratories were prohibited from immediately releasing their findings during a period when their announcements about the novel coronavirus could have informed health professionals and the public and stimulated spirited discussion about the virus's dangers (Chapter 6). Instead, the official press, as the mouthpiece of the party-state, amplified official messaging even when some reporters submitted internal warnings.[65] One cannot help but be reminded of the scenes in *The Plague*, where the Prefect equivocated about the plague with the public and delayed implementing rigorous prophylactic measures.[66]

The patterns outlined above were enhanced in the first half of January 2020 by political and seasonal calendars, which prompted officials to accentuate the positives and suppress the negatives. Nonetheless, it is still shocking to learn that, even with a growing number of new suspected cases and medical staff infections known internally by mid-January, those familiar with the situation in the Wuhan/Hubei health bureaucracy and major hospitals went to great lengths to conceal the infections. In hindsight, it wasn't a huge leap for these individuals to transition from not following through on early leads to actively restricting and suppressing the submission of new cases (Chapter 8) and preventing experts from Beijing from discovering in-hospital infections of healthcare workers (Chapter 9). Furthermore, they were able to do so by hiding behind rules and pleading innocence. In the meantime, key scientific and health leaders, who relied on honest reporting from Wuhan/Hubei, were lulled into a false sense of security, believing that they had made the right decisions and taken adequate actions to control the outbreak (Chapter 7).

Information, Cognition, and Overcoming Tunnel Vision in Organizational Cultures

In the context of organizational cultures, the Chinese political-administrative system, which involved multiple levels of health administrations, CDCs, and hospitals across the governing hierarchy, exhibited strong bureaucratic-pathological tendencies in handling early information about the outbreak. Rather than warning the public, the political-administrative complex in

Wuhan/Hubei, under the guidance of the NHC, insisted until January 20, 2020, that the outbreak was "preventable and controllable," suppressing those who raised concerns about viral contagion (Chapters 5, 6, and 8–10).

Rather than clearly communicating risks to the public, the official discourse was marked by ambiguity and evasion. Before the Wuhan lockdown, the WMHC's language downplayed the outbreak. Although health authorities were aware of the novel coronavirus and its potential for infectivity, they continued using the term "PUE" until January 9, when the official verification process was completed. The public was not informed of the partial knowledge and serious concerns held by leading experts (Chapters 6 and 7). This situation reflects Diane Vaughan's concept of disaster-prone organizational culture that "created a way of seeing that was simultaneously a way of not seeing."[67]

Various processes reinforced the official "no worries" and wait-and-see discourse, causing crucial cases pointing to human-to-human transmission of the novel coronavirus to be ignored or dismissed in Wuhan and Beijing (Chapters 8–10). If the virus had limited infectivity, as officially claimed, the multi-pronged efforts to isolate and treat patients in Wuhan might have succeeded (Chapter 7). If the outbreak had been contained, it would have been a minor event in global health history, showcasing the capabilities of China's public health system as part of the Chinese party-state.

Set against the official discourse, Dr. Zhong Nanshan's announcement of human-to-human transmission on January 20, 2020, sparked public outrage in China and worldwide. People questioned why it took the Chinese government so long to acknowledge the transmission and mobilize the public.[68]

In reality, experts, the Chinese CDC system, and health administration leaders had adopted a cognitive framework centered on zoonosis-in-Huanan-market, which led to the expectation of a small number of human-to-the-human transmission cases. Even though they had evidence pointing to cases of suspected human-to-human transmission from the very beginning (Chapters 3, 4, and 7–9), such evidence was seen as "limited transmission." The primary concern of Chinese public health leadership was not the presence of any human-to-human transmission, as the public had come to see, but rather the severity and extent of such transmission. Consequently, members of the second expert team and the Senior Advisory Panel, led by Dr. Zhong, sought evidence of medical staff infections as a key indicator of transmission severity (Chapters 9 and 11).

Simultaneously, from the end of December 2019, experts and health authorities created multiple obstacles to recognizing viral PUE cases without exposure to the Huanan Seafood Market in Wuhan. These included the initial case definition in the joint provincial–municipal–district epidemiological investigation, the inclusion-exclusion criteria in early January, deficiencies in epidemiological investigations, and testing delays (Chapters 3, 4, and 6–8). While Chinese authorities often deploy the stability maintenance regime to suppress incidents, using the same approach for a highly contagious virus proved counterproductive, akin to trying to wrap fire in paper.

Seventeen years after the SARS outbreak, once again key voices that effectively challenged the prevailing narrative and sounded the alarm during the health emergency in Wuhan/Hubei came from outside the established response regime. Taiwan CDC epidemiologists visited Wuhan and raised important questions regarding intra-family infections (Chapter 7). Though they were not part of the official government pathogen verification programs, virologists at the Shanghai Public Health Clinical Center sequenced the genome of the novel coronavirus and advocated for a more robust outbreak response (Chapter 6). Clinician-researchers in Thailand identified the first novel coronavirus-infected patient outside China (Chapter 10). Clinicians, public health specialists, and research scientists in Shenzhen and Hong Kong identified and sounded the alarm about patients who had not traveled to Wuhan but were nonetheless infected with the novel coronavirus (Chapter 10). The stalemate in Wuhan was resolved when national health policymakers enlisted 83-year-old Dr. Zhong Nanshan from Guangdong to lead the Senior Advisory Panel on a mission to Wuhan to recognize the severity and urgency of the epidemic situation (Chapter 11). Ultimately, General Secretary Xi Jinping made the difficult decision to seal off Wuhan following intense discussions as well as pressure from the WHO.

The contributions from experts based outside of Wuhan/Hubei played a pivotal role in counteracting the organizational dysfunctions and pathologies that led to the suppression and concealment of crucial epidemic information in Wuhan. Moreover, these contributions bring to light pressing and complex questions regarding leadership, decision-making, and missed opportunities in responding to the outbreak. Above all, they underscore the challenging issue of preventability.

Research using the SEIR (susceptible–exposed–infectious–removed [recovered]) model, co-led by Dr. Zhong Nanshan, found that if public epidemic control measures had been implemented merely 5 days earlier in January 2020, China's total COVID-19 cases would have decreased by a staggering two-thirds.[69] Another study, conducted by Xu-Sheng Zhang and his team, modeled the potential effects of putting such measures into action 1, 2, or 3 weeks earlier in Wuhan. They concluded that these hypothetical scenarios would have curtailed confirmed cases in China by approximately 57%,

81%, and 93%, respectively.[70] Findings of this magnitude inevitably lead us to the following question: Was there a genuine opportunity to contain the outbreak in its early stages in Wuhan/Hubei and thereby avert one of the most catastrophic pandemics in history?

By excavating and reconstructing the initial response to the outbreak in Wuhan, this study aims to help the global community of dedicated public health specialists and the public to draw their own conclusions on this pivotal issue. Such endeavors will also contribute to our understanding of effective strategies and best practices necessary for preventing and managing future pandemics.

The Politics of the Wuhan Lockdown

In its responses to the initial outbreak in Wuhan and the outbreak of SARS in 2003, China's public health emergency system, as part of the party-state, has found it difficult to promote accountability and earn public trust through transparency. In both cases, the outbreak spread beyond the origin city before authorities, with their command of the propaganda system, were willing to inform and mobilize the public to combat the epidemic outbreaks.

However, once the decision was made to lock down Wuhan and provide medical assistance to the region, the Chinese system rapidly transitioned into performance mode, showcasing its strengths in disaster response. With unwavering focus and determination, Xi and the Chinese leadership adopted a comprehensive approach involving the party, government, and society in their efforts to rescue Wuhan. They mobilized resources and manpower from across the country to alleviate the burden on overwhelmed hospitals and address community disarray and paralysis (Chapters 12 and 13).

Organizationally, the Chinese leadership established a special party-centered emergency leadership structure in late January 2020. Layered on the State Council Joint Prevention and Control Mechanism, this structure enabled the front-line leader, Politburo member and Vice Premier Sun Chunlan, to utilize the authority and organizational capabilities of the party-state to allocate resources and exert leadership over local authorities (Chapter 12). In February 2020, the national leadership replaced key leaders in Wuhan and Hubei toallay calm public anger, enhance political control, and enforce community-level lockdowns (Chapter 13).

I divide the emergency rescue operations in Wuhan/Hubei into two phases. The first phase focused on providing additional medical resources to treat infected patients when health centers were overwhelmed (Chapter 12). In what became the largest peacetime medical rescue mission ever, every province in China sent emergency medical teams to the region. Concurrently, Wuhan leaders repurposed existing hospitals and built temporary field hospitals to accommodate the surge in infected individuals. Moreover, under national guidance, Wuhan transformed large public spaces such as convention centers and stadiums into *fangcang* shelter hospitals to quarantine those with mild to moderate symptoms (Chapter 12).

Contrary to the conventional view emphasizing the importance of grassroots governance, the shock of the lockdown and the surge in infected individuals initially overwhelmed the grassroots governance structure. It wasn't until the middle of February 2020 that community-level actions gained traction, when treatment and quarantine capacities were significantly increased. Chapter 13 focuses on community-level struggles and, as the second phase of the Wuhan campaign, the efforts to enforce "enclosed management" of residential areas and home confinement of residents. Authorities relied on both "sent-down" staff of the party-state bureaucracy and the rank and file of grassroots governance structures to enforce community-level lockdowns and home confinement and provide essential services. Meanwhile, the rest of society was demobilized because of the community-level lockdowns and home confinement.

By the time the Wuhan lockdown was lifted on April 8, 2020, after 76 days, COVID-19 had already been declared a pandemic by the WHO, and the SARS-CoV-2 virus was rapidly spreading across the globe. China's ability to impose and strictly enforce the stringent lockdown in Wuhan/Hubei and throughout the rest of the country distinguished it from most other nations in terms of party-state dominance and societal compliance. It wasn't until late 2022 and early 2023 that China, weary from the costs and challenges of repeated lockdowns, finally transitioned away from its dynamic zero-COVID strategy and reopened its borders to the rest of the world. Meanwhile, the striking contrast in China's anti-epidemic performance before and after the Wuhan lockdown compels us to investigate and assess the causes of these variations in China's outbreak response, as well as explore their implications for both China's and global public health.

2

The Party-State, Fragmented Authoritarianism, and the Health Emergency Response Regime

The COVID-19 outbreak began in Wuhan almost exactly 17 years after the severe acute respiratory syndrome (SARS) epidemic started in Guangdong in December 2002. In the aftermath of the SARS crisis, the Chinese leadership, then with Hu Jintao as general secretary and Wen Jiabao as premier, placed heavy emphasis on building an institutionalized public health emergency response system.

By its very nature, public health emergencies, and especially infectious disease outbreaks, can quickly spiral out of control to disrupt and threaten the existing political, social, and economic order.[1] They require those involved to respond in a relatively short time with limited information. In these fog-of-war situations, the institutional and organizational parameters for responding to epidemics become critically important. Disaster research studies tend to see the causes of disasters as lying in the decisions made by individuals who are members of organizations with particular structures and cultures. These organizations, in turn, face competitive pressures to survive and expand in larger political, economic, and social contexts.

In this chapter, I situate China's public health emergency response system in the larger system of Chinese governance. China has a neo–Communist Party-state that combines Leninist organizational discipline, Maoist mobilizational capabilities, and twenty-first-century digital technologies. As articulated by every leader from Mao to Xi Jinping and summarized in a Chinese Communist Party (CCP) Central Committee decision adopted in October 2019, a major advantage of the Chinese system is its ability for China's leadership to pool forces and resources to "accomplish great things," officially translated as "to complete key national undertakings."[2] The stability maintenance regime has been a central component of this system. Acting in concert with the propaganda and censorship apparatus, these key elements make up a body politic that is primed to respond aggressively against elements deemed to pose a threat.[3]

Yet the Chinese body politic ruled by the CCP leadership is not a monolith but reflects the complexities and tensions of governing a vast country using multiple levels of party-government authorities organized into functional and territorial administrations. Scholars of China have used the fragmented authoritarianism model to describe and analyze the structural tendencies toward fragmentation and disjointedness in Chinese policymaking and implementation.[4] In behavioral terms, scholars have noted that central authorities have tended to adopt generalized language or rules that are ambiguous rather than spelled out in detail. Even though it compounds principal–agent problems, the deployment of ambiguity provides for greater local discretion and helps to promote flexible implementation suited to local conditions.[5] While giving play to divergent preferences and distinct interests, national leaders have also developed institutionalized mechanisms such as leading small groups and party commissions to coordinate, adjudicate, and make major decisions.[6]

The institutions of health governance, including the health emergency response regime, are nested in this complex political-administrative hierarchy. They performed woefully in handling the SARS outbreak in 2003 but received massive infusions of support afterward to develop significant capabilities for dealing with infectious disease emergencies. In this chapter I lay out the political and institutional context, beginning with the dominance of the CCP and its emphasis on maintaining stability. I then discuss the institutions of public health in this political-administrative context and present the contours of the public health emergency response regime, including the national disease reporting system, the pneumonia of uncertain etiology (PUE) and influenza surveillance programs, and efforts to enhance emergency preparedness.

Domination of the Neo-Communist Party-State

As the world's largest political organization, the CCP has recovered from the ravages of the Mao era, the shock of the Tiananmen Crisis, and the collapse of the Soviet Union. Since the late 1980s, CCP leaders have worked to sharpen the party's focus on its mission, bolster party organizations, train party elites, and expand the party's reach while the Chinese economy has rapidly grown.[7] They boast massive organizational and material resources, vigilantly protect the CCP's political monopoly, and unabashedly dominate the Chinese economy and society. The title of a collection of Xi Jinping's selected works says it all, "Adhere to the Party's Leadership of All Work."[8] Attributed to Mao, the refrain that "the party leads everything" was incorporated into the CCP Charter in October 2017.

The core components of the CCP's current governing philosophy, first laid out in the Deng Xiaoping era, are summarized as "One central task and two basic points"—taking economic development as the central task and the "Four Cardinal Principles" and "reform and opening up" as the two basic points. The Four Cardinal Principles, which Deng first enunciated in 1979, asserted the CCP's imprimatur to rule and pursue socialism through a "people's democratic dictatorship."[9] In practice, Deng's political successors as well as the party rank and file have taken to heart the following twin Deng catechisms: "Development is the hard truth" and "Stability overrides everything else."[10] Taken together, this set of tenets and catechisms—part of the canon of Deng Xiaoping theory in China—has provided for a grand bargain between the CCP and Chinese society.[11]

Within the confines of party-state domination, the relations between the center and localities in China have undergone major changes. The China of the 1980s was characterized by an emphasis on decentralization and responsibilities such that some economists began to describe the Chinese system as a form of "federalism or federalism, Chinese style."[12] Politically, however, there was little doubt that China remained a unitary state. In fact, since the Tiananmen Crisis and the breakup of the Soviet Union, China's leaders—Jiang Zemin and Hu Jintao (mid-1989 to late 2012), as well as Xi Jinping (2012 to present)—have introduced major initiatives to enhance central control.[13] Barry Naughton, an eminent political economist, describes these initiatives to strengthen the CCP-led political hierarchy as China's "counter reformation."[14]

Determined to prevent the CCP from succumbing to the fate of the Communist Party of the Soviet Union, Xi Jinping has been especially aggressive in pursuing manifold drives to strengthen the CCP and his personal power in the party. A massive and comprehensive war on corruption has ensnarled very large numbers of party and government officials.[15] Beginning with the Yan'an days under Mao Zedong, the CCP leadership has employed intra-party indoctrination and brainwashing to enhance organizational integrity, tighten ideological cohesion, and weed out the politically wayward. Every party leader in the post-Deng era has launched their own party-building drives and political education campaigns. Xi Jinping has made the revival of "red" political history a key strand of his party leadership and made the party rank and file relearn the original aspirations of the CCP and recommit to its mission.[16]

Even by the standards of Chinese political history, Xi Jinping's ability to concentrate power in his own hands as well as to use that power has been astonishing. During the times of Jiang Zemin and Hu Jintao, political authority and responsibilities were distributed to members of the Politburo Standing Committee; there thus existed a semblance of collective leadership among

China's top leaders.[17] In contrast, Xi Jinping formally obtained the designation "core leader" of the CCP Central Committee in 2016 (Hu Jintao never received that designation).[18] He got the national legislature to remake the Chinese Constitution in 2018 to allow him to serve as China's president (state chair) beyond the two-term limit. He also engineered a drastic overhaul of party institutions and created or elevated various "small leading groups" into formal central party commissions. Besides being general secretary of the CCP Central Committee and chair of the Central Military Commission and of the Chinese state, Xi has also assumed the chairmanship of central party commissions on finance and economy, national security, cybersecurity and informatization, foreign affairs, military–civilian integration, as well as ones for deepening reform, governing the country by law, and audit. By using these party commissions, Xi has made himself the hands-on supreme leader of the party-state and marginalized the premier's role.[19] Baogang Guo refers to this system as "partocracy with Chinese characteristics."[20] It is widely recognized that Xi is the most powerful Chinese leader since Mao Zedong.

The push to strengthen the CCP leadership under Xi reached a new height in early 2019 when the Party Central issued "CCP Regulations on Making Reports of and Requests for Instructions on Important Matters," which harked back to the 1950s Mao era.[21] Despite the administrative and organizational relationships specified in the Constitution and laws, the Party Central directed party members to report to and seek instructions from superordinate party leaders in localities and departments and, if necessary, from the Party Central Committee (through the General Office of the Central Committee) on important or major matters. These include "matters that are outside the remit of party organizations, party members, and leading cadres; as well as important things or circumstances that, although within their own remit, concern the overall situation or have widespread impact." The long list of matters for reporting and seeking instructions includes "major sensitive events, emergencies, and responses to mass incidents and disposal." "Suddenly emerging major events should be promptly reported, with good follow-up reporting depending on subsequent event development and handling."[22]

In view of the commanding role of the CCP leadership centered on Xi Jinping, these party regulations and the commanding role of Xi Jinping as the leader of the Chinese party-state are important to keep in mind when we seek to understand China's responses to a major health emergency like the novel coronavirus outbreak in Wuhan. In the provinces and municipalities, the Party Committee, led by the party secretary, is the nerve center for leadership and coordination on major initiatives. In this setup, the governor or the mayor serves typically as a deputy secretary. They are, in turn, joined by

Standing Committee members who oversee the political/legal affairs commission, propaganda, party discipline, organization, and so on.

Political Hierarchy and Territorial Administration

Including the national government, China has five levels of government within the same unitary structure—the State Council, provinces, prefectures, counties (districts), and towns/townships. The institutional structure for local governance administration is outlined in the People's Republic of China Constitution (1982, amended in 1988, 1993, 1999, 2004, 2018). The State Council is the highest administrative organ, and the tasks and responsibilities within it are technically distributed among constituent ministries and commissions, many of which report directly to the party leadership structure. The State Council leadership, consisting of the premier and his Executive Committee, "direct[s] all other administrative work of a national character that does not fall within the jurisdiction of the ministries and commissions" (Art. 89[3]).

The State Council leaders "exercise unified leadership over the work of local organs of State administration at various levels throughout the country, and . . . formulate the detailed division of functions and powers between the Central Government and the organs of State administration of provinces, autonomous regions, and municipalities directly under the Central Government" (Art. 89[4]). This hierarchical relationship is replicated within the provinces: "Local people's governments at all levels shall be responsible to state administrative organs at the next level up and shall report to them on their work. Local people's governments at all levels nationwide are state administrative organs under the unified leadership of the State Council; they shall all be subordinate to the State Council" (Art. 110).

Yet, leaving aside for the moment consideration of the role of the CCP leadership as noted above, the relationship between the national and subnational governments is more complicated than it appears because local governments are conferred dual roles: they are "the executive bodies of local organs of state power as well as the local organs of State administration at the corresponding levels" (Art. 105). In other words, local governments are not simply the extensions of superordinate levels of administrative authorities leading up to the State Council; they are also "executive bodies" for state power as embodied by the local people's congresses.

Moreover, local governments "within the limits of their authority as prescribed by law, conduct administrative work concerning the economy, education, science, culture, *public health* . . . issue decisions and orders; appoint or remove . . . administrative functionaries" in their respective jurisdictions (Art. 107, emphasis added). They "direct the work of their subordinate departments and of people's governments at lower levels and have the power to alter or annul inappropriate decisions of their subordinate departments and of the people's governments at lower levels" (Art. 108). Thus, the leader of a functional department such as health in a local government reports to the local leadership first when they need the help or guidance of the same functional department at the next higher level of the administrative hierarchy.

Yet, it would be gross negligence if we fail to note that local authorities are all under the leadership of the respective CCP committees. Generally, the party secretary of a locality also serves as the chair of the Standing Committee of the local people's congress. Therefore, when it comes to power, policy, and administration, it is all in the party. For example, the party secretary of the Provincial Party Committee is generally concurrently the chair of the Standing Committee of the Provincial People's Congress (PPC). The governor, usually a deputy party secretary, constitutionally reports to the PPC. Thus, the party secretary not only is senior to the governor in the provincial party committee but also has a legislative vis-à-vis executive relationship in his role as chair of the PPC Standing Committee. The same is true for most municipalities. As noted earlier in this chapter, the importance of CCP leadership has been enhanced in the era of Xi Jinping.

In summary, the multiple levels of government administration in the provinces and municipalities have complex identities. They are executive bodies with administrative powers and responsibilities over a broad range of areas such as the economy, education, health, the environment, order, and transportation. Nested within the multi-level dual hierarchies of the CCP and the government, the different levels of government administration in the provinces are responsible for reporting their work to the party-state organs at the next higher level in the hierarchy as well as nominally to the people's congresses at their corresponding levels. Scholars of Chinese politics frequently invoke the concept of "fragmented authoritarianism" when they try to make sense of the interactions and policy outcomes that emerge out of this complicated institutional setup.[23] As a result, under the principle of territorial responsibility and management, provincial leaders have outsized authority in their respective territories.[24]

The Stability Maintenance Regime

As noted above, the Chinese leadership has, in recent decades, pursued development alongside a constant concern with stability. The attention given to sensitive events, emergencies, and mass incidents in the party regulations mentioned earlier highlights the ongoing preoccupation of the Chinese leadership with stability maintenance. Whereas China during the Mao era was known for its fervor of revolutionary mobilization, the various levels of the Chinese party-state today are known for their focus on demobilizing civil society and for their unforgiving stance toward elements that are considered deviant, subversive, or threatening.

The stability maintenance regime has been an essential bulwark for China's hyper-developmentalism.[25] It has helped authorities requisition land for development projects, keep labor quiescent, and enrich the powerful and the well-connected. Land disputes have been a significant source of mass incidents. Local authorities facing such disputes have used their sway over the courts to deny those seeking redress the opportunity to even file lawsuits.[26] As the rate of economic growth has slowed down in recent years, the importance of stability maintenance to governance in China, both nationally and locally, has become more apparent.

Most institutions comprising the stability maintenance regime were rebuilt or established in the late 1980s and late 1990s, when the Chinese leadership, mostly with an engineering background, responded to various political exigencies, including the Tiananmen Crisis, the collapse of the Soviet Union, and the Asian Financial Crisis.[27] Central to this regime was the resurrection, in 1990, of the Central Political and Legal Affairs Commission (CPLAC). The CPLAC oversees the Supreme People's Court and Procuratorate; the Ministries of Public Security, State Security, and Justice; and, until 2018, the People's Armed Police. The Central Commission for the Comprehensive Management of Public Security (中央社会治安综合治理委员会), under the same leadership as the CPLAC, was created in 1991. It included representatives from a long list of party and government commissions, ministries, administrations, and the armed forces and represented a whole-of-party-government approach to stability. This was further complemented by the Central Small Leading Group for Stability Maintenance and the Leading Group for Dealing with the Falun Gong. This set of overlapping organizations was consolidated into the CPLAC in 2018.[28]

Luo Gan (2002–2007) and Zhou Yongkang (2007–2012) took charge of this set of powerful organizations, becoming China's czars for internal security as they faced protests and tensions resulting from the dislocations associated with rapid economic growth and restructuring.[29] The institutional structures and objectives of the stability maintenance regime are replicated in the provinces, municipalities, and counties/districts. By 2010, even townships had established amalgamated *zongzhiban* (offices for comprehensive public security) and *weiwenban* (stability maintenance offices).[30] An elaborate stability discourse has also been articulated, with official documents and some academic studies stressing the role of the stability maintenance regime in resolving conflicts and promoting harmony.[31]

Under the principle of territorial management and responsibility, local authorities are each responsible for maintaining stability in their respective territories (属地管理); and those leaders who perform poorly on stability are subject to "veto (一票否决)" on promotions and other benefits.[32] The "veto" elevates the importance of maintaining stability to a rarefied status in China's multi-level political hierarchy and reshapes the incentives and psychology of Chinese officials. Faced with the imperatives of development and the top-down assessments on stability, it is said that officials "may not get promotions for their failure to develop the economy, [they] will lose their posts if they fail to maintain stability."[33]

Preoccupied with stability maintenance, officials have been known to pursue apparent stability using whatever means possible, including high-handed political and extra-legal measures of repression as well as social welfare for the poor.[34] By deploying a combination of carrots and sticks, Chinese authorities can get away with using the stability maintenance regime to maintain control, preserve stability, and promote economic construction. These efforts to promote the veneer of harmony may and often do compound rather than resolve tensions and conflicts.[35]

The stability maintenance regime has been utilized to support China's hosting of high-profile mass spectacles such as the Beijing Summer Olympics (2008) and the World Expo (2010, Shanghai).[36] Xi Jinping, who was then China's vice president and a Politburo Standing Committee member, headed the leading group responsible for preparing for the Beijing Summer Olympics. Under Xi's leadership, the preparations for the 2008 Beijing Summer Olympics emphasized two themes: "Peaceful and Safe Olympics" and "Sci & Tech Olympics." Xi emphatically stated that "Without the 'Peaceful and Safe Olympics' [initiative], everything about [the Olympics] is out of the question."[37]

The hosting of these events has further enhanced monitoring and surveillance capabilities and reinforced the importance of stability maintenance operations for the party-state.[38] In preparation for the Beijing Summer Olympics, the Dongcheng District of Beijing combined the earlier practice of dividing urban spaces into grids for urban management with new technologies for monitoring and surveillance.[39] This practice, now known as "grid governance," has quickly spread, albeit unevenly, throughout China and become a central element of the "comprehensive management of public security."[40]

The whole-of-party-government approach of "comprehensive management" has also taken stability maintenance beyond coercion and surveillance to social assistance.[41] It would become a major pillar for China's pursuit of zero COVID.

For Chinese leaders accustomed to dialectical justifications, the contradictions of the stability maintenance regime are a necessary evil. These tensions and pathologies are further compounded by the political calendar.[42] There is much greater incentive by the Chinese leadership at all levels to keep a lid on petitions and protests in times of sensitivity such as the June 4 anniversary, National Day, May Day, the official CCP anniversary, New Year's Day and the Lunar New Year holidays, as well as major meetings for the National People's Congress and the CCP Central Committee. Subnational authorities in major cities or ethnic regions often have local occasions of significance to add to the calendar of "sensitive periods."

Stability as "Overall National Security" in the Xi Era

After he became general secretary, Xi Jinping pursued an intense effort to strengthen the CCP while guarding against potential risks. In response to fears of potential internal and external threats, Xi has repeatedly urged the party elite to engage in "bottom-line thinking" and to prevent and resolve major risks.[43]

Soon after becoming national leader, Xi established and has headed the long-mooted Central National Security Commission to provide unified leadership of domestic and international security under the principle of "overall national security."[44] As part of the 2018 party-state reforms, Xi has also led central party commissions on cybersecurity and others that deal with other new types of security risks. To consolidate and streamline the stability maintenance regime, three of the four institutions were merged into the CPLAC, which has been led by a Politburo member reporting to Xi since 2012.[45]

Under Xi Jinping's leadership, significant institutional reconfigurations and personnel changes have allowed him to exert personal control over the stability maintenance regime. He has repeatedly urged party leadership at all levels to prioritize both development and stability.[46] The CPLAC has promoted initiatives to develop an integrated system for the prevention and control of public security risks to reduce the incidence of crime and mass incidents and build a "peaceful and safe China."[47] Of particular note is the nationwide promotion of grid governance, which integrates digital technologies with community monitoring and surveillance of neighborhoods and villages.

The CPLAC has continued to employ detailed evaluations to assess the performance of both party and government authorities in "building peace and safety."[48]

Public Health and Chinese Governance

The Chinese public health system is part of the party-state. As the national party-state structure is replicated at the provincial and municipal levels, it is important to situate health emergency decision-making within the party-state structures at the national and subnational levels when we examine how decisions were made during the Wuhan outbreak. In this section, I provide an overview of the organizational landscape for health governance, particularly public health emergency management and response. I have two objectives in doing so. First, I delineate the evolution of the national health authority and its relationship with the health administrations in the provinces and subprovincial authorities. Although this is well known to specialists in Chinese health and governance, it is sometimes misunderstood by the public in China and by international observers. Second, I summarize the key elements of the health emergency response system that has been developed or enhanced since the SARS crisis of 2003. These include major laws and regulations pertaining to infectious disease prevention and control, especially public health emergency response. I give special attention to the crown jewel of this system, the world's largest online direct reporting system for infectious disease reporting and surveillance.

The Institutions for Health Governance

The core features of China's contemporary health governance took shape through two rounds of healthcare reforms, in 1997 and 2009.[49] The 1997 Decision on Healthcare Reforms and Development, announced during Chen Minzhang's tenure as health minister (1987–1998), outlined a vision of "healthcare for all" and aimed to establish a fairly comprehensive health system by 2010. The decision also defined the responsibilities of the national versus subnational governments in healthcare in accordance with the Chinese Constitution:

> The Central Government is responsible for leading the health work across the entire country. Its primary role is to formulate health laws, regulations, policies, and

> national health service plans, and to guide and coordinate the resolution of significant national or inter-provincial health issues. It employs various means to support localities in health development.
>
> Local governments of all levels are fully responsible for health work in their respective areas and must include health development as an important component of the leading cadres' target responsibility system and performance evaluation. Governments of all levels are also required to regularly report to and receive supervision and guidance from the People's Congresses at their respective levels on health reform and development.[50]

In China's constitutional framework, the National Health Commission (NHC) within the State Council serves as the national health authority. Previously known as the Ministry of Health (MOH) until March 2013, it underwent a merger with the National Population and Family Planning Commission in that year to form the National Health and Family Planning Commission. In 2018, it was renamed the "National Health Commission." It remains unclear to what extent these rounds of mergers and restructuring, including the absorption of population planning personnel into the NHC, may have impacted China's health emergency response leadership.

As of 2019–2020, Ma Xiaowei, an experienced health official, was the minister of health (NHC). He became the youngest vice minister of health in 2001 and was involved in the MOH's handling of the SARS outbreak in 2003. Minister Ma Xiaowei reported to a vice premier or state councilor overseeing health within the State Council, a position that had been held by a woman since 1993. As of 2020, Sun Chunlan, the only woman on the CCP's 25-person Politburo, served as the vice premier for health and education.

The provinces, municipalities, and counties/districts each have their own health commissions or bureaus. While Minister Ma Xiaowei serves as both the party secretary of the party group in the NHC and the minister of health, the provincial and subprovincial health commissions are typically led by a party secretary and a director general or director. These leaders report to a vice governor, vice mayor, or vice district head in their respective localities. Consequently, the health administrations in the localities are integrated into the *tiao-kuai* complex of administrative and CCP hierarchies.

The Chinese Centers for Disease Control and Prevention (CDC) system was reconstituted from the Chinese Academy of Preventive Medicine and local epidemic prevention stations in 2002. It consists of the China CDC in Beijing and CDCs in every province, municipality, prefecture, and county/district. We use the name "China CDC" throughout because it is used on the www.chinacdc.cn website. However, it should be kept in mind that the China

CDC in Beijing reports to the NHC and should properly be called the "CDC of the National Health Commission of China." The lower-level CDCs follow the technical or professional guidance of the China CDC, but they are public health institutions that belong to the respective provincial and subprovincial health administrations. As of 2020, China had a total of 3,385 CDCs across five administrative levels: the China CDC in Beijing for the NHC, 31 CDCs in province-level governments, 403 CDCs in prefecture-ranked (municipal) governments, 2,762 CDCs in district/county governments, and 188 others (including military).[51] In Hubei Province, for example, the Hubei Provincial Health Administration controls the Hubei Provincial CDC, while the Wuhan Municipal Health Administration controls the Wuhan Municipal CDC. Figure 2.1 presents the key political and administrative structure and organizations for health in Wuhan as of 2019–2020.

It is essential to differentiate between the China CDC, which is affiliated with and accountable to the NHC, and the Chinese CDC system, which includes the China CDC and provincial, municipal, and county/district CDCs. Even major international publications such as the *Wall Street Journal* sometimes use language such as "the Wuhan branch of the National Health Commission" and "the Wuhan office of the China CDC."[52] This language creates the impression that the NHC directly oversees the Wuhan Municipal Health Commission and that the China CDC in Beijing directly manages the Wuhan Municipal CDC. In reality, the local health commissions and their CDCs are part of the local authorities. They are components of the local political-administrative hierarchy.

China's Administrative-Political Hierarchy for Health (2019–2020)

Communist Party Central Committee
Politburo - Standing Committee
Xi Jinping, General Secretary
Propaganda Department
Central Political and Legal Affairs Commission

The State Council, Premier Li Keqiang, Vice Premier Sun Chunlan (with health portfolio)
- Ministries, Commissions, and National Administrations, such as Defense, Finance, Foreign Affairs, NDRC, Public Security, and
- National Health Commission (Ma Xiaowei, Minister; Departments)
  - China CDC (Gao Fu, Director General)
  - NHC Directly-controlled hospitals: Beijing Hospital, Peking Union Medical College Hospital, Sino-Japanese Hospital

Hubei Provincial Party Committee
Jiang Chaoliang, Secretary
Ma Guoqiang, Deputy Secretary
Wang Xiaodong, Deputy Secretary
Propaganda Department
Provincial Political and Legal Affairs Commission

Hubei Provincial Government, Gov. Wang Xiaodong, Vice Gov. Yang Yunyan (health)
- Commissions and Bureaus, including Public Security, Finance, and
- Hubei Provincial Health Commission (Zhang Jin, Liu Yingzi)
  - Hubei Provincial CDC (Liu Jiafa, Yang Bo)
  - Provincial Hospitals: Wuhan Tongji Hospital; Wuhan Union Hospital; Hubei People's Hospital; Wuhan University Zhongnan Hospital; Hubei Provincial Hospital of Integrated Chinese and Western Medicine

Wuhan Municipal Party Committee
Ma Guoqiang, Secretary
Propaganda Department
Municipal Political and Legal Affairs Commission
District Party Leadership

Wuhan Municipal Government, Mayor Zhou Xianwang, Vice Mayor Chen Xiexin (health)
- Commissions and Bureaus, including Public Security, Finance, and
- Wuhan Municipal Health Commission (Zhang Hongxing)
  - Wuhan Municipal CDC (Li Gang)
  - Municipal Hospitals: Wuhan Jinyintan Hospital (infectious diseases); Wuhan Pulmonary Hospital; Wuhan Central Hospital; Wuhan First Hospital; Wuhan Youfu Hospital
  - District health bureaus (13 district CDCs)

Figure 2.1 China's Administrative-Political Hierarchy for Health (2019–2020)
Note: NDRC, National Development and Reform Commission.

Provincial and subprovincial health commissions have authority over public hospitals within their respective territories. While the NHC directly funds and oversees three hospitals (Beijing Hospital, Peking Union Medical College Hospital, and Sino-Japanese Hospital), other major hospitals are entrusted to provincial health commissions. For instance, the Hubei Provincial Health Commission oversees 14 hospitals, including several that receive funding from the NHC. The Wuhan Municipal Health Commission has 13 hospitals, which include two specialized infectious disease hospitals (Jinyintan and Pulmonary), as well as hospitals for mental health, pediatrics, and traditional Chinese medicine.

In a major city such as Wuhan, public hospitals are not only essential medical service providers but also organizations with differentiated administrative rankings. Some hospitals have a "direct report" relationship with the provincial health commission, even though they also interact with the respective district and municipal bureaucracies. Some report to the municipal health commission, while others report to the district health bureau. Within each public hospital, the leadership structure includes the party secretary and the president, with the president being technically in charge but under the leadership of the CCP. The major public hospitals are not-for-profit organizations with complex internal structures in the form of departments, offices, and specialties. They also tend to have multiple campuses that are spatially spread out.

Xi, Political Campaigns, and Party Leadership in Hospitals

As we seek to understand what transpired at the end of December 2019 and in the following weeks, it's essential to consider the impact of the intensified political campaigns, particularly the Education Campaign on Communist Party Aspiration and Mission initiated by Xi Jinping in summer 2019.

Ideology and organization are of great importance to leaders of communist parties, and Xi Jinping is no exception. Fueled by the fear of decline that led to the collapse of the Soviet Union and the pride of China's achievements under CCP leadership, Xi Jinping has made the promotion of loyalty to the party and its leadership central to his political rule since becoming general secretary in 2012. He has initiated various campaigns to purge the party of corruption and disloyalty, strengthen his predominant role in the party and the armed forces, and instill faith in the CCP through political education and indoctrination.[53] This combination of ideological and disciplinary campaigns, along with stringent anti-corruption measures, has greatly enhanced Xi Jinping's power.[54] However, it has also produced a decline in morale among officials, making them more risk-averse than during the Jiang Zemin and Hu Jintao years.[55] Such risk aversion prompted even Xi Jinping to express his frustration in January 2021, a year after the Wuhan outbreak, that officials would not take action without his explicit instructions.[56]

Amid the highly contentious United States–China trade war in 2019, there was even greater emphasis on political education, with a digital twist. In January 2019, a digital app called "Xuexi Qiangguo" (学习强国) became mandatory for party members and those working in state-sponsored institutions, including universities and public hospitals. The app disseminates official news and discourses, especially those of Xi Jinping, and monitors the amount of effort users made on the app and on specific tasks. In June, Xi launched the Aspiration/Mission Campaign, a party-history study campaign with the goal of reminding party members to "remain true to the original aspiration and keep the mission firmly in mind." Initially aimed at cadres at the county-divisional rank or above, it was later extended to enterprises, organizations, and local communities in the second half of 2019.[57] The Aspiration/Mission Campaign emphasized upholding the leadership of Xi Jinping and the authority of party leadership. In universities and hospitals, among others, the campaign boosted the power and authority of party secretaries at the expense of the presidents.

The Aspiration/Mission Campaign was taken very seriously in the Hubei health sector. In July 2019, the leaders and senior staff of the Hubei Provincial Health Commission (then still known as the Health and Population Planning Commission) took on assigned roles to promote the campaign across the province.[58] In September 2019, the commission's leadership took leaders of public hospitals in Hubei to a training program at Qinghua University for "strengthening party building in public hospitals."[59] This initiative to enhance party leadership in major hospitals received praise from the NHC leadership and provided important institutional context for understanding the power of the health commission over hospitals and medical staff in Hubei, including Wuhan, the provincial capital, as we examine the situation in Wuhan in January 2020.[60]

The Aspiration/Mission Campaign was also used to promote public-spiritedness among the party rank and file. Xi urged them to solve problems that affected the "interests of the masses" and to win people's trust.[61] The campaign gave a big boost to demands by local party leaders in health administrations and hospitals to improve doctor–patient relations.[62] Most strikingly, despite the arrival of a strong flu season, party leaders of major hospitals in Wuhan promoted Operation Mask Removal, asking medical staff to refrain from wearing facemasks in most interactions with patients so as to "shorten the distance" between medical staff and patients.[63] Unfortunately, even when health officials knew of the coronavirus outbreak, major hospitals in Wuhan continued to insist on "no masks" in most departments. According to a doctor at Wuhan Central Hospital, the department chief sternly warned the staff not to wear masks: "Don't fight with the leaders, don't wear a mask, and don't talk nonsense."[64]

The SARS Crisis and the Health Emergency Response Regime

In this larger political-administrative setting, the SARS crisis marked a critical turning point for the development of China's health emergency response regime. Although Guangdong and the MOH began recognizing and treating cases of atypical viral pneumonia in early January 2003, the public was not informed of the outbreak until February 10, 2003, due to a culture of secrecy. This lack of transparency also left medical professionals across China unaware and unprepared. Despite the disease spreading to Hong Kong, Beijing, and other cities and countries, the MOH and the city of Beijing initially downplayed the severity of the situation.[65] The information blackout and control measures proved to be the virus's greatest ally.

The initial failures in responding to SARS were partly attributed to the political-legal structure for infectious disease prevention and control. Although Chinese politics allows for a significant amount of discretion for political leaders, a strict textual interpretation of the law is often enforced when it comes to accountability. The Law on Infectious Disease Prevention and Treatment (1989), along with its Implementing Regulations (1991), includes three categories of infectious diseases. However, it could not be activated until an emerging disease like SARS, referred to as "infectious atypical pneumonia" (传染性非典型肺炎) in Chinese, was officially recognized as an infectious disease by the MOH of the State Council. This system created delays and hindered an effective response to the outbreak.

Despite the identification of a coronavirus as the causative pathogen for the SARS cases in Hong Kong and other places in late March 2003, Health Minister Zhang Wenkang continued to argue that the atypical pneumonia cases in Guangdong were distinct from SARS during a visit to Hong Kong. According to Zhang, while a type of atypical pneumonia was first identified in Guangdong, it was unclear whether it was connected to the SARS cases in

Hong Kong and other locations. He even went on to state that he "didn't believe the infection cases in Hong Kong were imported from the Mainland."[66]

For many weeks, the World Health Organization (WHO) struggled to obtain data from China and send expert teams to Guangdong.[67] Finally, after the organization issued a travel advisory on Guangdong and Hong Kong and caught the attention of the top Chinese leadership, a WHO team in Beijing received approval to visit Guangdong on April 2, 2003. Dr. Gro Harlem Brundtland, the WHO director-general at the time, publicly criticized China for its secretive and uncooperative behavior in handling SARS, which was a rare step for the organization. She stated in exasperation that "this was the first time a disease had spread internationally in this way."[68] Two days later, on April 8, 2003, the MOH, with approval from the State Council, finally recognized infectious atypical pneumonia (SARS) as an infectious disease (Class B). From then on, Class A measures, including enforced isolation and quarantine of infected individuals, would be implemented in accordance with Article 24.1 of the Law on the Prevention and Treatment of Infectious Diseases (1989).[69]

Despite the official recognition of SARS as an infectious disease, the Chinese response continued to be plagued by shortcomings and cover-ups in Beijing. Zhang Wenkang, the health minister with close ties to former general secretary Jiang Zemin, persisted in stating that the outbreak was under control, even as the number of cases in major hospitals in Beijing surged. In mid-April 2003, hospital leaders, including those at the Sino-Japanese Friendship Hospital, resorted to putting some SARS patients in ambulances that drove around Beijing to avoid detection by a WHO expert team conducting site visits.[70]

The revelation of outright concealment by Dr. Jiang Yanyong and the WHO mission in China played a significant role in convincing national leaders of the urgent need to take decisive action against the epidemic in Beijing.[71] In the latter half of April 2003, Zhang Wenkang and Beijing mayor Meng Xuenong were dismissed, with Vice Premier Wu Yi taking over as health minister and Wang Qishan assuming the role of Beijing mayor. They launched a public campaign to quarantine SARS patients and control the outbreak, particularly in Beijing. With hard work, luck, and strong leadership from the WHO, SARS was declared contained in China and around the world by July 2003.[72] According to the WHO, between November 1, 2002, and July 31, 2003, a total of 8,096 people worldwide were affected by SARS, with 774 fatalities. Mainland China (349), Hong Kong (299), Canada (43), Taiwan (37), Singapore (33), Vietnam (5), and Thailand, the Philippines, and Malaysia (2 each) had the most significant numbers of deaths.[73] The struggles with SARS in the affected cities left indelible memories on policymakers and clinicians.

China was criticized for its handling of the SARS outbreak in 2003. However, national leaders at the time, including General Secretary Hu Jintao, Premier Wen Jiabao, and Vice Premier Wu Yi, readily acknowledged the deficiencies in China's response. It was widely recognized that China urgently needed a robust epidemic information system and an institutional framework for responding to health emergencies.[74] As a response, on April 24, 2003, the MOH required local CDCs to file daily reports on SARS cases via a secure website, and hospitals were incorporated into the reporting system a month later.[75] The State Council issued the Regulation on Handling Public Health Emergencies on May 9, 2003, which, with immediate effect, required the health ministry and province-level authorities to develop contingency plans for responding to such emergencies. The regulation had strict stipulations on the prompt reporting of infectious disease outbreaks. On May 12, the MOH promulgated a set of Rules for Managing the Prevention and Treatment of Infectious Atypical Pneumonia (SARS), which provided guidance on the management of SARS cases.[76]

Building a Public Health Emergency Response System

The Regulation on Handling Public Health Emergencies, first promulgated in May 2003 and revised in 2011, highlighted the urgent need for a unified health emergency response system. It emphasized the importance of reporting infectious disease situations promptly to the national health authority (MOH or NHC) in 1–2 hours. The health authority was also given the responsibility of disclosing epidemic information to the public and authorizing province-level health authorities to release epidemic information in their respective jurisdictions. Article 25 of the Regulation stressed the importance of "timely, accurate, and comprehensive" information dissemination, indicating strong dissatisfaction with China's performance prior to April 20, 2003.[77] This regulation, along with the revised Law on the Prevention and Treatment of Infectious Diseases (passed by the National People's Congress Standing Committee in August 2004) and the Emergency Response Law of 2007, forms the backbone of China's health emergency response regime.

In explaining the need to revamp the Law on the Prevention and Treatment of Infectious Diseases to legislators, MOH Vice Minister Gao Qiang candidly admitted China's failures in disease surveillance and reporting, treatment of infected individuals, control of cross-infections in hospitals, and implementation of emergency control measures. He acknowledged that "the channels for epidemic information reporting and notification are not smooth,"[78] which was a euphemistic way of referring to the serious concealment and cover-up of critical epidemic information during the SARS outbreak.[79]

Following the SARS crisis, the Chinese health leadership and public health community recognized the urgent need to improve disease surveillance, reporting, control, and emergency response. At the end of 2004, the MOH, together with the Ministry of Finance, announced a set of ambitious objectives for building a nationwide disease prevention and control system, covering national, provincial, municipal, and county levels.[80] MOH Order No. 40 aimed to establish "a well-functioning, responsive, and coordinated emergency mechanism for public health emergencies." Its key objectives (Art. 2) included enhancing disease prevention and control responsibilities for medical institutions, building an epidemic information network that covers both urban and rural areas, improving the infrastructure and laboratory equipment conditions of disease prevention and control institutions, and strengthening the building of professional teams for disease prevention and control, raising the capabilities for epidemiological investigation, on-site handling, and laboratory diagnosis. The order also included details on ensuring financial support for this initiative and laid out differentiated responsibilities and capabilities for national versus provincial and subprovincial disease prevention and control institutions in line with the Law on Infectious Disease Prevention and Treatment.[81] These initiatives created a palpable sense of optimism for the future of China's public health system.[82]

The National Disease Reporting System

Although the revised law on infectious diseases was approved, the experts and policy advisors I spoke with were well aware that Chinese institutions and regulations are deeply entwined with the wider political-administrative framework. Despite this, they recognized that their only option was to operate within the existing political-administrative structure. As a result, they turned to the emerging new information technology to overcome the deficiencies and flaws of the earlier disease reporting system, which relied on slow mail and was also susceptible to administrative bottlenecks.

Following the experience gained from case reporting during the SARS crisis, the MOH moved quickly to launch a national public health information system initiative. In early 2004, the National Notifiable Disease Surveillance

System (NNDSS), an internet-based platform, was officially launched.[83] This system enables lower-level CDCs and medical institutions to report infectious disease cases and public health events directly, as well as real-time monitoring of such information by the China CDC.[84] The NNDSS is designed for infectious diseases that are officially included in the Law on the Prevention and Control of Infectious Diseases. The revised 2004 law added infectious atypical pneumonia (internationally known as SARS) and human avian influenza (H5N1) as Class B infectious diseases. In 2014, H7N9 was added as a subtype of human avian influenza.

The implementation of the NNDSS significantly accelerated the reporting process for notifiable infectious diseases.[85] China CDC statistics showed that the NNDSS had expanded to encompass over 70,000 reporting units by 2013, covering all subnational CDCs, 98% of medical institutions at the county and above level and 94% of township-level healthcare units.[86] The system had 146,000 authorized real-name users by the end of 2016. Building on the NNDSS, the China CDC developed information systems to facilitate disease surveillance for specific illnesses, such as tuberculosis and HIV/AIDS, and established some data-sharing arrangements between the NNDSS and individual disease systems.[87]

PUE Surveillance

The NNDSS was intended to enhance China's preparedness for situations similar to the SARS crisis. However, paradoxically, the system was designed to be used only for legally notifiable infectious diseases rather than identifying newly emerging infectious diseases. Therefore, it would not have been useful for reporting infectious atypical pneumonia (SARS) cases until the disease was officially recognized and included in the list of notifiable infectious diseases.

Recognizing this significant gap, the MOH initiated a trial program for the surveillance of PUE in August 2004, before the revised Infectious Diseases Law was enacted. The national PUE surveillance program was established with the recognition that airborne pathogens are likely to spread rapidly, requiring a prompt response. It is designed to surveil and provide early warning of possible cases of SARS (infectious atypical pneumonia), human avian influenza, and other infectious respiratory diseases. The program requires prompt case reporting based on clinical, radiological, and laboratory criteria and stipulates follow-up clinical diagnosis and procedures for escalation to higher-level CDCs and health authorities as necessary.[88] Technically, the PUE cases are submitted through the same internet platform as the NNDSS. From 2005 to 2006, 236 PUE cases were reported and followed up, with 21 later confirmed to be cases of human avian influenza (H5N1) not linked to known outbreaks.[89]

In response to the lessons learned from the SARS crisis, the WHO adopted the *International Health Regulations* (2005), third edition.[90] These regulations raised the requirements on countries for reporting and responding to emerging infectious diseases, and China was eager to contribute to the worldwide surveillance and response network.[91]

Building on the encouraging results of the PUE trial program, the MOH upgraded and expanded the original PUE program into the National Program for the Surveillance, Screening, and Management of Cases of Pneumonia of Uncertain Etiology in May 2007. This program continues to focus on SARS, human avian influenza, and other cluster-like infectious respiratory diseases.[92] It provides detailed protocols for reporting, follow-up diagnosis, and case confirmation, as well as the corresponding prevention and control measures.

The PUE surveillance system was instrumental in identifying human avian influenza cases, especially the identification of the H7N9 avian flu in 2013.[93] In response to the emergence of Middle East respiratory syndrome (MERS) cases caused by the MERS coronavirus, China's national health authority established protocols between 2013 and 2015 to deal with MERS cases that might present as atypical PUE cases. As a result, screening for atypical PUEs has been a serious focus in public health training programs.

The Influenza Surveillance System

China began collaborating with the WHO on influenza surveillance in 2000 and has since strengthened its efforts following the SARS crisis.[94] Influenza is currently included in the NNDSS, and the China CDC has established the China National Influenza Center (CNIC) and the Chinese Influenza Surveillance Information System to enhance its participation in the WHO's Global Influenza Program. The CNIC has also collaborated with the US CDC on virology and epidemiology training. By 2014, the Chinese National Influenza Surveillance Network had reached a steady state of 554 sentinel hospitals and 408 laboratories, which have nucleic acid detection techniques and virus isolation capabilities. As of 2020, there were 410 laboratories in the network.[95]

Sentinel hospitals report cases of influenza-like illness to the Chinese National Influenza Surveillance Information System and send respiratory specimens to network laboratories for diagnostic testing using real-time reverse-transcription polymerase chain reaction. If the samples test positive for influenza virus, they are cultured using Madin-Darby canine kidney cells and/or embryonated chicken eggs. The network laboratories then send the virus isolates to the CNIC for further analysis.[96]

The NHC issues the annual Diagnosis and Treatment Plan for Seasonal Influenza, along with manuals for medical staff training. In October 2019, the NHC established the National Expert Team for Influenza Medical Treatment, led by Wang Chen, president of the Chinese Academy of Medical Sciences/ Peking Union Medical College, with Dr. Zhong Nanshan of SARS fame as advisor. The team was tasked with revising the Diagnosis and Treatment Plan and related guidelines, and the 2019 edition was released in mid-November.[97] Interestingly, the interactions among the medical experts and between them and NHC administrators proved valuable preparation for dealing with a different respiratory disease: most of the expert team members would later play important roles in responding to the novel coronavirus outbreak and ensuing COVID-19 pandemic that began in late 2019.

Health Emergency Preparedness Laws, Institutions, and Capabilities

The Regulation on Handling Public Health Emergencies has provided a framework for preparing the National Preparedness Plan for Public Health Emergencies and province-level preparedness plans. Health emergency response offices have been established in both the national and provincial health authorities, as well as in the Chinese CDC system.[98] In early 2006, the State Council released the national plan, which was quickly adapted by provincial authorities.[99] For instance, the Province of Hubei created the Hubei provincial health emergency preparedness plan in 2006 and updated it in 2010.[100] Notably, the Hubei preparedness plan was accompanied by a medical rescue preparedness plan for emergencies.[101]

The enactment of the Emergency Response Law in 2007 should have given a further boost to the health emergency response system. However, despite calls to update and amend the Regulation on Handling Public Health Emergencies to align it with the Emergency Response Law, this was not done until 2020.[102] Following the Wuhan outbreak, legal scholars debated whether Article 38 of the Law on the Prevention and Treatment of Infectious Diseases or Article 43 of the Emergency Response Law should have taken precedence in terms of disclosing epidemic information and issuing public alerts. The former, consistent with the Regulation on Handling Public Health Emergencies, gives the State Council health authority the responsibility to disclose information, while the latter empowers governments at the county level or higher to issue appropriate-level public alerts.[103] In fact, the national health authority, the MOH and its successors, granted province-level health authorities the right to "timely and accurately publicize epidemic information on statutory infectious disease outbreaks and information on public health emergencies in their respective jurisdictions" through Notice [2006] No. 79, in the event of infectious disease outbreaks, epidemics, and other public health emergencies in their administrative areas.[104]

Capabilities, Experiences, and Complications

Following the SARS crisis, China not only developed capabilities to combat infectious diseases but also gained experience dealing with emerging or recurring infectious diseases such as hand, foot, and mouth disease (HFMD), H5N1, H5N2, H1N1, and H7N9. China's identification and response to human avian influenza virus H7N9 outbreaks in 2013–2017 were particularly noteworthy. Unlike during the SARS crisis, Chinese scientists and epidemiologists earned international praise by taking the lead in virus identification, research, and prevention in addressing H7N9.[105]

China's increasing global prominence in combating infectious diseases was demonstrated in 2014 when a team led by George Gao Fu, then the deputy director general of the China CDC, and two infectious disease experts of the Academy of Military Medical Sciences, joined the fight against Ebola in Sierra Leone and a number of other countries.[106] President Xi Jinping placed "extreme importance" on the medical mission to Africa, insisting that the Chinese team also maintain a "zero infection" among its own members.[107] In 2017, China's drug regulatory authority became the first government body in the world to approve an Ebola vaccine, which was developed by the bioengineering institute of the Academy of Military Medical Sciences of China and CanSino Biologics.[108] Chinese scientists also made major progress identifying the source of the SARS coronavirus and the MERS coronavirus.[109]

Despite notable successes, China's responses to outbreaks between SARS and COVID-19 were not without flaws. During the HFMD outbreak, foot-dragging, concealment, and poor communication with the public were observed, including information blackouts and even misinformation.[110] While the H7N9 outbreaks were contained with modest prevention and control efforts, this success relative to SARS was partly due to the lower infectivity of H7N9.[111]

China has been aggressive in preventing pathogenic threats from abroad such as H1N1, Ebola, MERS, and Zika. For example, during the H1N1 outbreak in 2008–2009, China implemented strict measures to test and quarantine international travelers and suspected individuals.[112] While these measures received popular support and were touted as evidence of China's growing capabilities to handle all infectious diseases, Yanzhong Huang noted that officials across the country often adopted excessive responses to create the impression of a vigorous government response and that they were "acting differently this time around."[113]

The improvement of China's health emergency response capabilities was complicated by its multi-layered governing hierarchy, which can propel investment-driven growth but can also lead to feigned compliance, distortion, and subterfuge when central and local interests diverge. During the H1N1 outbreak, there were issues of upward information flow and transparency, and local officials were practiced in "secrecy and inaction."[114] Zhong Nanshan noted that some areas maintained zero fatalities from H1N1 by refusing to identify, let alone disclose, such deaths. He expressed doubt in the accuracy of the nationally reported number of influenza A (H1N1) deaths.[115]

The leadership of China's CDC was aware that local authorities and medical institutions may not always comply fully with disease reporting and could be motivated to conceal cases, despite the lessons learned from SARS. While the cases submitted through the NNDSS are technically observable at the China CDC, cases that are reported to the local CDCs but are not entered into the online system would not be known to the Beijing-based CDC team. According to Zeng Guang, who was the China CDC chief epidemiologist until January 2020, "I was in charge of national infectious disease epidemic reporting for 17 years. During those 17 years, the most common problem I encountered was that, when local outbreaks occurred, the local health administrations would not allow local medical institutions and even the local CDCs to make reports" in the national online reporting system.[116]

Although the PUE surveillance program was expanded to require reporting of PUE cases alongside statutory cases of SARS and human avian influenza, it was an administrative measure organized by the national health authority and was not incorporated into the Law on the Prevention and Control of Infectious Diseases. This legal distinction is not widely recognized but has had significant consequences for reporting and accountability.[117] Between 2004 and 2016, the PUE surveillance system received a total of 1,666 PUE cases, averaging 128 cases per year for the entire country. However, this number is significantly lower than the experiences of clinicians in respiratory medicine. After reviewing typical prefectural comprehensive hospitals, a China CDC team concluded that "the case reporting rate in the PUE surveillance system is quite low, and the system's performance is unsatisfactory."

To improve the rate and accuracy of infectious disease submission, the National Health (and Population Planning) Commission introduced an updated set of Rules for Managing Infectious Diseases Information Reporting in 2016. These rules aim to make health commissions responsible for the operation of the infectious disease reporting system and state that any medical institution, including rural doctors or those in private clinics, must report epidemic information if they encounter cases. The rules also grant staff in local CDCs the authority to review cases reported for accuracy and duplicates and direct them to delete incorrectly reported or duplicated cases promptly. These rules cover not only the notifiable infectious diseases specified in the Infectious Diseases Law (which require reporting within 2–24 hours) but also infectious diseases identified by provincial authorities, PUE cases, and deaths from unknown causes.[118] However, since these rules do not have the force of law, their impact has been limited, including for the initial novel coronavirus cases in December 2019.

Enhancement of Health Emergency Preparedness

As noted above, Xi Jinping has pursued a security-focused governing philosophy centered on the concept of "overall national security." This approach emphasizes the prevention and management of various risks. In the health sector, the national health leadership answered the call for "overall national security" with the issuance of extensive guidance in 2016 to province-level authorities on strengthening health emergency preparedness and response. The aim was to create, by the end of 2020, a health emergency response system that could effectively respond to domestic health emergencies while also raising China's profile in the global public health and safety arena. The guidance identified eight major tasks, including surveillance, preparedness planning, and emergency response, with the first two tasks focused on institutional development. Task 1 emphasized organizational and systems building based on the principle of territorial management and differentiated responsibilities across multiple levels of the functional and territorial hierarchy. Task 2 called for enhancing the Joint Prevention and Control Mechanism, a valuable legacy from the SARS crisis, through inter-departmental integration, coordination, and joint action, as well as military–civilian integration and regional cooperation. The guidance also encouraged international cooperation through joint action and participation in joint exercises, among other means.[119]

In 2018, Xi Jinping emphasized the need for "constant vigilance and strict precautions against major infectious diseases like SARS."[120] Marking the centennial year of the great influenza of 1918–1920, Feng Zijian of the China CDC, echoing other health leaders, warned that another pandemic was almost unavoidable.[121] In July 2019, the NHC, with assistance from the China CDC, conducted a National Emergency Response Exercise for Public Health Emergencies based on the health emergency preparedness plan. The exercise involved over 8,200 participants from all province-level health commissions and some subprovincial health commissions. In the scenario, a passenger arriving from an epidemic zone abroad was found to have a fever and tested positive for a known viral pathogen. Representatives from local health commissions were tested on critical components of the Joint Prevention and Control Mechanism during the exercise, including submitting reports of infectious disease cases, conducting contact tracing and quarantine, managing patient treatment, taking responsibility for biosafety, and effectively communicating with the public.[122]

Another health emergency response exercise was conducted at Wuhan Tianhe Airport on September 18, 2019, in anticipation of the World Military Games, also known as Wuhan 2019, which hosted over 9,300 athletes from 140 countries. The exercise scenario involved responding to a case of novel coronavirus infection at the airport, which was coincidentally similar to what would later become the reality with the outbreak of COVID-19. The exercise included epidemiological investigation, medical screening, quarantine and isolation, and case transfer and treatment.[123] Leaders and staff from Wuhan's health institutions, including the municipal health commission, the municipal CDC, and the Wuhan Jinyintan Hospital, participated in the exercise.

While Chinese preparedness exercises were focused on dealing with pathogens coming from foreign countries, the country engaged in international preparedness efforts. Gao Fu, the director general of the China CDC, participated in the "Exercise 201" public pandemic simulation held in New York in October 2019. This exercise brought together high-level decision makers to respond to a severe pandemic scenario involving the outbreak of a novel zoonotic coronavirus that transmitted from bats to pigs to people and then became efficiently transmissible. The fictional scenario was set in Brazil but modeled on SARS and involved a virus that is "more transmissible in the community setting by people with mild symptoms."[124]

Conclusion

In the aftermath of the SARS crisis, China has channeled resources to expand capacities for disease prevention and control, investing heavily in research and national reporting and building a health emergency regime of laws, institutions, and procedures. China's health leaders were especially proud of having built the world's largest national disease reporting system.

It has become commonplace in the aftermath of the COVID-19 pandemic for Chinese public health officials and experts—Gao Fu, Zeng Guang, and Gao Fu notably—to say that public health in China had suffered from relative neglect in the 2010s as the searing memory of SARS receded and that the public health sector has had difficulty retaining and attracting talent relative to clinical practice. One study noted that the language for medical and health reforms increasingly shifted from "prevention" to "service," thus diminishing the relative weight of prevention.[125] Yet such an assessment must be put in the context of the capacity building and real-world disease fighting experiences China had already acquired with SARS and subsequent infectious disease outbreaks. In the years between SARS and COVID-19, this political ecology for infectious disease prevention and control appeared to have served China well in responding to the various infectious diseases in China and from abroad, including human avian influenzas such as H1N1 and H7N9 as well as Ebola and MERS.

As China prepared to enhance its health emergency preparedness with training exercises in spring 2019, then China CDC director general Gao Fu was asked about China's capabilities for handling SARS-like epidemics. Gao responded with swagger: "SARS-like viruses can appear at any time. However, I am very confident to say that 'SARS-like events' will not occur again, because the infectious disease surveillance network system of our country is well established, and such events will not happen again."[126]

Yet health emergency response is not an isolated domain. It must operate within and is constrained by an ecology of institutions, organizations, individuals, as well as their interactions across multiple levels of the party-state structure and across time and space. Whereas the handling of infectious disease outbreaks typically requires a whole-of-government approach, it requires the different domains of the party-state to work together to further the goals of public health. Unfortunately, the imperatives of party-state domination may conflict with the principles for effective health emergency preparedness and response.[127] By the end of 2019, Gao's bravado was put to severe test by an outbreak of SARS-like pneumonia cases in the city of Wuhan.

3

The Wuhan Alarm

Unusual Pneumonia Cases and a SARS-Like Coronavirus

Despite China's public health community participating in health emergency exercises involving an imagined novel coronavirus coming from abroad earlier in 2019, hardly anyone anticipated a real coronavirus outbreak in Wuhan, the capital of the central Chinese province of Hubei (population 59.3 million in 2019).

In hindsight, early signals about hard-to-treat pneumonia patients began to circulate in the Wuhan medical community in mid-December 2019. At that time, Wuhan was in the midst of a serious influenza wave, and some schools even suspended classes to deal with the flu situation.[1] With so much attention on the influenza, the significance of unusual pneumonia cases being caused by something else was easily dismissed.

Wuhan Youfu Hospital (Figure 3.1) was very close to the Huanan Seafood Market, the epicenter of the initial outbreak. Doctors at Youfu Hospital started to treat patients with serious flu-like symptoms beginning on December 12. They wanted the patients to get computed tomographic (CT) scans so that they could know more about the cause of the symptoms, but the patients, who were mostly workers at the Huanan market, didn't think that their symptoms warranted paying for CT scans. According to a doctor at Youfu Hospital, hospital leaders requested and received guidance in mid-December 2019 from "superior levels," presumably the Wuhan Municipal Health Commission (WMHC), about scattered pneumonia cases in the Huanan Seafood Market. They were told that these cases "were not SARS, and no human-to-human transmission has been found."[2]

The early signals about the outbreak in Wuhan reached the international public health community, including Ian Lipkin, an eminent epidemiologist at Columbia University who had helped China combat severe acute respiratory syndrome (SARS) in 2003 and strengthen its public health system afterward. In mid-December 2019, he heard, via a member of his research staff, from a Chinese contact about an outbreak of unusual pneumonia cases in Wuhan and offered his help for diagnostic testing.[3] Sources reported that Lipkin wrote to China Centers for Disease Control and Prevention (China CDC) director

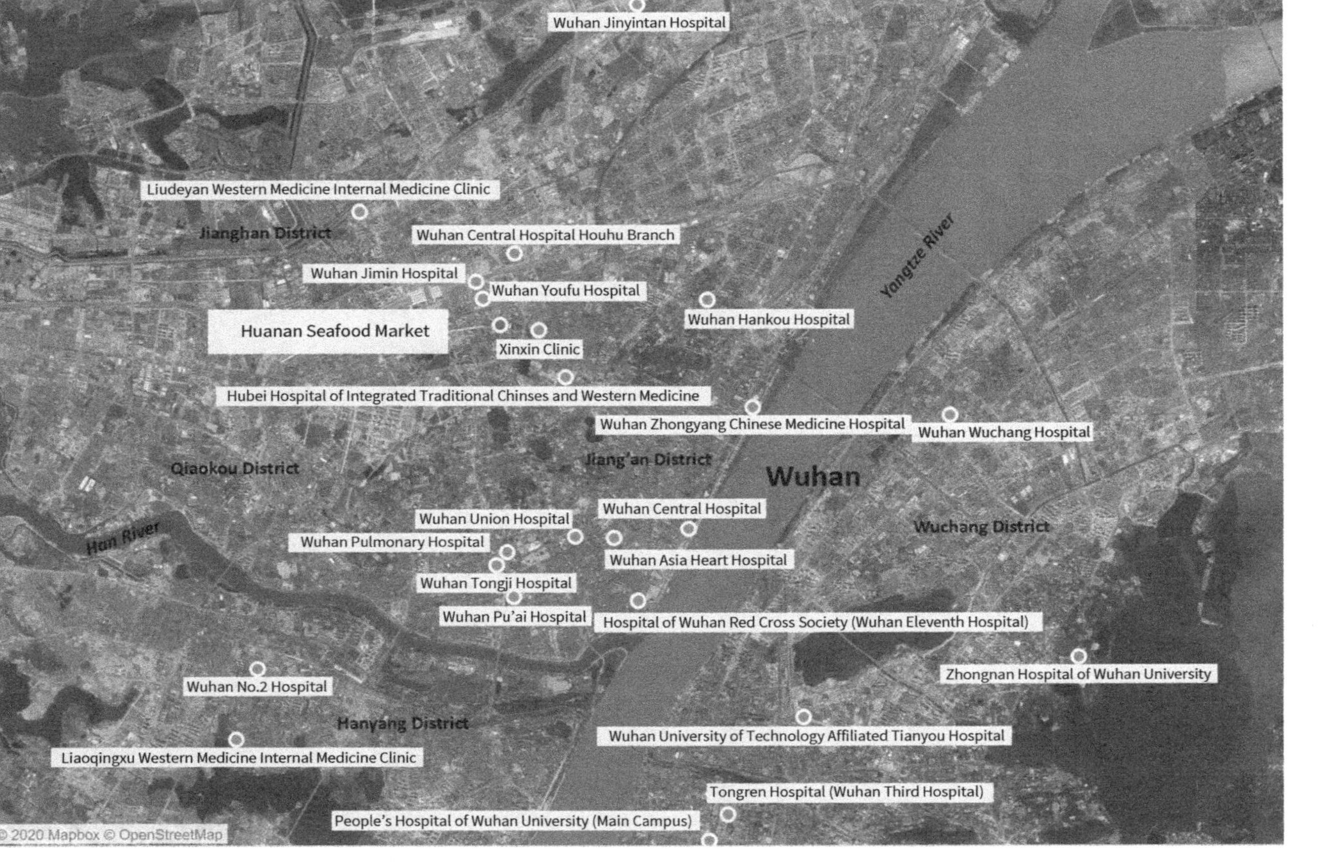

Figure 3.1 Map of Selected Hospitals in Wuhan

general Gao Fu to inquire about the outbreak but did not hear back from Gao until December 31, 2019.[4]

None of these early instances of unusual pneumonia cases, often referred to as PUE (pneumonia of uncertain etiology), were reported to the China CDC via the National Notifiable Disease Surveillance System (NNDSS). By December 25, 2019, a growing number of such pneumonia cases were treated by physicians in prominent hospitals in Wuhan. Dr. Lü Xiaohong, a physician at Wuhan No. 5 Hospital, noted that around December 25, 2019, healthcare workers in two Wuhan hospitals, including staff from the respiratory department, were rumored to have contracted the viral PUE and had been placed in isolation. Dr. Lü surmised that, since medical staff in the respiratory section typically took great care to protect themselves, this pneumonia must be highly contagious. Upon further investigation, she learned that the patients with this unusual PUE exhibited severe lung infections on their CT scans but displayed minimal coughing or fever symptoms.[5]

It is most likely that physicians and hospital administrators from some hospitals in the Wuhan area reported PUE cases to local CDCs between December 15 and 26, 2019. However, except for the inquiry made by Wuhan Youfu Hospital, these reports have not been made public. The first publicly documented report of such cases occurred on December 27, 2019.

This chapter recounts the response of clinicians, independent clinical laboratories, hospital administrators, and health leaders to the emergence of COVID-19 cases in Wuhan at the end of 2019. Contrary to popular belief, it was not a single doctor who first reported the cases. Instead, clinicians from several hospitals reported PUE cases to local CDCs in Wuhan from December 27 to 29, 2019. Despite some initial setbacks, the persistence of clinicians, notably Dr. Zhang Jixian, and hospital administrators eventually led to the Hubei provincial health commission launching a joint investigation on December 29, 2020. By then, an increasing number of health experts in Wuhan had learned that some of the pneumonia cases were caused by a SARS-like coronavirus. We give special attention to Patient A, whose transfer from one hospital to another facilitated the exchange of valuable disease information.

Furthermore, commercial diagnostic laboratories, such as Vision Medicals, played important yet officially unacknowledged roles in identifying the pathogen and alerting clinicians and health leaders to the dangers of the novel coronavirus. The chapter links the case of Patient A with the notable diagnostic tests conducted at Vision Medicals, which provided the first known genomic sequence pointing to a SARS-like coronavirus as the causative agent of Patient A's pneumonia.

Lastly, the chapter discusses the investigation and report conducted by a joint team of provincial, municipal, and district health officials and specialists. This unpublished joint investigation report was critical in shaping the public health community's understanding of the outbreak and significantly influenced the official response to the epidemic. It is therefore important to pay close attention to what it included and what it left out.

The First Reports to Local CDCs, December 27–29, 2019

China's official white paper on its COVID-19 response credits Dr. Zhang Jixian for being the first to report cases of what would be known as COVID-19 to health authorities in Wuhan/Hubei.[6] In reality, her peers at several other hospitals also filed reports of PUE cases with local CDCs and requested investigation during this time. These included Dr. Fan Zhongjie at the Red Cross Society Hospital, Dr. Zhang Jianping at Tongji Hospital, and Dr. Ai Fen and others at Wuhan Central Hospital (WCH; Houhu Branch). All of these hospitals, except for Tongji Hospital, were located near the Huanan Seafood Market. At the time, these doctors suspected that the unusual pneumonia cases they were treating were likely infectious, so they took necessary precautions.

Physicians from at least three Wuhan hospitals initially reported PUE cases to district CDCs on December 27, 2019. District CDC staff utilized standard testing kits to rule out a range of pathogens, but their investigations did not go beyond that. Judging by the inquiry the Youfu Hospital leadership made with health authorities about unusual flu-like pneumonia cases in mid-December 2019, it was likely that there had been earlier reports of similar PUE cases in Wuhan to district CDCs but, as was the case on December 27, the local CDCs did not identify something unusual.

Dr. Zhang Jixian

Dr. Zhang is the director of pulmonary and critical care medicine in the Hubei Provincial Hospital of Integrated Chinese and Western Medicine (hereafter "Hubei Integrated Medicine Hospital," also known as "Xinhua Hospital"). Between the afternoon of December 26, 2019, and the morning of December 27, 2019, her section admitted an elderly couple. The couple had fever, coughs, and breathing difficulty; and the husband, who had diabetes, tested negative for flu and other common viral and bacterial diseases. However, his CT scan showed multiple "ground glass opacities" in both lungs. Dr. Zhang became concerned as the two patients had highly similar CT scans and were a couple, and their lung infections looked "completely different from those we had seen of previous pneumonia patients."[7]

During the 2003 SARS crisis, Dr. Zhang served as a SARS expert team member in Wuhan's Jianghan District. She and her team members screened for suspected SARS cases by examining patients' chest X-rays and gathering information on their residency and occupation as part of epidemiological investigations. Dr. Zhang retained these practices like habits and instinctively looked for patient clusters.[8]

On December 27, 2019, Dr. Zhang also saw the elderly couple's son and encouraged the healthy-looking son to get tested. Around noontime, Dr. Zhang received the son's test results, which indicated a low blood count, a low lymphocyte count, and a CT scan showing milder lung infections similar to those of his parents.[9] "When a family of three all develop [lung infections], it would be highly unlikely for them not to have an infectious disease," Dr. Zhang recalled.[10]

It is important to note that China was particularly sensitive to SARS, officially called "infectious atypical pneumonia" (传染性非典型肺炎) in Chinese, following the 2003 SARS crisis. The Infectious Diseases Law classifies infectious atypical pneumonia, caused by the SARS coronavirus, as a Class B infectious disease but nonetheless stipulates Class A emergency responses for it.

Additionally, the national guidelines for monitoring, screening, and managing cases of atypical pneumonia of unknown or uncertain etiology (PUE) define PUE cases based on four criteria: fever (axillary body temperature ≥38°C), imaging features of pneumonia (CT scan or X-ray), reduced or normal total white blood cell count or a reduced lymphocyte count early in the onset of the disease, and non-response to antibiotic treatment. The guidelines specify that PUE clusters, defined as two or more related cases within 2 weeks, must be immediately reported to the district/county CDC as well as the national direct report system.[11] As noted in Chapter 2, the reporting of PUE cases is associated with the national disease reporting system but not governed by the Infectious Diseases Law.

Upon realizing that she had a family cluster of atypical PUE cases that looked like SARS, Dr. Zhang Jixian knew that she needed to report the cases. "This situation must be reported," she recalled telling herself.[12] While doctors and hospital administrators theoretically have direct access to the NNDSS to file cases, doing so would have immediately drawn attention from the China

CDC. Therefore, local health authorities typically prefer to first evaluate the situation on their own terms.

According to Wu Zunyou, who would become the China CDC chief epidemiologist in January 2020, when Dr. Zhang Jixian saw the CT scans of her patients and feared that SARS had returned, she "did not dare to file reports [on the cases] in the [NNDSS] system, so she reported [directly] to the local CDC" on December 27, 2019.[13]

To be more exact, Dr. Zhang reported the cluster of cases to the Hospital Infection Office and the Medical Affairs Department as well as Vice President Xia Wenguang, and they in turn informed staff at the district CDC. According to Dr. Xia, Zhang spoke to him with an emphatic tone, stating, "It's a disease we've never encountered before, it's also a family [cluster of] infections. Something is definitely wrong!"[14]

That afternoon, staff from the (Wuhan) Jianghan District CDC went to the hospital to take patient samples for testing and conducted epidemiological investigation. Dr. Zhang was present and spoke with the local CDC staff.[15]

Another patient with similar symptoms checked in that same afternoon. By Sunday, December 29, 2019, there were a total of seven patients with similar symptoms in Dr. Zhang's section. Unlike the family of three, the other four patients worked at the Huanan Seafood Market—a large marketplace with hundreds of stalls and shops that sold far more than seafood. The Huanan was located less than 2 miles away from Dr. Zhang's hospital.

By the time these patients were admitted to the Hubei Integrated Medicine Hospital, they had already received treatments in smaller hospitals or clinics. Several of them had severe symptoms and were not responsive to conventional antibiotic treatment. Facing these tough cases, Dr. Zhang sought help. At about 1 PM on that fateful Sunday, she implored Dr. Xia Wenguang, the vice president responsible for medical affairs, to bring together specialists from various sections and offices, including the Respiratory Medicine, Gastroenterology, Circulation, Endocrinology, Intensive Care, Radiology, Laboratory, Pharmacy, Infection, and Medical Affairs Departments, to review and examine the seven cases.[16]

In requesting assistance from these different specialties and offices throughout the hospital, Dr. Zhang indicated the daunting challenges she and her colleagues faced in treating these patients. Although she didn't anticipate an epidemic outbreak at this point, this gathering foreshadowed the forthcoming disaster in Wuhan and worldwide.[17]

Dr. Xia Wenguang, a prominent rehabilitation specialist, deferred to Dr. Zhang's assessment and immediately gathered 10 specialists to review the seven cases.[18] The collective consultation record clearly stated that the patients with severe symptoms had received antiviral and antibacterial treatments, but their conditions failed to improve. The family cluster was noted and cited as an indication of infectivity.[19] For the most severely ill patients, "CT scans of the lungs showed multiple infectious lesions in both lungs, with ground glass opacities." The gathered specialists were unanimous that the situation with the seven patients was concerning and required vigilance.[20]

During the consultation, Dr. Xia learned that there had been two additional patients with similar symptoms who were transferred to the more prestigious Tongji Hospital and Union Hospital. These two patients were also workers at the Huanan Seafood Market. This information further heightened Dr. Xia's concern.[21]

Two days earlier, hospital staff had reported the initial family cluster of three to the district CDC. The district CDC staff had essentially repeated the battery of tests performed at the hospital that had come out negative for common diseases.[22] With a heightened sense of urgency, Dr. Xia decided to escalate their request. While the Hubei Integrated Medicine Hospital is physically located in Jianghan District of Wuhan, it is administratively under the direct leadership of the Hubei Provincial Health Commission. On that Sunday, Dr. Xia and staff reported the seven PUE cases directly to the Disease Prevention and Control Departments of the provincial and municipal health commissions, requesting urgent expert consultation.[23]

Dr. Zhang Jixian deserves significant credit for first identifying the PUE cases, and she was later commended in Hubei and nationally for her persistence in sounding the alarm and successfully reporting the cases.[24] However, Dr. Xia Wenguang is the unsung hero who played a decisive role in getting the provincial and municipal health leadership to respond promptly at this juncture. That afternoon, the WMHC, in consultation with the provincial health commission, activated its emergency response protocol. It ordered the Wuhan Municipal CDC, Jinyintan Hospital (Wuhan's dedicated infectious disease hospital), and the Jianghan District CDC to dispatch a joint team of specialists to the Hubei Integrated Medicine Hospital to investigate the cases. We will discuss the joint team's findings later in this chapter.

"Patient A" of WCH

In fact, besides Dr. Zhang Jixian, clinicians and public health staff at three other hospitals also filed reports on SARS-like cases in Wuhan between December 27 and 29. Tongji Hospital and the Hospital of Wuhan Red Cross Society made reports on December 27. The WCH reported on December 29.

Dr. Zhao Jianping of the Tongji Hospital also made a report of PUE cases on December 27, 2019. In making the decision, Dr. Zhao relied on the diagnostic test results that had been done on a patient, hereafter "Patient A," at the WCH. Patient A was a 65-year-old retired male with diabetes. A former deliveryman at the Huanan Seafood Market, Patient A was retired but regularly visited the market to chat with friends and play cards. On December 13, he began experiencing chills and a fever of 39.1°C. He first visited the WCH Nanjing Road Campus as an outpatient on December 15 and was prescribed oral antibiotics and antiviral drugs such as amoxicillin & clavulanate potassium and oseltamivir.[25] He returned to WCH on December 18 with breathing difficulty and was admitted into the emergency ward with a diagnosis of "community-acquired pneumonia, severe." His CT scan revealed "multiple scattered patchy faint opacities in both lungs." Despite being administered carbapenems, a class of broad-spectrum antibiotics for treating severe bacterial infections, his condition did not improve.[26] He was transferred to the WCH respiratory ward for specialist treatment on December 22, 2019. Dr. Hu Yi served as the director of the Respiratory and Critical Care Medicine section.[27]

To identify the pathogenic cause of Patient A's infection, doctors obtained consent from Patient A's family to use genomic sequencing. On the evening of December 24, they performed a procedure called bronchoalveolar lavage (BAL) washing to collect BAL fluid from the patient's lungs. The BAL fluid sample was then sent to Guangzhou-based Vision Medicals (微远基因) for genomic sequencing using a metagenomic next-generation sequencing (mNGS) platform.[28] Founded in June 2018, Vision Medicals is one of many commercial diagnostic laboratories that have emerged in China, capable of producing genomic sequencing results in about 3 days for approximately 3,000 yuan (about US$450).

Meanwhile, Patient A's situation continued to worsen. "My husband couldn't take it anymore. [He was] running a high fever, couldn't breathe, his body couldn't stand it anymore," recalled Patient A's wife.[29] Hoping for better treatment, she transferred Patient A to Tongji Hospital. By then, other patients with similar symptoms, including a patient "Chen" who had visited the Huanan Seafood Market on December 16, were also being treated at Tongji Hospital.[30]

Dr. Zhao Jianping and Patient A at Tongji Hospital

Dr. Zhao Jianping was the deputy leader of the SARS Expert Team in Hubei Province during the SARS crisis in 2003. By 2019, he had become the director of Respiratory and Critical Care Medicine at the prestigious Wuhan Tongji Hospital, where he was widely regarded as one of China's leading experts in respiratory medicine. On or around December 27, 2019, Dr. Zhao was alerted by staff in his department about three patients, including a couple, who exhibited "very unusual CT imaging features, showing diffuse, infiltrative lesions in both lungs."[31] The patients also had low blood cells and reduced lymphocyte counts, which suggested a serious respiratory illness.

In a February 2020 interview that initially appeared on the website of the Wuhan Association for Science and Technology but has since been removed from other sites, Dr. Zhao described how he and his colleagues responded to the initial cases on December 27. "Starting on December 27, 2019," he said, "we identified some patients, family-cluster-like, with suspected (novel coronavirus) infections; they were basically clustered in families in disease onset. Based on the [observed] patient conditions at that time, none of us had expected [this disease] would be this severe like it is now. Yet, *what was clear then was that it possessed infectivity and there was 'human-to-human transmission'*" (italics added).[32]

Dr. Zhao further explained that one of the patients had already undergone mNGS testing done through another hospital: "the test results showed suspected infection with a novel coronavirus. Thus, there was human-to-human transmission and suspected infected patient(s); these two pieces of information made us immediately aware of the danger of this disease."[33]

Upon identifying the initial cases, Dr. Zhao and his team promptly reported them to the Qiaokou District CDC in Wuhan.[34] However, according to a source in Dr. Zhao's section, staff from the district CDC were initially reluctant to investigate, mistaking the illness for influenza A and B. They had to be informed that the disease under investigation was not the flu.[35] Similar to the initial cases reported by Dr. Zhang Jixian on December 27, Dr. Zhao's reporting did not lead to an effective response from the local CDC system.

Meanwhile, Dr. Zhao and his staff quarantined the patients. Dr. Zhao also ordered staff to adopt strict infection control measures and to screen patients in the respiratory wards for patients with similar symptoms. By the next day, they had identified 12 more patients with similar symptoms and connected to the Huanan Seafood Market. Thanks to Dr. Zhao's leading role in respiratory medicine in Wuhan and Tongji Hospital's direct administrative reporting relationship with the Hubei Provincial Health Commission, he was quickly brought into the center of the citywide effort to treat the unusual pneumonia cases.

Dr. Zhang Dingyu of Jinyintan Hospital

After learning that Patient A was diagnosed with a novel coronavirus infection, Dr. Zhao Jianping also took the initiative to contact the leadership of

Jinyintan Hospital, Wuhan's dedicated infectious disease hospital. Dr. Zhang Dingyu, president of Jinyintan Hospital, recalled that Dr. Huang Chaolin, his deputy, received a call from a professor at Tongji Hospital around 6:30 PM on December 27, who requested permission to transfer a patient to Jinyintan Hospital. Dr. Zhang vividly recalled that moment, as it had already turned very dark outside in Wuhan. Dr. Huang happened to be with Dr. Zhang at the time of the call and they inquired about the infectious disease affecting the patient. They were informed that the patient had tested positive for coronavirus.[36]

It is worth noting that Tongji Hospital is one of China's best comprehensive hospitals, and it is highly unusual for them to transfer difficult-to-treat patients to other hospitals. Dr. Zhang Dingyu recalled that the patient of concern had been transferred from the WCH to Tongji Hospital because of Tongji's strong reputation.[37] However, Jinyintan Hospital was the designated hospital for responding to public health emergency events in Hubei Province and the city of Wuhan. Therefore, it made sense for Dr. Zhao Jianping to request such a transfer in accordance with health emergency protocols. In the process, Dr. Zhao would likely have consulted with senior staff members in the provincial or municipal health commission.

Since they had participated in the September 2019 health emergency response exercise that involved responding to novel coronavirus infection, Dr. Zhang and Dr. Huang hesitated about accepting the transfer patient after hearing the reference to a coronavirus. They consulted experts at Beijing Ditan Hospital for infectious diseases. The experts in Beijing advised them to accept the transfer, stating that Jinyintan Hospital was an infectious disease hospital and that the patient required their attention.[38]

Vision Medicals and the Crucial Role of Commercial Diagnostic Laboratories

In preparation for the patient's arrival, Dr. Zhang Dingyu contacted Vision Medicals, the third-party commercial lab that had conducted mNGS testing on Patient A's sample. However, Dr. Zhang was quickly informed that the printed report Vision Medicals had provided to the hospitals indicated "RNA virus not tested."[39] This meant that, due to the sensitivity of the diagnostic results, Vision Medicals had not provided written confirmation of the positive test result for a SARS-like coronavirus to the patient's family or the hospital. Instead, it had only informed the hospitals of the positive test result by phone.

"Little Mountain Dog" and Genomic Sequencing at Vision Medicals

On a WeChat public account (Winjor001), a lab scientist writing under the moniker Xiaoshangou, or "Little Mountain Dog," posted a long account of how she analyzed the genomic sequence labeled "Bat SARS-like coronavirus" beginning on the morning of December 26, 2019.[40] The genome was obtained from the BAL fluid sample of Patient A and became one of the earliest registered on the Global Initiative on Sharing All Influenza Data (GISAID) database (BetaCoV/Wuhan/IPBCAMS-WH-01/2019, collection date: 2019-12-24).

Screen captures of Little Mountain Dog's conversations with her team leader and supervisor showed that they immediately recognized that this SARS-like coronavirus should be treated in the same class as the plague. China's Infectious Diseases Law only includes two diseases—plague and cholera—as Class A infectious diseases, but SARS, a Class B disease, was treated as a Class A infectious disease for prevention and control purposes. The lab supervisor instructed Little Mountain Dog not to let anyone else handle the sample.

After comparing with a database of genomic sequences using mNGS, Little Mountain Dog and the Vision Medicals team discovered that they were analyzing a novel coronavirus that was 81% similar to the SARS coronavirus of 2003. Recognizing the significance and potential consequences of their findings, the company's leadership proceeded with caution. They refrained from putting the result on paper for the time being because they did not want to alarm the doctors. Instead, they informed the doctors at the WCH and Wuhan Tongji Hospital of the diagnostic result by phone only.[41] Dr. Ai Fen, director of Emergency Medicine of WCH, recalled that a colleague at the Emergency Ward, apparently in shock upon learning of the lab test result, repeated several times to her that the testing lab had reported finding a coronavirus.[42]

Dr. Zhang Dingyu Enlisted the Help of the Wuhan Institute of Virology

On December 27, Dr. Zhang Dingyu of Jinyintan Hospital was able to convince the Vision Medicals team to share the genomic sequence data immediately to prepare for treating Patient A. Under Dr. Zhang's leadership, Jinyintan Hospital had entered into a cooperation agreement with the Wuhan Institute of Virology (WIV) to support a joint lab.[43] Dr. Zhang enlisted the help of WIV researchers to compare the genomic sequence from Vision Medicals with the WIV's genomic database. At around 10:30 PM, the WIV team informed the Jinyintan leadership by phone that it confirmed the diagnosis of a bat-borne SARS-like coronavirus.[44]

The following day, December 28, Dr. Zhang and Dr. Huang were informed that Patient A's family did not agree to have the patient transferred from Tongji to Jinyintan Hospital.[45] Nevertheless, Jinyintan Hospital's leadership learned about patients who were known to be infected with a SARS-like coronavirus, which turned out to be extremely important preparation for what came 2 days later. Similarly, doctors in Respiratory and Critical Care Medicine at WCH were proud that they had ordered the mNGS diagnostic test for Patient A. In retrospect, this was the earliest such test known to have been conducted on a COVID-19 patient.[46]

Alert from Vision Medicals

The scientists and leadership of Vision Medicals were extremely alarmed when they discovered that the sample they investigated contained a SARS-like novel coronavirus. Screen captures of the WeChat conversations between Little Mountain Dog and her team supervisors revealed that they quickly recognized the severity of the situation and decided to act: "This [virus] is worse than the plague," "might again result in a serious public health problem," "we should do our best to notify [policymakers] to isolate [the virus carriers] and prevent its spread among humans."[47]

On December 27, while communicating with doctors in Wuhan about the test results, the Vision Medicals leadership learned that Patient A was "gravely ill and quarantine measures were adopted" (the timestamp showed 2019-12-27 13:47).[48] They continued to maintain contact with Dr. Zhao Jianping or his team at Tongji Hospital. They also collaborated with researchers at the Institute of Pathogen Biology of the Chinese Academy of Medical Sciences for further genomic analyses.

As they learned more about the patient's condition and conducted additional analyses, the concern at Vision Medicals deepened. Besides interacting with Dr. Zhang Dingyu, the Vision Medicals leadership also reached out to the Wuhan Municipal CDC on December 27 and 28. They traveled to Wuhan on December 29–30 to "report to the leadership of the hospital and the CDC face-to-face about the results of analyses done by us and the Institute of Pathogen Biology of the Chinese Academy of Medical Sciences. Everything is under intense, confidential, and rigorous investigation."[49]

Separately, BGI, the largest Chinese genomic diagnostics company with a strong presence in Wuhan, detected a novel coronavirus on December 29, 2019, from a sample sent from Wuhan Union Hospital. The BGI team informed the Union Hospital staff of the novel coronavirus finding by phone on December 30 and suggested the hospital report the case to the health authority.[50] The GISAID database also shows that BGI investigated patient samples collected at the Central Theater Command General Hospital (a military hospital located a short distance from the Wuhan University Zhongnan Hospital) on December 26 and 31, 2019, and January 1, 2020.

The Health Administration Response and Joint Epidemiological Investigation

While little information has been disclosed about how the Wuhan CDC and Health Commission received Vision Medicals' findings regarding the SARS-like coronavirus, there is no doubt that the discovery caught the attention of Wuhan's health leadership. Consequently, the leaders of Vision Medicals were invited to Wuhan for a face-to-face briefing on their findings. On the afternoon of Sunday, December 29, officials from the Hubei and Wuhan Health Commissions received a report from Dr. Zhang Jixian and her hospital, detailing no fewer than seven PUE cases. This emergency request, coupled with another report from the WCH on the same day, prompted the Hubei and Wuhan health leadership to shift into emergency response mode.

Emergency Consultation at the Hubei Integrated Medicine Hospital

On the morning of December 29, Dr. Huang Chaolin made rounds at Jinyintan Hospital and then took the afternoon off. However, just 2 hours after returning home, he received a call from the WMHC. The WMHC official asked him to screen some suspected pneumonia cases at the Hubei Integrated Medicine Hospital. Dr. Huang invited Dr. Wu Wenjuan, the intensive care unit chief at Jinyintan Hospital, to join him. On their way, they learned that the patients included a family of three, which alerted Dr. Wu that they were dealing with an infectious disease.[51]

Dr. Huang and Dr. Wu arrived at Hubei Integrated Medicine Hospital around 4 PM and donned N95 facemasks for their visit.[52] Dr. Zhang Jixian met with them, showed them the patients, and reviewed the cases. The consultation meeting included these doctors and members of a joint epidemiological investigation team led by Dr. Guan Xuhua from the Hubei Provincial CDC.[53] Dr. Zhang Jixian recalled having minimal communication with the epidemiologists that day. No one mentioned the novel coronavirus situation that afternoon, and Dr. Zhang Jixian was not informed of the genomic sequencing results until January 7 or 8, 2020.[54] One can only wonder how the course of the COVID-19 pandemic might have changed if the epidemiologists had engaged in a more informative conversation with Dr. Zhang, who had clearly recognized that the first three of the seven patients had no connection to the Huanan Seafood Market.[55]

As the vice president of Jinyintan Hospital, Dr. Huang Chaolin held significant authority. After discussing the situation, Dr. Huang concluded that "these patients were probably infectious" and posed a risk to others if they remained in a general hospital. They "needed to be transferred to Jinyintan Hospital, which specializes in treating infectious patients."[56] At this point, Dr. Huang reported to Zhang Dingyu and a WMHC official by phone to update them on the situation and discuss patient transfer arrangements.[57] Zhang Dingyu recalled that their knowledge of the SARS-like coronavirus test results from Patient A had helped them prepare for that Sunday.[58] They instructed the staff handling the patient transfers to wear full protective suits and use the Jinyintan Hospital's negative pressure ambulance. Multiple trips were necessary to ensure proper isolation of the transfer patients, and the transfers were not completed until close to midnight.[59] Dr. Huang also discussed with Hubei Integrated Medicine Hospital leaders that evening about making a proposal to Wuhan/Hubei to call for shutting down the Huanan Seafood Market.[60]

The Joint Epidemiological Investigation Team Report

As mentioned earlier, a team of epidemiologists was present at the Hubei Integrated Medicine Hospital on December 29. In response to the emergency, leaders of the Hubei and Wuhan Health Commissions directed the Hubei Provincial CDC, the Wuhan Municipal CDC, and three district CDCs to form a joint investigation team to conduct emergency investigations. The team was led by Guan Xuhua, director of the Institute for Infectious Disease Prevention and Treatment at the Hubei Provincial CDC, and her deputy Tong Yeqing. Guan, who had a background in clinical practice and disease prevention, had played crucial roles in Hubei's efforts to address H5N1, H7N9, and H1N1 flu outbreaks and other health emergencies. She was credited with establishing Hubei's provincial disease surveillance information management system and training over 70 epidemiologists.[61] Yang Xiaobing, who was Guan Xuhua's counterpart in the Wuhan Municipal CDC and led the municipal contingent, was also a veteran of various outbreak investigations.

On December 29 and 30, 2019, Guan, Tong, and Yang led the joint team to interview patients and collect samples at the Hubei Integrated Medicine Hospital, Jinyintan Hospital, WCH (Houhu), and Tongji Hospital. Yang and his Wuhan CDC colleagues interviewed patients at Jinyintan Hospital to understand their exposure to risk factors, reviewed the cases with clinical experts overnight, and then went to the Huanan Seafood Market to conduct on-site investigations, including connecting the cases with the spatial distribution of stalls in the market.[62] The joint team quickly put together and submitted a report on December 30 titled *Investigation and Handling Report on the Situation of Multiple Hospital-Reported Pneumonia Cases of the Huanan Seafood Market*.[63]

The joint team's investigation report is significant because it helped frame and shape the thoughts, deliberations, and decisions of key decision makers at a critical juncture in the unfolding outbreak in Wuhan. The title of the investigation report highlighted the Huanan Seafood Market. The report itself began with a quick overview of the Huanan market and then offered the case definition, a vital step in an outbreak investigation: "Individuals with exposure to the Huanan Seafood Market and their family members who have been diagnosed as pneumonia cases in [Wuhan] hospitals since December 1, 2019, with infections by other pathogens not having been ruled out." Note that the "who" here refers to both the individuals and their family members.

A well-formulated case definition facilitates the consistent identification and counting of cases of interest; conversely, a poorly formulated case definition may harm the sensitivity and effectiveness of a disease surveillance system.[64] The case definition found in the Wuhan investigation report is difficult to read in the original Chinese language. While it is ill-defined in terms of the clinical and diagnostic features of "the case," the definition stands out for its emphasis on exposure to the Huanan market, which will have momentous implications in subsequent weeks.

According to the report, the investigation team was aware of a total of 25 cases across different hospitals. They conducted epidemiological investigations on 20 of these cases, including 14 males and 6 females. The disease onset dates were December 12–17 (8 cases) and 19–25 (12 cases). Of the 20 patients, 17 had worked at 13 stands/stalls at the Huanan market, primarily in the western section (12 stalls/stands), while 3 did not work at a specific stall/stand in the market. In other words, the report classified all 20 patients as having an exposure history to the Huanan market. The Wuhan Municipal

CDC conducted nucleic acid testing on throat swab samples from 17 of the 20 patients, and all samples tested negative for the flu and 20 upper respiratory pathogens; five samples tested positive for *Streptococcus pneumoniae*. The diagnostic results from hospitals for respiratory viral antibodies were all negative.

In retrospect, the report failed to address the issue of disease infectivity and the dangers of the outbreak. Section 2 of the report mentioned two families: one consisted of a husband (Lan), wife (Qi), Lan's brother, and Lan's father-in-law; the other included a patient (Chen) and Chen's mother (later identified as mother and son). However, the team report merely claimed that these family clusters were cases of "common exposure" to the Huanan market, thus excluding the possibility that the infection could have passed from one family member to another. In contrast, Dr. Ai Fen of the Wuhan Central Hospital saw the "mother and son" on December 28–29 and learned that the mother, who was seriously ill, had contracted the unusual pneumonia when she brought food to her son, a worker in the Huanan market, even though she did not touch anything in the market. Dr. Ai Fen immediately suspected that the disease was likely "transmissible from person to person."[65]

Since the investigation report was compiled within a 24-hour period, one might expect it to be somewhat tentative in its conclusions. However, it was quite the opposite. The report boasted that the team "carried out on-site verification and detailed epidemiological investigations to ascertain the disease onset, medical history, and suspicious exposures." Although the report acknowledged the two families and noted at one point that most patients were found at "only 13 stands/stalls" in the western section of the Huanan market (with more than 650 stands/stalls), it concluded that the only commonality among the 20 cases was "their history of exposure to the Huanan market." "At present, no clustered cases have been discovered in that market: the stands/stalls with cases were rather scattered, [the cases] have no obvious contact and crossover [with each other], and no clustering [aggregation (聚集性)] in time and space" (Section 4.3).

The report omitted or failed to discuss several important points worth noting. First, the report did not mention the additional five cases the team had not investigated, likely because these five patients were being transferred to Jinyintan Hospital.[66] Second, the family cluster that Dr. Zhang Jixian first encountered on December 26–27—an elderly couple and their asymptomatic son—was absent from the family clusters mentioned in the report. In hindsight, this omission is significant because members of this family had no exposure to the Huanan market, and their cases indicated viral spread outside the market. However, their cases were likely excluded because the case definition included exposure to the Huanan market. Third, although the report referred to pneumonia cases in both the title and the text, it did not discuss the pathogenic cause of the pneumonia except to attribute it to exposure to the Huanan market. While the case definition mentioned the need to rule out "infections by other pathogens," it appeared the authors had a specific, but unnamed, pathogen in mind for the pneumonia cases connected to the Huanan market. It is unclear whether the authors of the report chose to omit any mention of the SARS-like coronavirus in the written report, similar to the decisions made by leaders of Vision Medicals and BGI. However, by December 30, lab results showing SARS-like coronaviruses had become available to key individuals in several major hospitals, as well as the Wuhan Municipal CDC, the WMHC, and possibly others. It is almost certain that some members of the joint investigation team were aware of these results. Regardless of the reason for this omission, it will be evident in the next chapter that experts in Wuhan and Beijing considered the coronavirus-related diagnostic results when they met to assess the outbreak situation on the evening of December 31, 2019.

Dr. Zhang Dingyu, BAL Samples, and the WIV, December 30, 2019

On the morning of December 30, 2019, Dr. Zhang Dingyu checked with the doctors attending to the patients who were brought to Jinyintan Hospital overnight. He learned that Wuhan CDC staff had taken pharyngeal swabs from the patients, but the tests were negative for flu and 20 upper respiratory pathogens.[67]

At this point, the knowledge Dr. Zhang had gained on December 27, 2019, regarding Patient A's diagnostic results proved helpful. Recall that Dr. Zhang had obtained the genomic sequencing results from Vision Medicals and asked expert researchers at the WIV to review and confirm Vision Medicals' finding of a SARS-like coronavirus. Dr. Zhang suspected his patients had the same viral pneumonia. "The genomic sequencing by others had a positive result [of coronavirus]; why didn't our tests find it? The negative test results [from our tests] suggested there were problems [with our tests]," Dr. Zhang reminisced.[68]

Since the patient sample investigated at Vision Medicals was obtained using the BAL procedure, Dr. Zhang spoke with Dr. Huang Chaolin and ordered the collection of BAL fluids. "This is the most correct decision we made early [in the outbreak]," Dr. Zhang recalled with pride.[69]

BAL is an invasive procedure. It requires a medical practitioner to insert a bronchoscope into the patient's lungs through the mouth or nose; fluid is then squirted into a small part of the lung and recollected. Of the nine patients with unusual pneumonia, seven agreed to the procedure. The chief of endoscopy and a team of nurses completed it by around 4:40 PM. Under Dr. Zhang's direction, the BAL samples were divided into four portions each, resulting in four sets of samples.[70] This move showcased Dr. Zhang's tactical brilliance as a medical leader.

That late afternoon, two of the four sets of samples were sent to laboratories for investigation. One was provided to the Wuhan Municipal CDC, and one went to the WIV. The remaining two sets were stored at Jinyintan Hospital.[71]

According to Professor Shi Zhengli of the WIV, Zhang Dingyu personally delivered the samples to the WIV early that evening.[72] She also learned from the institute's director that the Wuhan Municipal CDC requested the WIV to investigate the samples after learning of two lab test results that indicated infections with SARS-like coronaviruses.[73] Having devoted 16 years of her research life to coronaviruses from other parts of China, Shi "had never expected this kind of thing [a novel coronavirus outbreak] to happen in Wuhan, in central China." Her team began working that evening.

Wuhan in Health Emergency Response

After receiving the information from the joint team, the Hubei/Wuhan health leadership sprang into action on the afternoon of December 30, 2019. At 3:10 PM and 6:50 PM, the WMHC, following "emergency instructions from higher authority," issued two urgent notices to select medical organizations in Wuhan.[74] The first notice asked hospitals to "immediately screen for PUE patients treated in the past week who possessed similar characteristics" to those from the Huanan Seafood Market. The hospitals were asked to submit the relevant information on an attached form by 4:00 PM.[75] The second notice directed hospital leaders to coordinate treatment for the so-called PUE patients and to submit patient information to the district CDC and the WMHC Medical Administration Division. It ended with a clear and ominous injunction: "Without authorization, no unit or individual shall willfully release rescue and treatment information to the public."[76]

By the evening of December 30, the WMHC had orchestrated the transfer of 27 patients to Jinyintan Hospital from major hospitals. These included the patients under Dr. Zhang Jixian's care—the son from the family of three had mild symptoms and chose not to leave for Jinyintan, but a relative of one of the other patients also had symptoms and took the opportunity for treatment at Jinyintan—plus others from the WCH, Tongji Hospital, and Union Hospital.

Among them was Patient A. Amid the health emergency response, Patient A's wife could not resist his transfer, even though Patient A was already intubated. Special efforts were made to transport Patient A to Jinyintan Hospital on December 30. This turned out to be the last time Patient A's wife saw him. Patient A died in Jinyintan Hospital on January 30, 2020. By then, Wuhan was already in lockdown. His wife wanted to bring some burial clothes for him but was denied.[77]

In a strong indication of intense official concern about the SARS-like coronavirus and Wuhan's rich medical and biological expertise, the WMHC organized clinical experts, epidemiologists, and virologists from Wuhan Tongji Hospital, Jinyintan Hospital, the Hubei Provincial and Wuhan Municipal CDCs, and the WIV to gather at Jinyintan Hospital to evaluate the unusual pneumonia cases. Dr. Zhao Jianping was among the clinical experts that evening and would later serve as the leader of the Hubei medical experts treatment group. He remembered December 30 as a pivotal moment and summed up the gravity of the situation with three numbers: "At that time, 28 experts went to Jinyintan to consult on 27 patients, of which 13 were critically or seriously ill."[78]

The "PUE" Patients at Jinyintan Hospital

Dr. Zhang Li, chief of the 3rd Ward in the South Building and chief physician in the Tuberculosis and Respiratory Department of Jinyintan Hospital, had previously worked at Wuhan TB Hospital, one of Jinyintan's predecessor hospitals, and cared for the first SARS patient at that hospital in 2003. On December 29, Zhang Li was tasked with leading her staff to set up an isolation area for the incoming PUE patients.[79]

Dr. Zhang Li recalled feeling "scared" upon seeing patients arriving on the evening of December 29. More patients were admitted on December 30, following the WMHC order. There was widespread fear among patients and medical staff that SARS had returned. Some patients were already experiencing breathing difficulties, including the intubated Patient A. According to Dr. Zhang Li, the entire ward, with over 40 beds, filled up quickly; and similar patients continued to arrive in the following days.[80]

The nursing staff at Jinyintan became increasingly alarmed. As an indication of the severity of the situation, the staff were instructed to use the highest Level III protection, which they had practiced during an epidemic preparedness exercise prior to the World Military Games in the fall. The chief nurse, after reviewing the patients' CT scans and based on her knowledge of SARS, felt that the situation was more complex than the WMHC had announced.[81]

Both Dr. Wu Wenjuan and Dr. Zhang Li noted the patient clusters on December 29–30. Dr. Wu Wenjuan vividly remembered her surprise at seeing the Fang brothers and their cousin among the "PUE" patients as she had difficulty telling them apart.[82] Dr. Zhang Li observed that "most of the patients knew each other. Some patients told [us] that their relatives [with the same symptoms] were hospitalized there and were dying. They were either of the same clan or were people who played mahjong together."[83] The patients either were directly connected to the Huanan Seafood Market or lived nearby, and it was evident that they had a contagious disease. "At the end of December, we had already determined that this contagious virus was related to the Huanan Seafood Market," she said.[84]

Dr. Huang Chaolin was particularly struck by the fact that three patients from Wuhan Union Hospital who arrived on December 31 were on ventilation. Another patient, Mr. Zeng, a 61-year-old male with chronic liver disease and other conditions, was in a coma and on ventilation when he arrived from Wuhan Puren Hospital on the same day. Mr. Zeng's condition worsened, and he was placed on an ECMO machine on January 1, 2020.[85] "ECMO" stands for extracorporeal membrane oxygenation, a life-support system that provides cardiac and respiratory support when the patient's heart and lungs cannot sustain life. Jinyintan Hospital had received four ECMO machines some years prior, but they had rarely been used until now.

Conclusion

In late December 2019, expert clinicians in Wuhan were alarmed by clusters of unusual pneumonia cases that failed to respond to treatment. Drawing on their experience with SARS, some clinicians recognized that the clinical symptoms of this mysterious disease, especially the lung images on CT scans, resembled those for SARS. Clinicians in several major hospitals in Wuhan reported the PUE cases to hospital administrators and district CDCs in the Chinese disease prevention and control system. Dr. Zhang Jixian and her colleagues at the Hubei Integrated Medicine Hospital were the most intrepid at reporting the cases, gaining the attention of the Hubei provincial and Wuhan municipal health leadership on December 29, 2019.

In this context, the Hubei provincial health leadership launched a joint provincial–municipal–district CDC team investigation on December 29, 2019. The investigation report by this team offered a case definition centered on exposure to the Huanan Seafood Market. It also made strong assessments that, in hindsight, clearly misjudged the infectivity of the causative pathogen and failed to consider the possibility that the pathogen was contagious. The assertions and emphatic statements of this report, offered at a critical moment in the unfolding pandemic, played an influential role in shaping the deliberations and decisions on the outbreak.

Whereas it took months before the medical and scientific communities in 2003 could ascertain that the SARS outbreak was caused by the SARS coronavirus, the situation was strikingly different in late 2019. With genomic sequencing as a leading diagnostic technique, the diagnostic results from Vision Medicals and other labs soon became available to clinical leaders at Wuhan Central, Jinyintan, and Tongji Hospitals, as well as members of the municipal and provincial health authorities. When they began to accept transfer patients on December 29, 2019, the Jinyintan Hospital leadership made key decisions based on their knowledge that Patient A had tested positive for a SARS-like coronavirus.

Front-line clinicians in multiple hospitals, mostly in respiratory or emergency medicine, recognized early on that the unusual pneumonia they were treating was likely infectious. Dr. Zhang Li of Jinyintan Hospital later led a highly influential *Lancet* study of the first 99 COVID-19 patients at Jinyintan.[86] Her recollection of the situation is especially valuable: "At the end of December, the signs of human-to-human transmission were already very obvious, and anyone with a little common sense could reach that assessment."[87] Recognizing the danger they faced, these clinicians adopted strong protective measures for their staff. When the Wuhan health leadership brought together 28 leading experts to review the cases and evaluate the situation on December 30, 2019, it was evident that the provincial and municipal health authorities and experts in Wuhan took the so-called PUE outbreak extremely seriously. This was partly because key decision makers in Wuhan/Hubei already knew about the SARS-like coronavirus diagnosis. In the meantime, the number and percentage of patients who were already seriously ill at that point—nearly half of the patients who had been transferred to Jinyintan—deeply impressed the leading clinical experts with the gravity of the situation.

Despite the sense of urgency surrounding the outbreak in Wuhan and the extensive information available to medical and community professionals, as well as China's post-SARS emphasis on national disease reporting, it was surprising to discover that the highly regarded NNDSS was not utilized for reporting the initial PUE or SARS-like pneumonia cases. These cases were encountered by front-line clinicians, infectious disease specialists, hospital administrators, and officials from district, municipal, and provincial CDCs and health commissions in Wuhan and Hubei in mid- to late December 2019.[88] In other words, a large number of individuals and organizations had the opportunity to report the unusual PUE cases to the China CDC via the NNDSS. Had the NNDSS been in effective use, some of the PUE cases in Wuhan might have been reported by mid-December 2019 if not earlier. Yet, none did. In a March 2021 interview with Phoenix Television, China CDC director general Gao Fu confirmed that doctors in Wuhan reported the early cases to local hospitals, but the cases "really didn't make it to our [national disease reporting] network."[89]

This lack of reporting or submission from Wuhan and Hubei to the central health authority starkly contrasted with the Hubei Provincial CDC's earlier declaration in December 2019 that Hubei would maintain its "national No. 1 ranking on comprehensive quality of infectious disease information." This discrepancy raises crucial questions about the politics of epidemic information flow within the Chinese party-state system, how these dynamics may have impacted the outbreak's handling during December 2019, and what other information may still be missing from public scrutiny that could have affected the outbreak's course. Additionally, it foreshadows the interactions between the National Health Commission/China CDC, Hubei Province, and Wuhan municipality in the subsequent weeks.

4

The New Year's Eve Meeting

The Huanan Seafood Market and the Health Emergency Action Program

We do not know whether and how soon the Hubei/Wuhan health authorities would have reported the outbreak to the China Centers for Disease Control and Prevention (China CDC) and the National Health Commission (NHC). However, on the evening of December 30, 2019, Gao Fu, the director general of the China CDC, learned of the outbreak in Wuhan through posts on social media. He swiftly reported to the NHC leadership, setting in motion a series of emergency responses by the NHC and the China CDC. This chapter traces the events that led to this critical development and examines the New Year's Eve meeting that resulted in the implementation of emergency prevention and control measures. These measures, including the closure of the Huanan Seafood Market due to its suspected role as the source of the infections, established the foundation for subsequent policies and actions in the first half of January 2020.

When considering these developments, it is important to bear in mind the hierarchical party-government structure that exists in China, which involves interactions between central, provincial, and municipal authorities. Institutional hierarchy and official rank play crucial roles in determining how individuals interact within this system. When officials representing the central government arrive, it is customary and significant for local officials to show deference. In this instance, NHC officials and China CDC experts arrived in Wuhan uninvited to offer guidance and assistance. In practice, the central officials and experts quickly assumed leadership roles and exerted significant influence over key decision-making related to the epidemic, such as the closure of the Huanan Seafood Market, the development of an epidemic response action plan, and the vetting of public releases about the outbreak. Despite NHC officials' assertion that they would abide by the principle of territorial management and their obtaining of consent from the Hubei/Wuhan leadership for crucial decisions, such as the closure of the Huanan market, the implementation of these decisions made it clear to local officials that national authorities had assumed ultimate authority and, consequently, relieved them of the burden of making the most significant decisions.

The Alarm from Wuhan on Social Media

Although the Wuhan Municipal Health Commission (WMHC) issued an emergency notice to medical institutions on December 30 prohibiting the unauthorized disclosure of information about the outbreak, the ban quickly proved ineffective due to social media. That same evening, the WMHC's emergency notices and information about the severe acute respiratory syndrome (SARS)–like coronavirus began to spread rapidly on major social media platforms.

Chinese individuals use a wide variety of WeChat groups to connect with others, whether for work, family, friendship, or simply conversation. For instance, Wan Ying, a chief nurse for Pediatrics at Wuhan Central Hospital (WCH), was a member of over 40 work-related WeChat groups.[1] To facilitate rapid distribution, the WMHC emergency notices were initially shared with key staff members in medical institutions via WeChat. Soon, however, the circulation of these notices extended beyond the immediate WeChat work groups to the overlapping public health/medical communities in China. Some have speculated that a mysterious whistleblower shared the emergency notices within WeChat networks, but the existence of numerous social and professional networks on WeChat, as well as the tendency among many to share information of compelling public interest, was enough to quickly spread the information from Wuhan to professional colleagues in Beijing.

On the morning of December 30, Dr. Ai Fen, head of the Emergency Department at WCH, examined another patient who had worked at the Huanan Seafood Market and exhibited symptoms of "typical lung infections" associated with the unusual pneumonia cases. Later that afternoon, around 4 PM, Dr. Ai's colleague shared with her the lab test results and analysis of a patient (Patient B) who had been admitted on December 27, 2019, and subsequently moved to the respiratory ward. These results and analysis came from CapitalBio MedLab (北京博奥医学检验所有限公司), a diagnostic lab based in Beijing. Dr. Ai was startled to see the words "SARS coronavirus" in the analysis and promptly reported the case to the Public Health Section of the hospital, as well as alerting Dr. Hu Yi, director of Respiratory Medicine. To inform her colleagues in the Emergency Care department, Dr. Ai highlighted the words "SARS coronavirus" on Patient B's test results in red and shared the image of the page in her WeChat group. Dr. Ai also forwarded the same image to a WeChat group comprising her Tongji Medical School classmates.[2]

At 10:20 PM, Dr. Ai Fen received the WMHC notice from the hospital leadership, which banned the disclosure of treatment information about the pneumonia cases. However, it was already too late.[3] The image that Dr. Ai shared, with the words "SARS coronavirus," struck a nerve and immediately went viral, being reshared millions of times and generating an enormous amount of discussion. Among those who reshared the image was Dr. Li Wenliang, an ophthalmologist at WCH who did not know Dr. Ai personally. Dr. Li saw the image in one WeChat group and then shared it with his Wuhan University Medical School classmates in another WeChat group, adding that seven confirmed SARS cases from the Huanan market were being quarantined in the Emergency Ward at the WCH Houhu Branch (picture on the left in Figure 4.1).[4] He cautioned, "Don't circulate [this message] outside [this group]. Make your family and loved ones take precautions."[5]

Gao Fu and Intervention from the NHC/China CDC

Dr. Ai Fen and those who shared her post with the words "SARS coronavirus" played a crucial role in sounding the alarm about the new pneumonia cases in Wuhan. Wu Zunyou, who became the China CDC chief epidemiologist in January 2020, recalled that Dr. Ai's post "had gone crazy in WeChat groups."[6] Among those who learned of the outbreak through WeChat were staff members of the China CDC in Beijing, including Director General Gao Fu.

Surveillance of emerging disease outbreaks was a critical responsibility of the China CDC, and a major outbreak was always a cause for concern for the director general, according to an interviewee with in-depth knowledge of the organization. The director general is comparable to a commanding general, and the online National Notifiable Diseases Surveillance System serves as the communication system. At the end of 2019, the China CDC director general was Gao Fu, an accomplished virologist and immunologist who has conducted significant research on zoonotic diseases (diseases transmitted from animals or insects to humans). As only the third director general of the China CDC, Gao Fu, known in English as "George," is renowned for having made an extraordinary journey from veterinary training in backwater Shanxi to earning his PhD in microbiology at Oxford University, carrying out research and teaching at Harvard and Oxford, and being inducted into the Chinese Academy of Sciences as an academician. Gao's training, research, and

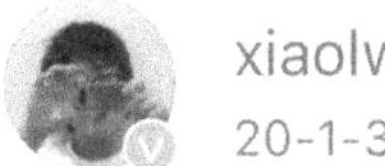

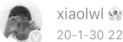

xiaolwl

20-1-30 22:14 from 贫困家庭 iPhone...

大家好，我是武汉市中心医院眼科医生李文亮。12月30日，我看到一份病人的检测报告，检出SARS冠状病毒高置信度阳性指标，出于提醒同学注意防护的角度，因为我同学也都是临床医生，所以在群里发布了消息说“确诊了7例SARS”。消息发出后，1月3日，公安局找到我并签了训诫书。之后我一直正常工作，在接诊了新冠病毒肺炎患者后，1月10号我开始出现咳嗽症状，11号发热，12号住院。

那时候我还在想通报怎么还在说没有人传人，没有医护感染，后来住进了ICU，之前做了一次核酸检测，但一直没出结果。经过治疗最近又进行一次检测，我的核酸显示为阴性了，但目前仍然呼吸困难，无法活动。我的父母也在住院中。

在病房里，我也看到很多网友对我的支持和鼓励，我的心情也会轻松一些，谢谢大家的支持。在此我想特别澄清，我没有被吊销执照，请大家放心，我一定积极配合治疗，争取早日出院！

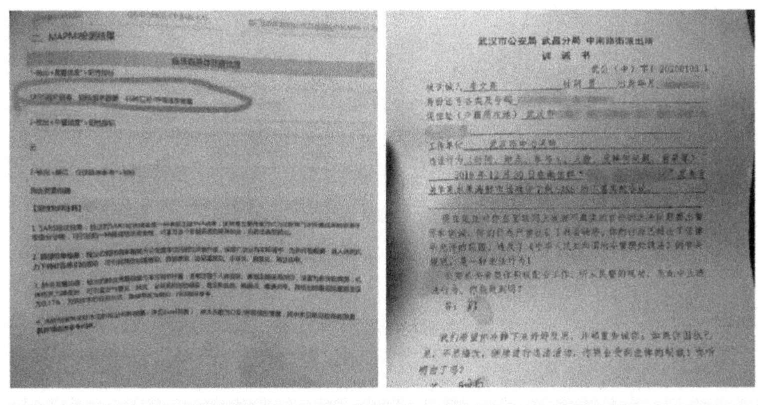

Figure 4.1 Screen Capture of Dr. Li Wenliang's Weibo Post on January 30, 2020

Screen capture by Dali Yang from the public Weibo account of Dr. Li Wenliang, @xiaolwl 2020-01-30, https://weibo.com/1139098205/Is0XboARR.

institutional role made him particularly attuned to the possibility of emerging microbes and infections.

As previously mentioned, the China CDC operates a national disease direct reporting system that is monitored 24/7 in Beijing, as well as a dedicated team that produces a daily surveillance report on infectious diseases and emergency public health events. As of December 2019, the report contained categories for avian–human influenza, pneumonia of uncertain etiology or cause (PUE), and influenza outbreaks. Influenza outbreaks were further divided into seasonal influenza outbreaks and outbreaks of influenza-like illnesses, for which China had recently increased monitoring. Given that it was flu season, the daily reports in December 2019 included a lengthy list of influenza-related information each day. Toward the end of the month, the report occasionally noted PUE cases: two in Shandong on December 24 and one in Guizhou on December 27, with specific hospitals or locations provided. None were reported in Wuhan/Hubei.

The Public Health Emergency Center (also known as the Emergency Operations Center) of the China CDC produces a health surveillance risks assessment report that draws on information from the surveillance network (daily report), internet searches, and information from "other departments," such as the foreign ministry. This report is submitted to the NHC and distributed to all provincial CDCs and includes a running list of public health events being monitored.

For the December 30, 2019, report, which covered December 27–29, the top item on the list was the Ebola epidemic in Congo and Uganda. In China, there were outbreaks of brucellosis, dengue, measles, and tuberculosis; but the biggest category was the nationwide influenza outbreak. Jingmen and Suizhou, two cities in Hubei Province, were listed as having reported flu cases. With the benefit of hindsight, it is noteworthy that Wuhan was conspicuously absent from the December 30, 2019, health surveillance risks assessment report.

Late in the evening of December 30, 2019, Gao Fu read various social media postings from Wuhan about SARS or SARS-like pneumonia cases. Without intending to do so, some staff members of the WMHC, as well as Dr. Ai Fen, Dr. Li Wenliang, and others, became whistleblowers, drawing attention to a situation that the local authorities in Wuhan appeared to have been trying to keep under wraps. Since Wuhan had not reported any cases using the national disease reporting network, Gao himself played the role of a scout on December 30, 2019. For the NHC leadership, Gao was a hero who helped them seize the initiative and take control of the situation.[7]

Gao Fu recalled reading online that the WMHC had issued a "red-letter-headed document asking for immediate submission of unexplained pneumonia cases."[8] This alarmed him because the Wuhan pneumonia cases had not been reported through the national direct reporting system. Gao or his deputy Feng Zijian, an epidemiologist, called the head of the Wuhan CDC to verify the situation. They learned that the number of cases in Wuhan was well above the threshold of three cases for reporting to the China CDC. Unsurprisingly, Gao expressed exasperation with the Wuhan CDC for failing to report through the national disease reporting system.[9] Gao remembered that he and Feng Zijian "kept discussing the situation until 2:30 or 3 AM."[10]

Troubled by what he heard, or didn't hear, and the information he gathered from social media, Gao Fu deduced that the Wuhan situation required immediate attention. He reached out to the NHC leadership, including Minister Ma Xiaowei and the two vice ministers responsible for health emergency response (Yu Xuejun) and disease prevention/control (Li Bin).[11]

Ma Xiaowei, appointed health minister in 2018, had been the youngest vice minister of health during the SARS crisis in 2003. He bore some responsibility for the misjudgments and errors in the Ministry of Health's response to SARS at the time. The saying "soldiers are always preparing to fight the last war" is relevant here as Ma's experience with SARS had made him highly vigilant to any mention of SARS and coronavirus.[12]

When Gao Fu called late at night on December 30 about the unusual pneumonia cases and suspected coronavirus in Wuhan, Minister Ma required no convincing to take action. They quickly agreed to dispatch an NHC work team, including a group of six leading experts in epidemiology, virology, and respiratory medicine, to Wuhan for emergency management. These experts (see Table 4.1) had all participated in combating the SARS outbreak in 2003 and were members of the National Expert Advisory Committee on Public Health Emergencies.[13] The China CDC, a subordinate organization of the NHC, operates the Public Health Emergency Center and would send its emergency response team as well. Feng Zijian and Li Qun, the China CDC deputy director general and the director of the Public Health Emergency Center, respectively, boarded the 6:30 AM flight from Beijing to Wuhan.[14]

As an academician and leader of the State Key Lab at the China CDC, Xu Jianguo held the most senior position among this group of experts and served as the head of this ad hoc team. Notably absent was Zeng Guang, who, at the time, was China CDC's chief epidemiologist and had played a significant role during the SARS epidemic in Beijing 17 years prior. The astute Zeng was well acquainted with Director General Liang Wannian from the NHC and would have made an excellent partner for Liang (more below).

Although the NHC staff and the China CDC had assembled an impressive group of experts, Ma Xiaowei, who had faced serious health issues in previous

Table 4.1 NHC Ad Hoc Expert Team for Emergency Visit to Wuhan, December 31, 2019

China CDC Experts:
Xu Jianguo, Director of the State Key Laboratory of Infectious Disease Prevention and Control, China CDC. Academician of the Chinese Academy of Engineering (2011); former director of the Institute of Communicable Disease Control and Prevention of the China CDC (2003–2015)
Feng Zijian (epidemiologist), Deputy Director General of the China CDC, and former Director of the China CDC Public Health Emergency Center
Li Qun (epidemiologist), Director, Public Health Emergency Center, China CDC
Clinical Experts:
Cao Bin, Vice President and Director of the Respiratory and Critical Care Medicine Division, Sino-Japanese Friendship Hospital[a]
Li Xingwang, Lead Specialist, Infectious Disease Treatment Center, Beijing Ditan Hospital

[a]Cao's other affiliations are with the Department of Pulmonary and Critical Care Medicine, Center of Respiratory Medicine, National Clinical Research Center for Respiratory Diseases; Institute of Respiratory Medicine, Chinese Academy of Medical Sciences, Peking Union Medical College, Beijing; Department of Respiratory Medicine, Capital Medical University, Beijing.

years, remained uneasy. Given his experiences during the SARS crisis and the fact that Wuhan/Hubei had not reported the outbreak to the central government, he likely viewed the situation in Wuhan/Hubei as both urgent and politically complex. Historically, Hubei was known for its independent streak, and more than technical expertise might be needed to manage the outbreak in Wuhan. If Ma had adhered to bureaucratic protocol, he would have dispatched Yu Xuejun, the vice minister responsible for health emergencies, and Xu Shuqiang, the director general of the NHC Health Emergency Response Office. However, Yu specialized in population and development and lacked experience leading a major health emergency response; Xu Shuqiang, trained in traditional Chinese medicine, was known for his courage during the 1998 flood and the SARS crisis when he served as a vice president at the Sino–Japanese Friendship Hospital but not his expertise in responding to infectious disease outbreaks.

Instead of turning to Yu or Xu, Minister Ma sought the expertise of SARS veteran Liang Wannian, who had just returned from a refresher training course at the Central Party School, an exclusive training center for the party elite. During the 2003 SARS crisis, Liang Wannian served as vice president and dean of the School of Public Health at Capital Medical University. He was recruited by Beijing mayor Wang Qishan to join the Beijing Municipal Health Bureau and help contain the SARS outbreak in Beijing. Since 2009, Liang had held positions as director general of the Health Emergency Office and of the

Department of Healthcare Reforms in the Health Ministry/NHC. As a battle-tested troubleshooter, Liang was expected to be experienced in handling public health crises within their political bureaucratic contexts. Thus, Ma had good reason to ask Liang for assistance on this occasion.

"Wannian," Minister Ma reportedly said to Liang that morning, "you've got to go to Wuhan."[15] Entrusted by Minister Ma, Liang was on the flight to Wuhan around noon.[16]

The National Teams' Visit to Wuhan

The NHC experts from Beijing arrived in Wuhan at around 2 PM on December 31, 2019. After a brief meeting with health leaders at the WMHC, they divided into two separate teams for field visits, accompanied by local experts and staff. The clinicians went to Wuhan Jinyintan Hospital to examine pneumonia patients and learn about the treatment being administered. Meanwhile, experts from the China CDC visited the Huanan Seafood Market to conduct epidemiological investigations.[17] This division of labor has, over time, led to a divide between clinicians and public health professionals.

At Jinyintan Hospital, Cao Bin and Li Xingwang met with Zhao Jianping, other doctors, and hospital leadership, including Zhang Dingyu, Huang Chaolin, and Wu Wenjuan. Cao Bin recalled that he and Li Xingwang saw patients in the intensive care unit (ICU) and "discussed every patient" with the Wuhan experts. Together, they "made a very detailed description of these patients' clinical characteristics."[18]

The China CDC's emergency response team focused on epidemiological and etiological investigations. They went to Wuhan Jinyintan Hospital and then the Huanan Seafood Market.[19] With the market still in operation, members of the epidemiology team had a unique and brief opportunity to observe the Huanan market during normal operating hours and gather epidemiological information. The Huanan market, a gigantic bazaar with a damp and crowded environment in the winter, was particularly conducive to the survival and spread of the novel coronavirus.[20]

According to Zhang Dingyu's recollection, national and provincial experts, including clinicians, epidemiologists, and virologists, filled a large conference room at Jinyintan Hospital. "We went over all the patients. After that, we concluded: First, the pictures of these patients looked all the same, so they must have the same illness; Second, this was probably a viral infection, not some other kind of infection."[21] The reference to viral infection suggests that the experts gathered at Jinyintan Hospital took into account the available diagnostic test results showing a SARS-like coronavirus.

The NHC Team and the WMHC "Situation Update" of December 31, 2019

In the preceding days, the Wuhan/Hubei health leadership had prioritized maintaining stability within the provincial-local framework and opted not to disclose the outbreak to the public, particularly at the end of the year. However, as the outbreak began to attract national and international attention, there was mounting pressure on the Wuhan/Hubei leadership to address the heightened public concern. With the NHC work team in the city, the Hubei and Wuhan health leadership received guidance and approval from the NHC regarding their first public release on the outbreak. According to Xu Shuqiang, "the National Health Commission guided the Wuhan Municipal Health Commission of Hubei Province to release epidemic prevention and control information on December 31, 2019."[22]

The meticulously worded situation update or advisory, issued under the name of the WMHC, was published on the WMHC website at 1:38 PM. It announced that through a citywide hospital screening effort, 27 pneumonia cases linked to the Huanan Seafood Market had been identified. Of the 27 cases, seven were classified as "serious," while the rest were deemed "stable and controllable," with two patients healthy enough to be discharged soon.[23]

It is important to note that the number 27 referred to cases with exposure to the Huanan market (including through family association) and did not include cases with no history of exposure to the market. Furthermore, the WMHC update provided a more reassuring set of figures concerning serious cases, while Dr. Zhao Jianping clearly remembered that 13 of the 27 patients were "critically ill" on December 30, 2019.[24] The update also stated, "So far, the investigation has not found any obvious human-to-human transmission, and no medical staff infection has been found." This statement marked the beginning of a series of official announcements from Wuhan that conveyed reassuring messages or, in other words, downplayed the severity of the situation.

According to the WMHC update, experts from multiple hospitals and research institutes reviewed the cases and concluded that the patients had a form of "viral pneumonia." Without disclosing the diagnostic results indicating a SARS-like coronavirus as the cause of the disease, the update stated that viral pneumonia could be caused by various pathogens, including coronavirus. In remarkably accurate language, it advised the public "to maintain indoor air circulation, avoid going to enclosed and poorly ventilated public places and crowded areas; consider wearing a facemask when going out."[25]

Diagnostic Results from Genomic Sequencing as of December 31, 2019

After receiving the seven samples on the evening of December 30, researchers at the Wuhan Institute of Virology worked tirelessly and sequenced a novel SARS-related coronavirus on December 31, 2019.[26] As of December 31, at least four commercial and research laboratories had identified this novel SARS-related coronavirus as the causative pathogen for the unusual pneumonia cases in Wuhan. Table 4.2 lists the four labs and the hospitals that requested the lab analyses.

Table 4.2 Laboratories That Had Identified SARS-Like Coronaviruses, December 31, 2019

a. Vision Medicals (Wuhan Central Hospital | Wuhan Tongji Hospital Respiratory Section), December 29–30, 2019
(Wuhan CDC received heads-up on December 27–28 by phone.)

b. CapitalBio MedLab (Wuhan Central Hospital Respiratory Section), December 30, 2019
(The results were circulated on social media. Dr. Zhang Dingyu saw the results on December 30 and noted a discrepancy between the English ["SARS-related coronavirus"] and Chinese ["SARS coronavirus"] terms used.)[27]

c. BGI (Wuhan Union Hospital), December 30, 2019
(BGI recommended that Wuhan Union Hospital report to WMHC. On January 1, 2020, BGI provided a whole genome of the novel coronavirus to the China CDC and submitted the diagnostic test reports on three patients to WMHC.)[28]

d. Wuhan Institute of Virology (Wuhan Jinyintan Hospital), December 31, 2019
(Maintained close contact with the Wuhan Municipal CDC and later the China CDC.)

In one way or another, these diagnostic results became available to the leading experts and health authorities gathered in Wuhan to treat the unusual pneumonia patients and review the outbreak situation. Of special interest was the role of BGI, the largest Chinese genomic diagnostics company, with a strong presence in Wuhan. On December 29, 2019, BGI researchers identified a coronavirus that was approximately 80% similar to the SARS coronavirus. The BGI team informed Union Hospital staff of the results by phone the following day. On December 31, 2019, BGI assembled a whole genome of the coronavirus from three samples.[29]

China CDC Director General Gao Fu stayed in Beijing on December 31, 2019, starting the morning by orchestrating the China CDC's plan for sequencing and isolating the novel coronavirus. He then "went to a third-party genomic sequencing firm to analyze the sequence fragments [of the novel coronavirus] it had obtained in its sequencing services."[30] That third-party firm was BGI, with which Gao had maintained strong ties for many years.[31] Gao's analysis of the genomic sequences of the novel coronavirus lent significant weight to his assessment of the viral pathogen and the outbreak in Wuhan at this critical juncture. The next morning (around dinnertime on New Year's Eve in New York), Gao informed Ian Lipkin of Columbia University by a voicemail left on Lipkin's phone that a novel coronavirus had been identified, and it was "not highly transmissible because the number of family clusters were very small."[32]

The New Year's Eve Meeting, December 31, 2019

The national experts and health administrators, including leaders from the Hubei Provincial and Wuhan Municipal Health Commissions and CDCs, met that evening to assess the outbreak situation and determine the necessary responses.[33] There was much to digest and, most importantly, to act on. No amount of planning for public health emergencies can abolish the severe time constraint.

As noted in the WMHC update earlier in the day, the experts and health administrators had a good amount of clinical information, preliminary epidemiological investigations, and "preliminary results from laboratory tests"—likely referring to the results from the Wuhan Institute of Virology and other labs that had detected a SARS-related coronavirus. We can assume that details of the joint investigation team report, emphasizing infection by exposure to the Huanan Seafood Market, were also available to key participants at the meeting.

At the request of the provincial health leadership, Dr. Zhao Jianping of Tongji Hospital presented on the clinical situation, including some cases he had personally treated for several days.[34] The clinical experts from Beijing and Wuhan unanimously recognized the patients' characteristics, which Dr. Cao Bin summarized as generally rapid disease onset, fever, dyspnea (difficult breathing), dry cough, and no sputum production. Seriously ill patients experienced not only dyspnea but also ARDS (acute respiratory distress syndrome), and some also had sepsis. Patients had "shockingly similar" chest computed tomographic (CT) scans, displaying bilateral ground glass opacities that indicated widespread lung damage; mild areas might represent hypoxia (oxygen deficiency), while severe areas indicated respiratory failure. Their lab test results showed a normal or low white blood cell count, especially a low lymphocyte count.[35]

Cao Bin, Li Xingwang, and Zhao Jianping, among others, had treated SARS patients in 2003 and were intimately familiar with the symptoms and characteristics of SARS patients. They observed strong similarities between the new pneumonia and SARS. In their co-authored article in *The Lancet*, published in January 2020, they emphatically stated, "Clinical presentations greatly resemble SARS-CoV. Patients with severe illness developed ARDS and required ICU admission and oxygen therapy."[36] By highlighting the strong similarities between SARS and the viral PUE they were now confronting, these leading clinicians would have advocated for a vigorous public response.[37]

The Huanan Seafood Market as the Source of Infections

The emphasis on SARS-like symptoms and the knowledge of a SARS-related or SARS-like coronavirus reinforced each other. It was widely known in China that the SARS coronavirus in 2003 was later traced to civets and other animals as intermediate hosts and ultimately to a colony of bats as natural reservoirs.[38] On December 31, 2019, the key pieces of information at hand included SARS-like symptoms, laboratory findings of a SARS-related coronavirus, and the singular focus in the joint investigation team report on the Huanan Seafood Market as the source of infections. All of these pieces of information led meeting participants to see a strong link between the SARS-like pneumonia patients, most of whom worked at the Huanan Seafood Market, and the wildlife sold there.

For the Wuhan-based epidemiological community, the Huanan Seafood Market, located close to the bustling Hankou Railway Station, was all too familiar because it was less than a 10-minute walk from the Wuhan Municipal CDC. Wuhan CDC staff members, some of whom were researchers on zoonotic spillovers, had taken guests to the market to observe the variety of wildlife on sale there as potential disease transmitters. Edward Holmes, an evolutionary biologist and virologist at the University of Sydney, made such a visit in 2014. He recalled that the Huanan market was larger than others he had seen in China. The pictures he took showed live animals, such as bamboo rats and raccoon dogs, in cages stacked on top of each other.[39] "It felt like a disease incubator, exactly the sort of place you would expect a disease to emerge," he noted.[40]

Periodic efforts were made by the Hubei Forestry Bureau to enforce wildlife and natural resource protection. For example, prior to the World Military Games, the Forestry Bureau launched the Mt. Kunlun No. 5 Action in Hubei to crack down on wildlife trade and consumption.[41] On September 25, 2019, the forest force, together with staff from the Wuhan market regulation administration, undertook joint enforcement action at the Huanan Seafood Market, focusing on eight stalls that were licensed to sell wildlife. In practice, it was likely that enforcers and sellers engaged in a cat-and-mouse game. Once the World Military Games enforcement action ended, enforcement became more relaxed. A *Beijing News* reporting team discovered that some of the stalls sold unlicensed wildlife.[42] Reminiscent of Shenzhen during the SARS outbreak in 2003, there were restaurants in Wuhan and particularly in outlying areas that had "game" in their names or business descriptions in late 2019.

In the aftermath of the Wuhan lockdown, Wuhan authorities denied the presence of illegal wildlife at the Huanan Seafood Market. The Wuhan Bureau of Landscape and Forestry (WBLF), perhaps to avoid blame and protect Wuhan's reputation, later claimed that the stalls selling wildlife at the market were all licensed and that no illegal wildlife was sold there.[43] However, such official denials were contradicted by public notices on the WBLF website announcing the imposition of fines on vendors who illegally sold wildlife such as hedgehogs in May 2019.[44]

According to a study published in *Nature Scientific Reports*, between May 2017 and November 2019 (after the World Military Games), monthly surveys of 17 shops in four major markets in Wuhan, including the Huanan Seafood Market, found that these shops sold 47,381 animals from 38 species, including 31 protected species, during the study period. The mammals on sale were wild-caught or farmed "non-domesticated" animals, including badgers, hedgehogs, masked palm civets, minks, bamboo rats, raccoon dogs, and marmots. Some of these species are now known to be susceptible to SARS-like coronaviruses and were sold in unhygienic conditions.[45] Separately, 2 months after the Huanan market was closed and most of its products had been removed and repeatedly disinfected, sanitation workers at the Huanan market continued to see badgers, snakes, hedgehogs, and weasels around.[46]

The China CDC origins tracing team conducted extensive sampling operations in the Huanan Seafood Market between January and March 2020. However, the sampling took place after the market was visited by the joint investigation team, which may have prompted vendors to remove illegal wildlife.[47] In a highly anticipated article published in *Nature*, China CDC researchers reported the prevalence of SARS-coronavirus 2 (SARS-CoV-2) in the environmental samples. Their analyses confirmed the presence of

SARS-CoV-2-susceptible animals in the Huanan market. However, they noted that there was no evidence proving these animals were infected with SARS-CoV-2, nor could they demonstrate that zoonotic spillover occurred in the Huanan market.[48] In contrast, other researchers have used the evidence from the China CDC database to support the zoonotic spillover theory.[49]

The Debate about the Source and Transmission of Infections

As we learned earlier, the Hubei–Wuhan joint investigation report, led by Guan Xuhua, highlighted that exposure to the Huanan Seafood Market was a common factor among the initial cases investigated and thus implied that the Huanan market was the source of infections. In early 2018, Dr. Guan Xuhua of the Hubei CDC led an epidemiological investigation of human H7N9 cases in Hubei. Under immense pressure, she recommended that the provincial government close live poultry markets as the source of infections, despite acknowledging that she and her colleagues could not be 100% certain that the H7N9 virus originated solely from these markets.[50] The Huanan market situation, therefore, was not an unfamiliar one.

On December 31, 2019, epidemiologists and virologists, including those from Beijing, used the findings from the joint investigation team to identify the Huanan market as the source of the outbreak and advocated for its closure. Feng Zijian of the China CDC, who was one of the lead participants at the meeting, recalled, "Of the 27 initial cases we obtained, 26 had a history of exposure to the Huanan Seafood Market, and only one did not, so the inference that the patients became 'infected from exposure to the Huanan Seafood Market' took the lead."[51] In a high-profile interview, Director General Gao Fu expressed doubts about the case that had no apparent exposure to the Huanan market: "I remember one of the patients, from [December] 27th, no clue [of connection]. But you talk to the patient, when you do this investigation, it looks like there might be some clue, he or she might have some connections [with the Huanan market]."[52] In a March 2020 interview with *Science*, Gao Fu stated succinctly, "From the very beginning, everybody thought the origin was the [Huanan] market."[53]

For the China CDC experts, it was crucial that multiple diagnostic results had identified a SARS-related coronavirus, and all the patients, as they had learned, were connected with the Huanan market. Based on the virtually identical genomic sequences of the coronavirus from nine patients, China CDC virologists, including Gao Fu, later suggested that "bats might be the original host of this virus, and an animal sold at the seafood market in Wuhan might represent an intermediate host facilitating the emergence of the virus in humans."[54] Gao Fu's research includes cross-species transmission of viruses. Since Gao reviewed the genomic sequence of the novel coronavirus earlier in the day on December 31, 2019, and thought that the virus "was not highly transmissible,"[55] his input carried significant weight.

Since the culling of civets and the slaughtering of poultry had become standard operating procedures for dealing with SARS and avian influenza in the post-SARS-crisis years, it was natural for epidemiologists and virologists who believed the Huanan market to be the source of SARS-like pneumonia infections to call for disinfecting and closing the Huanan market as an emergency response. As noted in Chapter 3, Dr. Huang Chaolin also discussed the need to shut down the Huanan Seafood Market early on.

While details remain limited, the discussion about the Huanan Seafood Market turned into a prolonged debate during the New Year's Eve meeting. The epidemiologists and virologists faced opposition. The Wuhan-based experts, particularly the clinicians, were not as certain about the Huanan market being the sole source of infections and were, therefore, skeptical about the effectiveness of the proposed shutdown. Wu Zunyou, who later became the China CDC chief epidemiologist, noted that Wuhan, along with Beijing and Shanghai, was a city with a high concentration of intellectual talent. It "had many prominent figures in medicine; in the field of respiratory systems particularly, the experts [from Wuhan] are not only nationally but also internationally renowned."[56] In other words, the Wuhan experts needed convincing.

As noted in Chapter 3, the clinicians who reported the unusual pneumonia cases to the local CDCs and health commissions also believed the disease to be contagious and took precautions accordingly. Since the clinical experts gathered at Jinyintan Hospital on December 31 had seen and treated the patients and reviewed the details of every case, they were also familiar with patients who had no exposure to the Huanan market and with the family clusters. Consider the elderly couple first seen by Dr. Zhang Jixian on December 26–27. The Hubei joint investigation report did not mention the couple as they had no exposure to the Huanan market by the case definition of the joint team. However, we know the elderly couple were transferred to Jinyintan Hospital on December 29, while their son chose to stay at the Hubei Integrated Medicine Hospital. As a result, the clinicians had a different and more comprehensive set of cases and patients in mind, based on clinical symptoms and CT scans.

When Feng Zijian spoke of the first 27 cases, he failed to mention that the criteria for these cases included exposure to the Huanan market (except for family members). For the epidemiologists and the China CDC leadership, the elderly couple (and their son) who were first seen by Dr. Zhang Jixian simply did not exist as cases of pneumonia with exposure to the Huanan market, according to the case definition. Even on the eve of the Wuhan lockdown, the Outbreak Joint Field Epidemiology Investigation Team led by Li Qun of the China CDC began its description of the initial outbreak in Wuhan by reporting only four of the seven cases that Dr. Zhang Jixian and the Hubei Provincial Hospital of Integrated Chinese and Western Medicine had reported: "On December 29, 2019, a hospital in Wuhan admitted *four* individuals with pneumonia and recognized that *all four* had worked in the Huanan Seafood Wholesale Market, which sells live poultry, aquatic products, and several kinds of wild animals to the public" (italics added).[57]

According to Wu Zunyou, the local clinical experts pointed to the cases that did not have exposure to the Huanan market.[58] Were these clinical experts not convinced the Huanan market was the source of the outbreak? Or were they suggesting the possibility that the virus had already spread beyond the market? These are questions with fundamental implications for the trajectory of the unfolding pandemic. In any case, the clinical experts disagreed with the joint investigation report and the epidemiologists that the virus infected only humans working in the market. Consequently, in the words of Wu Zunyou, their stance was, "So why shut down the Huanan Seafood Market? It would be making a big fuss over a minor issue."[59] Wu conceded that "there was indeed no adequate basis" for closing the Huanan market as the source of the outbreak and dealing a devastating blow to the people who made a living at that market.[60] Instead, as the WMHC update issued earlier in the day on December 31, 2019, indicated, the Wuhan-based experts supported getting the public to take preventive measures, "to maintain indoor air circulation, avoid going to enclosed and poorly ventilated public places and crowded areas; consider wearing a facemask when going out."[61]

In subsequent days and weeks, the clinician–epidemiologist divide persisted. Following the New Year's Eve meeting, the clinicians developed the Diagnosis and Treatment Protocol under the leadership of Cao Bin and Li Xingwang. Their description of the epidemiological characteristics of the outbreak stated, "[m]ost of the admitted cases have a history of exposure to the Wuhan Huanan Seafood Market, with some cases showing characteristics of family clusters, and most of these cases in clusters had a history of exposure to this market."[62] This language suggests that the clinicians were not only attentive to the possibility of family clusters but, by using "most" as a modifier, they were also open to cases not having exposure to the Huanan market. The leading clinical experts, including Cao Bin, Huang Chaolin, Li Xingwang,

Zhang Li, and Zhao Jianping, among others, would also conduct their own epidemiological investigations of inpatients at Jinyintan Hospital as part of their clinical study of disease characteristics (published in *The Lancet*).[63] Their data on exposure to the Huanan Seafood Market among the early patients would later provide compelling evidence that the virus was already spreading outside the Huanan Seafood Market at the time of the New Year's Eve meeting.

The Decision to Shut Down the Huanan Seafood Market

As the discussions extended into the wee hours of January 1, 2020, Director General Liang Wannian, who had recently returned from a training program at the Central Party School and thus carried with him an aura of political reanointment, made a "killer" political argument:

> We should think about this issue using the bottom-line thinking approach [prescribed by] General Secretary [Xi Jinping]. If we were wrong to close the market today, we could correct the mistake in a few days, and let it reopen. If we don't close [the market] today, we miss this opportunity, [and if] it is an opportunity we can't afford to lose, we won't be able to regain this opportunity.[64]

By invoking Xi Jinping's authority, Liang, representing the NHC and thus the central government, was able to bring the discussion to a close. Afterward, the health leadership at the meeting presented the decisions as recommendations to the Hubei provincial leadership, especially Jiang Chaoliang and Ma Guoqiang. It was in the early hours of January 1, 2020, when the provincial leadership approved the closure of the Huanan Seafood Market as part of a package of measures for controlling the outbreak and ensuring social stability.

It was already New Year's Day when the physical shutdown of the Huanan Seafood Market occurred just a few hours later. That morning, on what would normally have been a busy day for the market, "urban enforcers" arrived at the sprawling market and ordered the surprised sellers—who had been trying to dispel rumors of infections the day before—to suspend operations and close their stalls.[65] This was not the time for the legal niceties of discussing rents and compensation for the businesses—those discussions would have to wait for a later time.[66]

Wu Zunyou later claimed that the closure of the Huanan market "fixed [定格] the scale of the Wuhan outbreak" and defended the decisions to limit information sharing with the public.[67] However, in light of what we now know about subsequent developments, Wu's positive assessment, which represented the position of the Chinese CDC system, is clearly open to challenge and debate. The market shutdown stopped the transmission within the market but dispersed some virus carriers into the communities. Without corresponding actions to warn the public and urge public action, it may well have accelerated the spread of the virus beyond the Huanan market. Yet the fixation on the Huanan Seafood Market as the source of infections and the failure to recognize the severity of human-to-human transmission blinded the decision makers to such consequences.

For now, news of the market closure, along with police actions against alleged rumormongers about the outbreak, were repeatedly broadcast on Chinese television and widely disseminated online. This gave people—from officials to the public—a sense of security that the Huanan market—the alleged source of the virus—had been closed and thus dealt with.

The NHC Leadership and the Action Program for Epidemic Prevention and Control

It is worth noting that there was ongoing communication with the NHC leadership, particularly Minister Ma Xiaowei, and with the China CDC leadership in Beijing. During the SARS crisis, it took 3 months from the initial outbreak in Guangdong for the Ministry of Health to establish the National Leading Group on the Prevention and Control of Atypical Pneumonia. In contrast, recognizing the outbreak in Wuhan as an immediate threat, Minister Ma Xiaowei set up and activated the NHC Leading Group on Epidemic Response and Handling on January 1, 2020. Despite personal health issues, Ma Xiaowei personally headed this leading group, which met daily in the following days.

It is crucial to keep in mind that while the provincial and municipal health commissions are below the NHC in rank, they are first of all constituent agencies of the local authorities. As the provincial government ranks equally with the central ministry administratively, a central ministry or commission like the NHC cannot impose its will just by issuing documents. Therefore, Minister Ma, with his extensive experience in government service and bureaucratic infighting, quickly decided to station his own lieutenants in Wuhan. He first dispatched Vice Minister Li Bin, whose responsibilities include disease prevention and control and finance, to Wuhan on the evening of January 1, 2020.[68] A few days later, he replaced Li Bin with Yu Xuejun, the vice minister whose portfolio included the Health Emergency Office.[69] Minister Ma thus established a command post at the front line, leading the NHC working staff on the front to coordinate, supervise, and guide the epidemic prevention and control work in Hubei.[70]

As Minister Ma Xiaowei activated the NHC emergency response, he reported to and consulted with Vice Premier Sun Chunlan, whose portfolio included health.[71] By extension, the top national leadership was informed. In fact, news of the Wuhan outbreak was widespread and hard to miss, with reports of how the Wuhan authorities were handling the outbreak on the air every half an hour on New Year's Day.

In addition to the decision to close the Huanan Seafood Market, the New Year's Eve meeting established plans for several follow-up tasks. By January 2, the NHC had formulated an action program titled " 'Three Earlys' for the Prevention and Control of Viral Pneumonia of Uncertain Etiology."[72]

Multiple sources suggest that the action program was based on existing documents or protocols for handling respiratory outbreaks, particularly the H1N1 pandemic and the H7N9 avian flu.[73] The program called for "three earlys," which are early detection, early diagnosis, and early quarantine, classic tools from the infectious disease prevention and control toolkit that anyone who has taken a course in public health in China knows by heart. The purpose and objectives of the action program were to gain control over the outbreak and stop the viral spread, with "early treatment" added in later editions when it became apparent that COVID-19 patients faced long delays in receiving medical care, leading to severe illness.

It is worth noting that the action program had "viral pneumonia of uncertain etiology," or PUE, in its title, indicating that, unlike in 2003, the preparers of the document were certain that the PUE was caused by a virus. However, this and other documents produced for public consumption during this period avoided associating the disease with SARS or a SARS-like coronavirus. Later, when the International Committee on Taxonomy of Viruses decided to name the virus SARS-CoV-2, Chinese virologists including Gao Fu and other China CDC experts publicly opposed this decision and advocated for an alternative name to differentiate SARS-CoV-2 from SARS-CoV.[74]

The action program was accompanied by at least eight other documents that offered detailed guidelines and forms for carrying out specific tasks such as contact tracing. Li Qun and Liu Jun from the China CDC, along with specialists from the Hubei and Wuhan CDCs, led in putting together the protocols for emergency surveillance and managing close contacts of confirmed patients with the so-called viral PUE.[75] One crucial decision Li Qun made was to adopt the 14-day medical observation standard for close contacts, borrowing from the 2003 SARS protocol.[76] Over the following weeks, specialists from the China CDC collaborated with staff from the Hubei and Wuhan CDCs to guide and conduct epidemiological investigations of patients, trace contacts, and place close contacts under medical observation.[77]

Formulation of the Diagnosis and Treatment Protocol and the Treatment Program

At the New Year's Eve meeting, an urgent task was set to develop a diagnosis and treatment protocol that would be both professional and accessible to the average physician. On New Year's Day, clinical experts from Beijing and Hubei/Wuhan convened again, including chiefs of respiratory medicine and infectious diseases from some of the leading hospitals in Wuhan. Given the unknowns about the disease, some clinicians were "emotionally charged."[78] The atmosphere was filled with agitation and disquiet.

Dr. Cao Bin and Li Xingwang took command of the room, urging the clinical experts to focus on producing the protocol. Cao Bin had led the formulation of the Diagnosis and Treatment Protocol for community-acquired pneumonia in adults in 2016 and was the principal convener for developing the 2017 revised edition of the protocol for human-infected avian influenza A (H7N9).[79] In addition, he had consulted and reviewed patients at Jinyintan Hospital the day before. He was thus well equipped to sum up and describe the symptoms of the "viral PUE." The completion of this task in turn served as the starting point for formulating the Diagnosis and Treatment Protocol.[80]

Given their emphasis on clinical observation and inspection and their knowledge of a SARS-like coronavirus detected in diagnostic tests, the physicians present did not raise serious objections to the description of disease symptoms and agreed that the disease was likely a viral pneumonia caused by a type of coronavirus.[81] Following the action program, the clinicians settled on the language of the "Diagnostic and Treatment Protocol for Viral Pneumonia of Uncertain Etiology (Trial)" in the early afternoon of January 3, 2020.[82] As noted earlier, the clinicians used language that left open the possibility that patients of concern may not have had exposure to the Huanan Seafood Market. For clinicians such as Dr. Lu Jiatao, president of Wuhan Hankou Hospital, the reference to "viral PUE" evoked memories of the 2003 SARS crisis when he oversaw a fever clinic.[83]

Meanwhile, the principle of "four concentrations" of patients, resources, experts, and treatment was adopted for treating patients with the "viral PUE." The Wuhan Jinyintan Hospital was designated as the principal hospital for admitting and treating patients with the "viral PUE." Newly confirmed patients were transferred to Jinyintan Hospital and treated by the National and

Provincial Medical Rescue and Treatment Expert Team.[84] This team included 26 experts from the Hubei–Wuhan Joint Medical Treatment Expert Team led by Dr. Zhao Jianping and five medical experts sent to Wuhan by the NHC.

Wuhan Pulmonary Hospital and Hankou Hospital were initially designated as reserve hospitals for treating the so-called viral PUE patients. The Pulmonary Hospital specializes in infectious diseases, while the modest-sized Hankou Hospital (formerly Railway Hospital), located only 4 kilometers (2.5 miles) from the Huanan Seafood Market, is not an infectious disease hospital but had spare capacity. Dr. Peng Peng and Dr. Lu Jiatao, presidents of the two hospitals, quickly organized their staff to procure large quantities of N95 facemasks, protective suits, and other protective and disinfecting devices. Later, the Pulmonary Hospital was able to provide assistance to other hospitals in dire need.[85]

The Huanan Seafood Market and the Virus Origins Search

Given the strong suspicion that the virus likely came from wildlife sold at the Huanan Seafood Market, the China CDC team, led by Liu Jun, developed the "Protocol for Environmental Origins Tracing/Investigation" on January 1, 2020.[86] Liu Jun, a senior research fellow and trusted collaborator of Gao Fu at the China CDC, then led the Origins Tracing Working Team.[87]

As the Huanan market was being shut down and disinfected, it was urgent for the China CDC to sample the market immediately. The Working Team/taskforce started at the Huanan market at 8 AM on January 1, 2020. Liu and his team made about 20 trips to the marketplace and altogether collected more than 2,000 samples in operations that lasted through March. They submitted detailed progress reports to the health administration throughout this process.[88] A joint World Health Organization (WHO)–China study listed three categories of samples: environmental, animal (swabs and tissue), and sewage. Researchers at the Hubei provincial CDC were tasked with preparing and packaging the collected samples in the Biosafety Level 3 Lab for shipping and transfer to the China CDC and other research labs.

Outreach and Reassurance

As the NHC put the viral PUE action program in place, it also began to respond to inquiries from the WHO and authorized China CDC leadership to engage with the international public health community and overseas Chinese through the Hong Kong media. These efforts aimed to convey a message of reassurance.

According to the timeline compiled by the WHO, the WHO Country Office in China first learned of a viral pneumonia outbreak in Wuhan on December 31, 2019, from a public release on the WMHC website.[89] Dr. Gauden Galea, the WHO representative in China, contacted the NHC for information on January 1, 2020, and then again on January 3, 2020. On January 4 (January 3 in Geneva), the NHC provided information on the cases that the WMHC announced on January 3. In other words, similar to the SARS outbreak in 2003, China did not initiate reporting to the WHO in accordance with the International Health Regulations (2005).

On January 4 (the evening of January 3 in the United States), Gao Fu and US CDC director Robert Redfield, also a virologist, had their first phone call on the outbreak after Redfield had emailed Gao Fu earlier. Before speaking with Gao Fu, Redfield had been in touch with Anthony Fauci, director of the US National Institute of Allergy and Infectious Diseases. Fauci and Redfield were skeptical that all 27 of the first reported cases in Wuhan had been directly infected from animals in the Huanan market.[90] By the time of the Gao–Redfield call, the number of reported cases had risen to 44.

During the call, Gao stated that the initial cases had exposure to the Huanan Seafood Market. Since both were virologists, the idea of zoonosis was easily understood. Redfield pressed Gao on the suspected family clusters in the cases and raised the question of possible human-to-human transmission. In line with a WMHC release on January 3, 2020, that was approved by the NHC and reflected the assessment of the China CDC, Gao told Redfield he was "pretty confident there was no evidence of human-to-human transmission."[91] Gao and Redfield had more phone calls in the following days, and, according to Redfield, there was "not a sense of urgency" from Gao about the novel coronavirus between January 3 and January 6, 2020.[92]

As part of a coordinated messaging effort by the NHC, Xu Jianguo gave an interview to the mainland-controlled *Ta Kung Pao* in Hong Kong on January 4, 2020. Adhering to the January 3 WMHC release, he stated that "no obvious evidence of human-to-human transmission has been found, no medical staff infections have been found, and no death has occurred; [these facts] indicate that the threat level of the virus is limited."[93] Much like Gao Fu in his international messaging, Xu Jianguo projected calm. He urged the public "to remain rational," a discourse strategy that subtly implied that those who disagreed with him might be irrational. He saw no immediate need for the implementation of specific preventive measures until the virus investigation was fully completed. When questioned about the potential spread of the outbreak during the imminent Spring Festival (lunar New Year holidays), Xu confidently stated, "China has amassed years of experience in infectious disease control, and there will absolutely not be a significant spread due to the Spring Festival."[94]

Conclusion

Despite the initial failure to use the national disease reporting system in the initial handling of the unusual pneumonia cases in Wuhan, leaders of China's national health authority (NHC/China CDC) were able to discover the outbreak in Wuhan on December 30, 2019, and mount a rapid health emergency response the following day. As health administrators and experts from multiple disciplines gathered in Wuhan, they had a good grasp of clinical symptoms and access to diagnostic results from genomic sequencing that indicated that a SARS-like coronavirus was the causative agent. Compared with the stumbles of Chinese scientists during the SARS crisis, it was night and day between 2003 and 2019 when it came to the initial identification of the pathogen.[95] It was especially telling that China CDC director general Gao Fu was able to read the genomic sequence of the novel coronavirus on December 31, 2019. By January 1–2, 2020, BGI and the Wuhan Institute of Virology had obtained separate whole genomes of the novel coronavirus. All of this testified to China's improved capacity in disease surveillance and identification.

With the outbreak still relatively confined to Wuhan, China's public health leaders were thus dealt a strong hand of cards. This would have been an enormously opportune moment to intervene decisively and cut off the chains of transmission. Even though it is not possible to be 100% certain, there was a meaningful chance that the outbreak could have been contained in Wuhan/Hubei.

As this chapter has documented, the experts and health administrators built on the work already done in the previous 2 days by the Hubei and Wuhan health authorities and experts and developed a multi-faceted action program for containing the outbreak, as they had done to effectively deal with SARS, avian flu, and other outbreaks in the past. As the new year of 2020 turned and the Huanan Seafood Market was being shut down, they had good reason to think their hard work would result in another success.

However, this collective effort relied on a pair of faulty assumptions and judgments. First, the Hubei joint investigation team had prioritized exposure to the Huanan market as the key criterion for case definition rather than case identification based on symptoms. This emphasis on exposure history to the Huanan market was supported by the China CDC epidemiologists. Feng Zijian later explained that, due to the high prevalence of respiratory diseases, "failure to prioritize exposure history at the outset could result in a lot of 'misclassifications.'"[96] While an approach that emphasized exposure history saved time and effort for the Chinese CDC system, it overlooked cases, such as the first family cluster identified by Dr. Zhang Jixian, that were in retrospect harbingers of viral spread beyond those exposed to the Huanan market. This first assumption could only have been effective if a second assumption/judgment held, namely that the more than two dozen cases had all contracted the virus from one or more sources in the Huanan market, *not* from each other, and that the virus was not yet transmissible from human to human. From the perspective of disaster studies, these assumptions and judgments were a colossal intelligence failure.

These assumptions of the epidemiologists and virologists did not go unquestioned in the New Year's Eve discussion. After all, the clinicians participating in the discussion had already seen and treated patients with the same clinical symptoms but without the requisite exposure history. Clinicians with experience of treating SARS patients remembered the ground glass opacities on patients' CT scans that were characteristic of SARS patients. Likewise, international experts were not convinced that all these cases could have contracted the virus directly from animals.

Yet under pressure to decide, the Chinese health leadership, especially Liang Wannian from the NHC, invoked political considerations in closing the discussion and deciding on the closure of the Huanan market as the source of infections. On this occasion, the epidemiologists and virologists in the Chinese CDC system prevailed against the clinicians. Unfortunately, whereas Liang invoked Xi Jinping's bottom-line thinking, the one bottom-line risk the New Year's Eve meeting failed to prepare for was that the SARS-like coronavirus was already spreading from person to person beyond the confines of the Huanan Seafood Market.

In the ensuing days, news of the Huanan Seafood Market closure, together with police actions against alleged rumormongers about the outbreak, were repeatedly broadcast on Chinese television and widely disseminated. It thus gave officials and the public a false sense of security that the source of the virus had been closed and thus addressed. The public and international outreach and appeals by Gao Fu and Xu Jianguo, issued in their authoritative scientific leadership roles, became part of a repertoire of measures to maintain social stability under the well-known principle of "being intense inside and being relaxed outside."

5

The Stability Imperative and the Silencing of Doctors

From the perspective of organizational cultures in handling crises and disasters, the Chinese political-administrative system is characterized by features that tend to favor bureaucratic-pathological approaches to managing information. For the Communist Party and government leadership in China, moments of crisis and disaster demand information control and public opinion guidance. The party apparatuses for propaganda and stability provide institutionalized systems for guiding public opinion and maintaining social stability.

At the onset of the outbreak of unusual pneumonia cases in Wuhan, the Hubei/Wuhan authorities were highly alarmed by the severe acute respiratory syndrome (SARS)–like symptoms and the discovery of a SARS-like coronavirus. Despite mounting an emergency response to the outbreak, the leadership of the Hubei/Wuhan health administrations failed to report it to the central authorities. Moreover, on December 30, 2019, the Wuhan Municipal Health Commission (WMHC) attempted to prohibit the leaking of outbreak information.

This chapter begins by examining the factors that led the Wuhan/Hubei leadership to opt for employing local resources to control the outbreak, rather than informing and seeking the help of the national government. When the National Health Commission (NHC) did intervene, the local authorities deployed the full power of the local party-state to silence the whistle-blowing doctors and control the official discourse.

The second half of the chapter delves into the investigations and punishments of the doctors, particularly Dr. Ai Fen and Dr. Li Wenliang, as the local authorities implemented the epidemic prevention and control (*fangkong*) action program. Just when the authorities would have benefited from the discovery of new epidemic information about infections and openness to different opinions, the highly publicized efforts to punish the leakers, or "rumormongers," combined with strict censorship of online information on the Wuhan outbreak, had a doubly deleterious effect: they shut down critical information channels necessary for informed decision-making and failed to inform and prepare the public for the epidemic outbreak, unlike in Hong Kong where the people were better prepared.

Political Leadership and the Resurgence of Wuhan

Located in central China, Wuhan is the capital of Hubei Province, with a population of nearly 11 million residents. Situated at the intersection of the Han River and the mighty Yangtze River, it is a major transportation hub. Once referred to as the "Chicago of China," Wuhan's prominence diminished when the Chinese leadership shifted its focus to developing the coastal region during the 1980s and 1990s.[1]

However, with the national leadership's renewed attention to promoting the rise of the central region after 2006, Hubei Province, especially Wuhan, has become a significant beneficiary of this shift in regional development strategy.[2] Recognizing Hubei's importance in central China, two of the party secretaries for Hubei, Yu Zhengsheng (2002–2012; previously construction minister) and Li Hongzhong (2012–2017; previously party secretary of Shenzhen), were known for their development leadership before they were appointed to lead Hubei Province. Both were inducted into the Politburo, with Yu later becoming party secretary of Shanghai and a member of the powerful Politburo Standing Committee.

Under Yu's leadership, significant initiatives were launched in rail and air transportation to revitalize Wuhan's historic role as a transportation hub. Thanks to a creative shareholding arrangement, Wuhan Tianhe Airport Terminal 2 began operations in 2008, and its International Terminal was completed in 2012.[3] Wuhan also benefited from Liu Zhijun, China's minister of railways from 2003 to 2011, who was a Hubei native with strong ties to Wuhan and is known as the father of China's world-leading high-speed rail system. Liu upgraded the Wuhan Railway Bureau, making Wuhan an undisputed railway hub city by the time his career ended (in jail). According to one calculation for November 1, 2017, Wuhan's four major railway stations handled 29 passenger trains each hour, ranking Wuhan in the top five (behind Guangzhou, Shanghai, and Beijing) in China.[4] The acceleration in transportation development has, in turn, helped to speed up Wuhan's push into industry.

As Wuhan has regained much of its vibrancy among China's metropolitan areas, it has also lifted the rest of Hubei Province along with it. In 2019, Wuhan was ranked eighth among China's top 10 cities by gross domestic product (GDP) and was one of only three inland cities on that list.[5] According to the subnational human development index, which factors in per capita GDP, health, and education, Hubei Province moved up dramatically among 30 provincial units in mainland China. Its absolute ranking rose from 22 in 1990 to 20 in 2000, 15 in 2007, and 12 for 2012–2018.[6]

As its standing has improved, Wuhan has also gained more national attention and opportunities. For instance, President Xi Jinping held his summit with Indian prime minister Narendra Modi in Wuhan in April 2018, and Wuhan was the host city for the World Military Games in October 2019. In various policy domains, including social governance, health, and industrial development, Wuhan has been recognized for its exemplary performance within China.

As of 2019 and January 2020, the party leaders for Hubei/Wuhan were Jiang Chaoliang, the Hubei provincial party secretary, and Ma Guoqiang, the Wuhan municipal party secretary. Ma also served as one of the two deputy party secretaries for Hubei, alongside Hubei governor Wang Xiaodong.

The pairing of Jiang Chaoliang and Ma Guoqiang underscored the Party Central's emphasis on economic development. Jiang Chaoliang was one of the most distinguished bankers of his generation, having served as chair of the Bank of Communications and of China Agricultural Bank in the decade spanning 2004–2014, as well as president of the State Development Bank. He then served as governor of Jilin Province before his appointment as Hubei party secretary in 2016. In 2017–2018, Jiang was reportedly one of the leading candidates to succeed Zhou Xiaochuan as the governor of the People's Bank of China.[7] However, at the age of 63 in 2020, Jiang was approaching the retirement age of 65 for top provincial leaders. Hubei was likely to be the last significant stage for Jiang's political career before he would be given membership in the National People's Congress or the People's Political Consultative Conference.[8]

In contrast, Ma Guoqiang's was a rising star. Born in 1963, Ma hails from Hebei (not Hubei). He attended college in Wuhan before studying finance in Germany. He began his corporate career in 1995 with state-owned Baosteel, eventually serving as the chair of China Baowu Steel Group, one of the world's largest steel makers (2016–2018), before his appointment as deputy party secretary of Hubei and party secretary of Wuhan in 2018. As the Wuhan party chief, Ma drew on his corporate experience to urge party and government officials to prioritize making Wuhan business-friendly. In spring 2019, he vowed to "smash the 'rice bowls' of those who damage Wuhan's business environment." Ma also made four vice mayors pledge publicly to implement measures that would create a favorable business environment in Wuhan.[9]

In fall 2019, as Wuhan made its final preparations to host the World Military Games in October, Ma Guoqiang, working in tandem with Wuhan mayor Zhou Xianwang, put forth an ambitious vision for elevating Wuhan's status as an international economic, commercial, and technological center.[10] Following the success of the World Military Games, there was a sense of euphoria about Wuhan's growing prospects. The city had made massive improvements in infrastructure, including new subways, to prepare for the games; and news reports lauded Wuhan's "China speed" in constructing new facilities.[11] According to an interviewee whose spouse worked in the provincial party committee, Wuhan officials were brimming with pride as they basked in their own publicity campaign about Wuhan's rising stature.[12]

For Party Secretary Ma Guoqiang, there was much to look forward to in the year ahead. In the first week of January, he would be stepping down from his position as chair of the Wuhan Municipal People's Congress Standing Committee.[13] Though the Chinese political machinery can be opaque, this move was widely interpreted as a sign that he would soon be up for a promotion. Ma's predecessors as party secretary of Wuhan had a history of receiving promotions to national positions; moreover, between 2019 and 2021, two-thirds of the deputy provincial party secretaries in China were promoted to ministerial rank.[14] The promotion statistics for deputy provincial secretaries alone suggested that Ma would likely be considered for an upward move soon. This also meant that he was particularly motivated to present a positive image of Wuhan's situation.

The Calculus of Outbreak Response and Disease Reporting

It was against the backdrop of growing capabilities and soaring ambitions, combined with a sense of trepidation, that municipal and provincial health leaders in Wuhan initially responded to the outbreak of SARS-like pneumonia by pooling medical resources for emergency response efforts while refraining from reporting the outbreak to the national health authority, such as the China Centers for Disease Control and Prevention (China CDC) or NHC. While the China CDC had urged local CDCs to improve their reporting of infectious disease cases through the National Notifiable Disease Surveillance System, honest reporting of outbreaks could potentially harm a city's standing on other metrics. The incentive to avoid or conceal an epidemic outbreak during one's tenure would be especially powerful if a city could face penalties for having an outbreak in a given calendar year.

Chinese municipal leaders place great importance on achieving various city honors, such as being designated a National Healthy City or a National Civilized City, among others. Studies of these city ranking initiatives have found that cities receiving these designations have shown significant improvements in metrics such as the proportion of treated domestic sewage and the proportion of qualified farmers' markets.[15] Of particular interest to Wuhan was the National Healthy City designation, a competition sponsored by the National Patriotic Health Campaign Committee under the NHC. The standards for the National Healthy City designation include multiple infectious disease control indicators that may have incentivized local authorities to manipulate infectious disease reporting statistics and conceal outbreaks. Even after these requirements were toned down, the National Healthy Cities standards (2014) still include the requirement that "in the recent three years, there were no major laboratory biosafety accidents and epidemic outbreaks of Class A and B infectious diseases caused by ineffective prevention and control measures."[16]

As the provincial capital of Hubei and a city with a proud history, Wuhan had repeatedly failed to win the honor of being designated a "National Healthy City." It finally succeeded in 2015, a full 15 years after the inception of the honor, following a comprehensive "building national healthy city" campaign.[17] Achieving the National Healthy City designation was a hard-fought and hard-won struggle for Wuhan, and the hometown newspaper headlined it as "a dream come true" in 2015.[18] As a result, the municipal leaders of Wuhan would be especially reluctant to lose the National Healthy City designation due to a pneumonia outbreak at the end of the year.

In fact, one of the main initiatives on the agenda of the Wuhan leadership was obtaining the "National Ecological and Garden City" designation. This designation required meeting qualifications such as urban environment and health indicators, as well as having appropriate crisis response mechanisms.[19] On the final day of 2019, when the NHC and China CDC emergency response teams had arrived in Wuhan, Mayor Zhou Xianwang chaired a municipal government executive meeting to discuss preparations for launching a bid for this designation.[20]

Imagine you are a provincial or municipal official in a major city faced with a pneumonia of uncertain etiology (PUE) outbreak with only a few days left in the current year. You must decide whether to report the outbreak to the central government, which could not only damage the city's reputation but also jeopardize its designation as a "National Healthy City" and other status designations for several years to come. Given Party Secretary Ma Guoqiang's ambitious push to improve Wuhan's business environment, risking the loss of such a prestigious designation was like putting Wuhan's future at risk. In such circumstances, would you be tempted to conceal the outbreak and contain it with the resources at your disposal? In an interview that has since been removed from Chinese websites, Zeng Guang, who oversaw disease reporting at the China CDC for many years, acknowledged that "concealment and non-reporting of some infectious diseases is very common." Local authorities are afraid that reporting epidemic information to the central authorities would "negatively impact and harm the image of the city."[21]

Given these considerations, it is quite likely that officials in Wuhan/Hubei were hesitant to report the outbreak to the central government in late December 2019. Wuhan is a major center for health and medicine, with hospitals such as Tongji and Union Hospitals that are among China's very best, a top-level biosafety lab (Wuhan Institute of Virology), and a provincial CDC that proudly wears its research prowess as the Hubei Academy of Preventive Medicine. These resources allowed Hubei/Wuhan to field strong expert teams to investigate the outbreak, as well as to treat and quarantine the sick, as discussed in previous chapters. Thus, the health leadership of Hubei/Wuhan had good reason to attempt to handle and contain the outbreak with local resources before involving the central government.

Ironically, while the Hubei/Wuhan leadership did not rush to seek the involvement of the NHC at the end of December 2019, their considerations changed after the NHC deployed a working group and experts in Wuhan. With the formulation and implementation of the action program, which included the closure of the Huanan Seafood Market, the Hubei/Wuhan health leadership appeared to believe that the outbreak situation was under control. On the evening of December 31, 2019, the WMHC held a meeting of "main leaders" from municipal hospitals. The municipal health leaders shared information on the measures being taken and the efforts to investigate the causative pathogen. They advised the hospital leaders present to continue their normal medical work and "not panic."[22] However, it should be noted that some hospital leaders had already learned about the SARS-like coronavirus and did not take the reassurance from the WMHC leadership at face value.[23]

Less than a week after the closure of the Huanan market, Zhang Jin, party secretary of the Hubei Provincial Health Commission, attended the NHC-convened annual national health work conference in Beijing on January 6, 2020. During his speech, Zhang praised the Hubei provincial leadership for promoting the Healthy Hubei initiative and for giving the provincial health commission a more prominent role in policymaking. He also announced with pride that "there was zero importation and zero spread of infectious diseases during the World Military Games."[24] It is unlikely that he would have made such a statement in front of NHC leaders and his peers from across the country if he did not believe that the outbreak linked to the Huanan market in Wuhan was already under control or would be soon.

Stability Maintenance and the Silencing of Doctors

As the Hubei/Wuhan health authorities coordinated the emergency response to the so-called PUE outbreak on December 29–30, 2019, they had not expected that WMHC emergency notices and WeChat posts from doctors would go viral, prompting the NHC and the China CDC to send emergency teams to Wuhan the following day. As the national teams assumed leadership of the health emergency response, Hubei/Wuhan authorities prioritized stability maintenance and focused on identifying and punishing those who leaked information about the outbreak. Consequently, a mission to suppress leaks and exact revenge unfolded. In this context, Dr. Ai Fen and Dr. Li Wenliang of Wuhan Central Hospital (WCH), along with other doctors, faced punishment or reprimand.

The silencing and subsequent death of 34-year-old Dr. Li Wenliang from COVID-19 garnered immense attention in China and globally, even inspiring an English children's book.[25] His call for a healthy society to tolerate different voices, made public the day he died (see epigraph for Chapter 1), resonated strongly with the public. To appease widespread public anger, China's National Supervisory Commission initiated a highly publicized investigation. Authorities later honored Dr. Li as a martyr and, to a significant extent, managed to defuse tension with the general public by co-opting Dr. Li's identity.

Some argue that if social media posts by Ai Fen, Li Wenliang, and other health workers had not resulted in punishment in early January 2020, it would likely not have changed the epidemic's course.[26] While there is some merit to this argument, these authors may not fully appreciate the alarm that the doctors' postings about the SARS-like coronavirus generated. The punishment of these doctors, publicized and amplified through the official propaganda system—including repeated national television broadcasts—created a chilling effect on medical professionals who might have spoken out about human-to-human transmission of the novel coronavirus. The silence of the medical professions was compounded by a gag order on laboratories, discussed in the following chapter. The delay in recognizing human-to-human transmission was not merely a judgment error but had deep political-organizational roots.

As discussed in Chapter 4, the WeChat posts and messages from Dr. Ai Fen and Dr. Li Wenliang went viral on the evening of December 30, 2019. The mention of SARS(-like) pneumonia was too potent to ignore. A subsequent National Supervisory Commission investigation revealed that similar messages appeared in other WeChat groups, while the two WMHC orders issued earlier that afternoon were also circulated on WeChat, garnering attention from, among others, China CDC director general Gao Fu.[27]

Late that evening (around 10 PM), Dr. Ai and an unnamed colleague of Dr. Li's received a message from the WCH hospital administration, stating that the WMHC had instructed hospital staff *not* to share information about the so-called PUE with the public to avoid causing mass panic. The WMHC notice, marked with three exclamation points, sternly warned that "Those in serious breach will be held responsible."[28] However, the admonition came too late to prevent information about the outbreak from reaching the China CDC leadership and many other people.

Late that night, the WMHC leadership held an emergency meeting with hospital leaders to prepare for the arrival of NHC experts and the China CDC emergency response team on the morning of December 31, 2019. The meeting's agenda included addressing the social media leaks about the outbreak that drew the attention of the NHC leadership. Dr. Li Wenliang's name was identified.[29]

The WCH leadership, including the medical affairs director, attended the meeting and felt the WMHC leaders' fury. At around 1:30 AM on December 31, the medical affairs director called Dr. Li Wenliang and instructed him to go to the WMHC immediately. Upon arriving, Dr. Li was asked to wait in another room while the WMHC and hospital leaders continued their meeting. Around 4 AM, the WCH leadership met with Dr. Li to inquire about the sources of his WeChat messages.[30]

That marked the beginning of Li Wenliang's ordeal. Later that day, Dr. Li, a Communist Party member, was summoned to the WCH Supervision Section for questioning two or three more times. His interrogators, tasked with identifying the individuals behind the leaks, repeatedly pressed him about the sources of his WeChat messages. Dr. Li was eventually released after writing a self-criticism admitting that he had shared "untruthful information," "caused public panic," and violated relevant laws and regulations regarding the disclosure of infectious disease outbreaks.[31] At that point, he was informed that he would receive some form of internal sanction within the hospital.[32] A WCH source revealed that "many people at our hospital were called in by the hospital administration for [such] 'talks.' "[33]

Dr. Ai Fen was on duty on New Year's Day. Early that morning, a 65-year-old male patient was transferred from the Wuhan Red Cross Society Hospital to the Emergency Ward of the WCH Houhu Branch, which she oversaw. The patient was critically ill. Dr. Ai Fen discovered that the patient was a practicing doctor at a private clinic near the Huanan Seafood Market and had treated many patients with fever in recent days. She concluded that the doctor who was now her patient had likely contracted the unusual pneumonia caused by the suspected coronavirus. Concerned about the patient's contagiousness, she informed the WCH Medical Affairs Department and Public Health Section.[34]

In the meantime, WCH administrators searching for the sources of the social media leaks about the outbreak traced the messages containing the SARS-like coronavirus diagnostic result to Dr. Ai Fen. Just before midnight on New Year's Day, staff from the WCH Supervision Section instructed Dr. Ai to meet with the hospital leadership.[35]

Dr. Ai went early the next morning. Citing the WMHC leadership, the WCH official in charge of discipline delivered an "unprecedented, very harsh rebuke" to Dr. Ai:[36]

> You disregard the results of Wuhan's urban construction since the [World] Military Games; you are a sinner affecting Wuhan's stability and unity; you are the culprit undermining the city of Wuhan's forward development.[37]

The scolding continued:

> As the Chief of Emergency Care at Wuhan Central Hospital and a professional, how can you spread rumors and cause trouble in defiance of principles and organizational discipline?[38]

It is important to note that Dr. Ai Fen was not being criticized for the quality of her medical work or patient care. Instead, she was made to feel as if she was single-handedly sabotaging Wuhan's prospects as a city. The tone of the rebuke is reminiscent of Party Secretary Ma Guoqiang's strident demand to protect Wuhan's business environment. It is likely that the WMHC leadership had relayed remarks from one or more of Wuhan's municipal leaders. Dr. Ai Fen was taken aback. "That meeting hit me very hard, very big. When I came back, I felt like my whole heart was broken."[39]

During the peak of the Wuhan crisis and lockdown, Chinese media heavily criticized the WCH leadership, particularly Party Secretary Cai Li, for their poor leadership and harsh treatment of Ai Fen, Li Wenliang, and others. Meanwhile, Cai Li took careful measures to protect herself from the coronavirus. However, even a brief review suggests that Cai Li acted on orders from her superiors at the WMHC and higher levels.[40] In fact, considering the parallel developments involving the police and the propaganda apparatus (see the following section), Cai Li and the WMHC leadership were all part of a much larger political calculus centered on the party leadership in Wuhan.

While Dr. Ai Fen received a stern rebuke, she was also protected from even harsher punishment due to her decade-long service as the chief of the Emergency Care Department. For the time being, she was instructed to ensure that everyone in her department of over 200 remained quiet about the "atypical pneumonia" cases. She complied as ordered and did not even tell her husband about the rebuke she received on January 2 until January 20, 2020.[41] The logic of the party-dominated system prevailed.

The Punishment of Dr. Li Wenliang and Other Doctors and Its Chilling Effect on Medical Professionals

In the meantime, the party-state mobilized the power of the stability maintenance regime, targeting more junior doctors such as Dr. Li Wenliang and at least seven others from different hospitals who shared information in three separate WeChat groups for medical school alumni and practicing doctors.[42] A Wuhan police official later explained, "In the circumstances of that time, most people could not imagine the epidemic would get this severe later. The stability of social sentiments was the priority consideration for the authorities."[43]

As mentioned earlier, Dr. Li Wenliang was summoned to the WCH Supervision Section and required to make a self-criticism. He was given the impression that he would receive an internal sanction and that would be the end of it. To his surprise, on January 3, police officers from the local precinct ordered Dr. Li Wenliang to go to the police station.[44] He went accompanied by a colleague but without legal counsel. The two officers questioned him about the messages he posted. It is unclear how long Dr. Li was subjected to questioning or interrogation, but the political and psychological pressure on him was evident from the writ of admonition he signed.

According to the writ, which Dr. Li shared with the public in a Weibo post later on, Dr. Li pledged to stop "the unlawful spreading of untruthful opinion."[45] It further stated, "We hope you calm down and seriously reflect on your actions, and we solemnly warn you: If you stubbornly adhere to your views, fail to repent, and continue to engage in illegal activities, you will be punished by the law! Do you understand?" Dr. Li answered "Understand" and put down thumbprints on his answers and his own name (picture on the right in Figure 4.1).

For citizens living under the rule of law, it is striking that precinct police officers could humiliate a doctor from a major hospital and order him to sign a degrading writ of admonition without the benefit of legal counsel. In China, however, police routinely invoke the Public Security Administration Punishment Law (2005, amended 2012) to mete out a large number of punishments for infractions against public order, ranging from illegal drug use, prostitution, and hooliganism to petty thefts, gambling, and unauthorized use of virtual private networks (VPN) to access overseas websites.[46] The admonition is one of four categories of penalties that can be deployed by police and is, in fact, considered a lighter form of punishment among the four (the other three are fines, administrative detention, and cancellation of a permit issued by the Public Security Bureau).

Dr. Li Wenliang was one of at least eight doctors pursued by the police at the time for sharing information about the outbreak.[47] Dr. Liu Wen of the Wuhan Red Cross Society Hospital was also asked to go to the police station but was not asked to sign a writ of admonition.[48] Others were warned about their WeChat postings over the phone.[49] Because Wuhan police announced the action against "rumormongers" on January 1, 2020, but did not contact Dr. Li and other doctors until January 2–3, it was likely that the Wuhan municipal police leadership had not wanted to take enforcement action against the doctors until more senior political leaders pressed the matter. Police later tried to downplay the admonitions and warnings given to the doctors.[50]

The police admonitions and warnings, coupled with stern criticisms of the doctors within the healthcare system, were devastatingly effective at stifling the voices of medical doctors in Wuhan and the rest of Hubei. It is well known that, when campaigning for National Healthy City and other designations, city leaders in China would prep residents for possible questioning by visiting evaluators. One informed source in Wuhan suggested to me that, since the national health leadership had discovered the outbreak in Wuhan on their own and had sent experts and investigators, the leadership in Wuhan/Hubei was strongly motivated to warn the local population, especially the healthcare workers, not to reveal information to the investigators.

Many doctors in the Wuhan medical community were alarmed to learn that patients had been diagnosed with SARS-like coronavirus infections and would have been more forthcoming in providing information to decision makers and informing the public had they been given the chance. However, the injunctions and police warnings quickly silenced these doctors. At the Wuhan University Zhongnan Hospital, Dr. Zhang Xiaochun of the Radiology

Department reviewed the computed tomographic (CT) images of some pneumonia cases on December 27–28 and recognized their similarity to the CT images of patients afflicted with SARS. Members of her department then prepared and posted an article about the unusual pneumonia cases on their department's public WeChat account just before midnight on December 31, 2019. Late that evening, after they received the WMHC prohibition against unauthorized release of information about the outbreak, they promptly removed the WeChat public post.[51] As we report in subsequent chapters, the chilling effect of the doctors' punishment lasted well beyond the initial days and remained in effect when additional expert teams visited Wuhan in January 2020.

Party Leadership of Stability Work

What authority could get both the major hospitals and the police to silence doctors in a major city like Wuhan? We know the hospitals, depending on their administrative ranking, report to different levels of the government (provincial, municipal, and district). We also know separately that a joint Hubei provincial–Wuhan municipal team was put together to diagnose and care for patients with the unusual pneumonia at Jinyintan Hospital. Furthermore, we know that police were mobilized to reach doctors in hospitals located in different districts. Finally, as we report below, an intense propaganda campaign reaching the entire country was also underway.

For all these to occur, the central involvement of the Communist Party leadership in Wuhan municipality plus Hubei Province was needed to coordinate the health commission on the government side, propaganda in the party apparatus, and public security (police), which is overseen by the secretary of the Legal and Political Affairs Commission of Hubei as well as of Wuhan. Two of the leaders are of special interest. Ma Guoqiang, who was both the party secretary of Wuhan and one of two deputy secretaries for Hubei Province, was uniquely positioned in both Wuhan and Hubei Province to provide leadership as circumstances quickly evolved. As mentioned earlier, Ma Guoqiang was in early January 2020 preparing for further promotions. He was thus especially motivated to have Wuhan look good. To jump ahead of our story, this decision was also one he would come to deeply regret. Here, we quote from an interview Ma gave at the end of January 2020:

> I am now laden with self-shame, remorse, and self-blame. . . . I've been thinking that, if I had made the decision earlier to adopt draconian controls that are adopted

> now, the results would be better than the present. Then we would probably have had less impact on the rest of the country and would have caused the Party Central and the State Council less worry.[52]

This quote may sound like an attempt at self-protection through self-criticism by Ma. However, in Chapters 9 and 10 I'll explain that Ma's regret was tied to a specific date he had in mind, most likely due to the information and policy recommendations he received on that date.

Another important figure in the Hubei party leadership was Liang Weinian, the secretary general of the Hubei Provincial Communist Party Committee and a member of its standing committee. In his role as secretary general, he was the chief coordinator for the Hubei Communist Party leadership. He was concurrently the director of the National Security Office and, prior to becoming secretary general, had been the head of the Hubei provincial Propaganda Department (2015–2017).[53] Liang's previous experiences, coupled with his positions at the turn of 2020, made him a particularly potent player in the rough-and-tumble politics of this unfolding drama.

Preemptive Propaganda as Persuasion and Deterrence

Scholars of China's propaganda and censorship have noted that the motivations for censorship among the different levels of authorities in China vary. Local levels tend to be especially focused on hiding news or information that may hurt the careers of local officials.[54] In the case of the unusual pneumonia cases in Wuhan, however, the central propaganda apparatus joined hands with the leadership of Hubei and Wuhan to deliver an extremely powerful cautionary message in not just Wuhan but the entire country against sharing information about the pneumonia cases or the outbreak. On December 31, 2019, a coordinated effort was made to persuade the public to discount any rumors about SARS-like pneumonia cases in Wuhan. One widely shared report reminded readers that "official news releases by the government must be verified by specialists and screened for accuracy before they are released, hence it is normal they are delayed."[55]

At 5:38 PM on January 1, 2020, the Wuhan Public Security Bureau (police), using its Weibo account Ping'an Wuhan (Safe Wuhan, 平安武汉), announced that it had dealt with eight netizens for "unlawful acts" of spreading rumors about the unexplained pneumonia cases in Wuhan: "some netizens, without verifying [the facts], posted or shared untrue information and caused adverse social impact." It warned that police will "absolutely use the law to deal with and absolutely not tolerate unlawful behavior, namely fabricating and spreading rumors to disturb social order."[56]

Note that when the Wuhan police made the Weibo post on New Year's Day, they had not yet asked Dr. Li Wenliang and Dr. Liu Wen to come to the police station for investigation or to sign the admonition. The leadership in charge of orchestrating the different operations didn't wait for such details to be worked out. In a striking display of the Hubei/Wuhan leaders' urgency to exert control over information about the outbreak, they leveraged the propaganda system to have the punishment of eight "rumormongers" publicized in all major media outlets across the country.

While the initial reports were confined to the print and online media, just before noon on January 2, 2020, news programs on China Central Television began to broadcast that eight "rumormongers" had been punished in Wuhan for spreading false information about the Wuhan outbreak. Cycling the item throughout the day, the anchors also announced that the police would punish and absolutely not tolerate those who spread rumors and disturbed social order.[57] Even though the police and the official media avoided mentioning that the alleged "rumormongers" were all medical doctors, information about such punishment quickly spread in the medical community.

In broadcasting the punishment of doctors for "spreading rumors," the party and state media outlets, especially China Central Television, vastly amplified the impact of police warnings and admonition.[58] In effect, they delivered heavy doses of crude, hard propaganda that is known to stifle disagreement and deter dissent.[59] The repeated broadcasts served to dissuade people, particularly medical professionals in Wuhan, from sharing information on the SARS-like atypical pneumonia outbreak. It was like wielding a gigantic axe over the head of medical professionals. It also meant that the leadership of Hubei/Wuhan had the strong support of the central propaganda apparatus and thus the Party Central.

Doctors from across the country took note of the Wuhan police announcement. Many administrative and medical staff, not directly involved in treating the unusual pneumonia cases, were convinced that the party-state was genuinely cracking down on rumors. Among these medical staff was Dr. Cai Yi, the chief of Pain Medicine at the WCH. He recalled, "After Dr. Li Wenliang spoke out, we all initially thought [he] did make a rumor, and there were leaders who said so."[60] Dr. Cai finally realized the severity of the situation when he encountered a patient with the unusual pneumonia symptoms.

In a February 2020 interview with Reuters, Dr. Zhong Nanshan noted that behind Dr. Li Wenliang "stood hundreds of other doctors all wanting to tell the truth."[61] However, fearing repercussions, doctors and nurses who were aware of the outbreak could not inform their patients about the outbreak during early to mid-January 2020. According to a Wuhan Union Hospital doctor, all they could do was to urge patients to wear facemasks and half-jokingly advise them to avoid the Huanan market because "the items on sale there are not fresh."[62]

The concerted actions to control information release about the outbreak in Wuhan, euphemistically referred to as "cold treatment," were devastatingly effective. In the words of the Wuhan Union Hospital doctor, the official injunction was "don't tell," whether in official media or on social media. This directive applied to clinicians, including those in infection control, with the degree of information control in the CDC system being particularly strict.[63] The situation was similar at the Hubei Provincial Hospital of Integrated Chinese and Western Medicine. Hospital leadership instructed department directors to tell staff not to disclose information about cases of medical staff infections and especially to stay away from the media. Through January 20, 2020, doctors were repeatedly reminded "not to create or spread rumors, and to avoid causing social panic."[64] At WCH, which gained notoriety for maltreating medical staff, hospital leadership began warning staff not to share information about the unexplained pneumonia outbreak on December 30, 2019. They also asked staff "not to wear facemasks, for fear of causing panic."[65] For the next 3 weeks, even staff at community service centers were told to "neither trust nor spread the rumors [about the outbreak]." They in turn told residents that "the epidemic outbreak isn't that serious."[66]

However, the fear of official punishment spread far beyond Wuhan. A Zhejiang doctor with a substantial social media following recalls that the punishment of the eight doctors "made us doctors feel we were all in danger. . . . [I] believe doctors across the entire country shared the same feeling. The Wuhan police got to them and made a big splash on Central Television. After all that, no doctor dared to give an early warning!"[67]

While the official prohibitions prevented information leaks, they also dramatically curtailed a major channel that could have supplied valuable information on the epidemic to authorities and provided some warning to the public. During the SARS crisis in 2003, "rumors" of the mysterious and deadly disease prompted many people to wear facemasks and take other precautions. In Wuhan, this informal warning mechanism was not only shut down in the early weeks but reversed, as authorities initially refrained from disclosing information about the novel coronavirus and later emphasized that the novel coronavirus wasn't contagious from human to human. Liao Jun, senior reporter of the Hubei branch of Xinhua News Agency, led the charge for Xinhua News Agency and would later be rewarded by the authorities—and criticized by detractors—for her role in promoting the official line.[68]

The reach of the official media also extended to social media. On December 30, 2019, *People's Daily* reporter Cheng Yuanzhou sent out a widely shared message on Weibo. Citing multiple hospital sources, Cheng stated that the disease of concern was more likely a different serious pneumonia rather than the much-dreaded SARS. "Even if it is the SARS virus," he asserted, "there is a mature prevention and control treatment system in place, so the public need not panic."[69]

The local media—dominated by the *Hubei Daily* group and the *Changjiang Daily* group—are under the control of the Hubei and Wuhan party leadership, respectively. While the novel coronavirus spread, the front pages of newspapers published by these two groups increasingly took on the celebratory red color to lend support to the annual meetings of the Wuhan and then Hubei authorities while the Chinese lunar New Year drew closer.[70] In short, official media in China joined hands with the police and played a powerful role at the end of 2019 and early 2020 in silencing the medical profession in Wuhan while lulling most of the public into a false sense of safety. In the view of Ye Qing (叶青), a deputy director general of the Hubei Provincial Bureau of statistics, "people weren't worried, because, as is well known, [it was announced that there was] no human-to-human transmission . . . so it didn't worry us."[71]

In his review of the Chinese media, Guobin Yang, the eminent scholar of communication and sociology at the University of Pennsylvania, notes that it is the modus operandi for Chinese official media to behave as they did in January 2020.[72] Likewise, it is not surprising that the machinery of censorship was activated to remove social media postings that diverged from the official discourse on the outbreak. Some of the most notable messages and conversations censored were from the Wuhan Weibo user "雯_雯小妖."[73] A little after noon on January 5, 2020, she wrote, "This pneumonia in Wuhan is truly scary, two members of my family are infected. One has been taken to Jinyintan [Hospital] for isolation till now, situation unclear, but [we've been] asked to repeatedly sign on [notices of critical illness to authorize continued treatment]." In conversations with Weibo users within 20 minutes of her original post, she received 38 comments and answered several queries. She described the symptoms and noted that the patient at Jinyintan Hospital "is already having organ failure." Because the patient was in isolation, she noted, "even family members are not able to know what's going on." However, her exchanges with Weibo users showed she was quite certain about the contagiousness of the disease:

Q: Are your family from the Huanan Seafood [Market]?
A: No.
Q: Have your family members been to the Huanan Seafood Market?
A: Never been there.
Q: [Does your family live] close to the Huanan Seafood Market?
A: [Patient who] first went to hospital(s) near the Huanan market, and as a result [sentence cut off].
Q: May I ask, [does the disease] transmit from person to person?
A: You can be sure that it's contagious.

Shortly after she shared the above information, her Weibo account "雯_雯小妖" disappeared.[74] Due to the aggressive censorship, it is not possible to know how much more of such information was posted at the time. However, it is clear that much valuable information would have been available to the public and decision makers from medical professionals, patients, and their families had authorities permitted the sharing of information about the outbreak.

The Hong Kong Contrast

Before describing the events of the following weeks, it is useful to briefly note how the response in Hong Kong differed from that in Wuhan. Hong Kong experienced 299 deaths from SARS in 2003, compared to 349 on mainland China.[75] Like on the mainland, and in Taiwan and Singapore, the severity of SARS left enduring memories and generated strong lessons for dealing with respiratory infectious diseases in Hong Kong.[76] However, unlike in Wuhan, the Hong Kong leadership responded to the threat of the viral PUE outbreak by combining the lessons from dealing with SARS and other infectious diseases with respect for experts and policy transparency.

On January 4, the same day Xu Jianguo told Hong Kong–based Ta Kung Pao not to worry, Dr. Ho Pak-leung of the University of Hong Kong suspected human-to-human transmission had occurred in Wuhan and called for officials to adopt "the most stringent" precautionary measures.[77] The Hong Kong government, acting on expert advice, determined that the viral pneumonia cases in Wuhan had the potential for efficient human-to-human transmission that could lead to international spread and a public health emergency.

It quickly activated the Preparedness and Response Plan for Novel Infectious Disease of Public Health Significance ("The Plan") at the "Serious" response level with immediate effect.[78] In addition to strengthening temperature surveillance at ports of entry, procedures were in place for the isolation and treatment of individuals with fever and acute respiratory or pneumonia symptoms who had visited Wuhan within 14 days before the onset of the illness.[79] Similar actions took place in Singapore and Taiwan.

As noted earlier, authorities in Wuhan cracked down on doctors who shared information on the outbreak and severely restricted information suggesting the outbreak was severe. Despite the WMHC statement on December 31, 2019, staff at airlines, subways, and even hospitals in Wuhan were explicitly discouraged from wearing facemasks for fear of causing social anxiety and panic.[80]

In contrast, Carrie Lam, the Hong Kong chief executive, said on January 3, 2020, that the Hong Kong government would announce any cases of infection daily and urged members of the public to take appropriate personal hygiene measures. Flight attendants on a Dragon Airlines flight into Wuhan on January 3 wore facemasks and warned travelers to seek medical attention if they experienced a fever or respiratory symptoms.[81] The free flow of information, coupled with news of 21 suspected infections in Hong Kong (which turned out to be false alarms), prompted Hong Kong residents to stock up on N95 facemasks and other provisions.[82] What appeared to be an overreaction to some people at the time turned out to be good preparedness as Hong Kong would fare extremely well in coping with the first wave of SARS-CoV-2 infections in 2020. As of April 30, 2020, Hong Kong had a cumulative total of 1,039 confirmed COVID-19 cases, with 4 deaths and 843 recoveries.[83]

Conclusion

Multiple factors—from how cities are evaluated and the personal career considerations of Party Secretary Ma Guoqiang to the national political environment and political and holiday calendars—provided incentives for the Hubei/Wuhan leadership to quickly downplay the so-called PUE outbreak at the end of 2019. After the unexpected and forceful intervention of the NHC, marked by the closure of the Huanan Seafood Market, the Hubei and Wuhan authorities focused on cracking down on whistleblowing doctors in efforts to control the official discourse. In what appeared as revenge for leaking information, the Hubei/Wuhan authorities adopted strong-arm tactics to punish and silence doctors who shared information about the outbreak. Social media postings on individual patients and the outbreak in general were strictly censored. According to a Beijing-based commentator writing for an authorized overseas outlet, the official media, both national and local, were "truly 'dead'" prior to January 20, 2020, when it came to informing the public of the dangers of the outbreak.[84]

The crackdown on doctors who shared information and social media postings about the contagiousness of the so-called viral PUE was intensified by the national propaganda system, and as I will describe in the next chapter, it was combined with and exacerbated by information control measures imposed by the NHC. Taken together, these information control measures marked a pathological turn from the perspective of emergency response and information flows. If there had been no highly publicized police admonishment of Dr. Li Wenliang and other medical professionals, more information about cases in Wuhan and significant discussions of similarities to SARS would have been available.[85] Many people would have acted on the information to take precautions, as people did in Hong Kong. Decision makers would have been exposed to more signals that showed that the novel coronavirus was contagious. In the view of a commentary recommended by China's Supreme People's Court on January 28, 2020: "If the public had heard this 'rumor' [about the SARS-like pneumonia] at that time and, due to their concerns about SARS, took to wearing facemasks, practiced strict disinfection, and avoided the wildlife market, it would have been beneficial for us in terms of improving prevention and control efforts against the new type of pneumonia today."[86]

6
The National Health Commission, Laboratory Regulation, and Pathogen Verification

Until the SARS crisis of 2003, China's leadership and health system routinely treated information on epidemic outbreaks as state secrets on the premise that publicizing initial outbreak information or data would lead to unnecessary social panic.[1] However, the severe acute respiratory syndrome (SARS) disaster prompted Chinese leadership to recognize the importance of transparency in handling public health emergencies. Consequently, they introduced mechanisms to improve information disclosure as part of China's open government initiative.[2] For numerous cities grappling with SARS in China and around the world, a crucial lesson learned was the need to trust the public with information, enabling their participation in combating the epidemic.[3] As a result, some researchers argued that China transitioned from secrecy during SARS to openness when faced with the H1N1 pandemic in 2009.[4] In practice, the Chinese response to H1N1 was exceptional as the H1N1 pandemic was an external threat, easily framed as the common enemy for the health administration and the public. When an infectious disease outbreak originated within China, managing disease information could quickly become politically complex. Although Chinese authorities have been more open in handling disease outbreaks since the post-SARS years, the inclination and habits for information control and management have persisted.[5] This was apparent when the Hubei/Wuhan authorities employed harsh tactics to suppress information leaks about the SARS-like viral pneumonia of uncertain etiology (PUE) disease at the end of 2019 and in January 2020.

In a postmortem of the Wuhan outbreak, Wu Zunyou, by then China CDC chief epidemiologist, quickly cited the familiar paternalist rationale for controlling outbreak information: "When an issue is not clear, we will cause panic in society if we release it to the public."[6] Upon the central authorities' involvement in managing the Wuhan outbreak on December 31, 2019, they also embraced this paternalist rationale. The central propaganda system backed the Hubei/Wuhan authorities in censoring unwelcome information and used China Central Television to amplify the crackdown on doctors accused of spreading rumors. The National Health Commission (NHC) guided the issuance of public updates by the Hubei/Wuhan authorities. Altogether, from the perspective of organizations and information flows during a crisis, these measures would greatly thwart the discovery of epidemic information from among clinicians and severely curtail the availability of outbreak information to the public.

During an outbreak, prompt and accurate identification and verification of the pathogen causing the disease are crucial. The commercial laboratory Vision Medicals was the first to identify the novel coronavirus in a patient sample. However, after the NHC and China Centers for Disease Control and Prevention (China CDC) teams took over the outbreak investigation on December 31, 2019, they did not acknowledge the significant role played by Vision Medicals and other commercial laboratories. Instead, the NHC initiated and organized a four-laboratory pathogen identification project. In practice, the mission of the national laboratories was to verify and validate the preliminary findings about the SARS-like coronavirus made by commercial laboratories.

This chapter also reports that, despite official restrictions on laboratories studying the novel coronavirus, two other laboratories that were not part of the national pathogen verification project conducted their own analyses and presented their findings and assessments of the dangers from the novel coronavirus to the national health leadership. The Zhang Yongzhen team was especially noteworthy because Zhang not only made major efforts to alert authorities of the dangers from the coronavirus but also shared the genomic sequence of the coronavirus internationally.

While the NHC organized the pathogen identification project, it also implemented restrictive regulations on the types of laboratories authorized to handle patient samples from Wuhan and imposed a “gag order” on laboratory disclosures of information throughout the pathogen verification process. The measures by the NHC to restrict the disclosure of novel coronavirus research findings by laboratory scientists thus paralleled what the Hubei/Wuhan authorities did in suppressing medical professionals for sharing epidemic information. Altogether, central–provincial–municipal authorities worked in unison to create a pathological environment for epidemic information discovery, sharing, and analysis, thus negatively affecting the quality of information available and the decisions made to respond to the outbreak.

NHC Guidance on Epidemic Information Disclosure

In early January 2020, the NHC worked together with provincial and municipal authorities to restrict the unauthorized disclosure of information. As previously mentioned, the Wuhan Municipal Health Commission (WMHC) posted its first public release on December 31 with approval from the NHC. Xu Shuqiang, director general of the NHC Emergency Response Office, elaborated that the NHC "guided the Wuhan Municipal Health Commission of Hubei Province to release epidemic and prevention & control information on December 31, 2019 and on January 3rd, 5th, 9th; and, based on changes in the epidemic situation, to provide daily updates and public releases from January 11."[7] It is worth noting that the Chinese CDC system, including the national, provincial, and municipal CDCs, had no independent authority to issue such public releases; they supported and deferred to the respective health administrations.[8]

As the text of the December 31 WMHC release demonstrated, these public releases were carefully curated and designed to provide a positive spin in guiding public expectations. While the information available to public health officials is always partial and, given the incubation period of the disease, delayed during the initial days of an infectious disease outbreak, the health authorities had genomic sequencing results from multiple laboratories, including the Wuhan Institute of Virology (WIV), by December 31, 2019. In retrospect, the WMHC update not only significantly underreported the number of serious cases in treatment but also failed to mention what the WIV and other commercial laboratories had already achieved in preliminarily identifying a novel coronavirus as the pathogen. The health authorities could have stated that the results still required further verification, but by doing so, the China CDC laboratory in Beijing would have received much less credit for identifying and verifying the novel coronavirus.

According to Feng Zijian, deputy director general of the China CDC, senior experts recognized the severity of the disease and were concerned about human-to-human transmission from very early on; but "it always required prudence when releasing [epidemic] information." When pressed, he conceded that the official approach to information management was "conservative, but of course prudent."[9] As Wuhan was put under lockdown, the public quickly countered Feng's statement, noting that true prudence in the face of the SARS-like coronavirus would have involved taking serious public measures to respond to the outbreak, rather than downplaying its dangers.[10]

This understatement of severity and delay in announcing the novel coronavirus had significant cognitive, policy, and epidemic consequences. Even though key health decision makers knew that a novel coronavirus had been detected, official releases and reporting continued to use terms like "viral pneumonia of uncertain etiology" (不明原因病毒性肺炎), or simply PUE, through January 10, 2020. This language served to obscure the situation and contributed to the downplaying of the outbreak's severity among medical professionals in Wuhan and the general public.

Strict Control over Laboratories and the January 3 NHC "Gag Order"

Although commercial diagnostic labs played pivotal roles in the initial discovery of the novel coronavirus, the circulation of diagnostic results from these labs greatly disconcerted officials. The NHC leadership quickly took action to limit unauthorized handling and analysis of patient samples and impose restrictions on the release of diagnostic results and analyses by both commercial and state laboratories.

Prompted by the NHC, staff in Hubei swiftly contacted the commercial diagnostic labs, issuing what amounted to "cease and desist" orders following the New Year's Eve meeting. On January 1, 2020, an official from the Hubei Provincial Health Commission called the leadership of Vision Medicals, the first laboratory to identify and sequence the novel coronavirus. Vision Medicals' leadership was instructed to not conduct any additional tests on "atypical pneumonia" samples from Wuhan but to inform the authorities if they found new cases of the SARS-like atypical pneumonia during regular testing of patient samples. The company was also told not to share any information about the samples or test results, including disclosure in academic papers.[11] Other labs were similarly contacted.

The WIV, which is part of the Chinese Academy of Sciences, received such a call directly from an official representing the NHC on January 1, 2020. Wang Yan-Yi, director general of the WIV, emailed WIV staff the next morning to relay the NHC requirement. Noting that there was heightened public attention to the "pneumonia of uncertain etiology in Wuhan," she stated that "the dissemination of some inappropriate and inaccurate information in the previous period has caused a certain degree of public panic." She then shared her summary of the phone call from the NHC that essentially banned any media contact and asked all to "please make sure to strictly comply!":

> The National Health Commission clearly requires: all testing and experimental data, as well as results and conclusions related to this outbreak, shall not be

> released in self-media [such as web blogs] and on social media, and shall not be disclosed to the media (including official media) and collaborating organizations (including technical service companies).[12]

The efforts to rein in specific labs were followed by the issuance of a confidential NHC General Office "Communication (No. 3)" on January 3, prepared by the NHC Department of Science & Technology and Education. Entitled "Strengthening the Management of Bio-sample Resources and Related Research Activities in the Work of Preventing and Controlling Major Outbreaks of Infectious Disease," this directive was issued to province-level health commissions and laboratories with biosafety certifications for handling "human-transmitted pathogenic microorganisms."[13]

"Communication No. 3" stipulated that "samples from the Wuhan pneumonia cases" "be treated on an interim basis as highly pathogenic microorganisms (Class II)." This required that samples in and from Wuhan be handled in laboratories with the appropriate biosafety rating, authorization/designation by the province-level health commissions, and certification from the NHC. In other words, laboratories would be banned from investigating or testing samples of pneumonia patients in or from Wuhan unless they received specific authorization. On the same day, by "Communication No. 4" from the NHC Department of Science & Technology and Education, the NHC invoked biosafety management regulations and an assessment by experts to approve an application by the Hubei Provincial CDC biosafety level-3 (BSL-3) lab to conduct experimental work on the virus that causes the so-called PUE. It noted that the Hubei CDC BSL-3 lab already had the qualification to work with the Middle East respiratory syndrome coronavirus.[14] In this early phase of the outbreak, the Hubei CDC BSL-3 lab became the first and only province-level CDC laboratory to receive permission to handle samples of patients with the unusual viral pneumonia.

The NHC Communication No. 3 essentially served as an administrative gag order. It directed that non-designated "organizations and individuals that have obtained bio-samples . . . prior to the release of this notice shall immediately destroy the samples in situ or submit [the samples] to the state-designated preservation institutions for safekeeping, and also properly preserve the records and results of the relevant experimental activities." To the detriment of science, some hospitals that had such samples and were the first to report cases, such as the Hubei Provincial Hospital of Integrated Chinese and Western Medicine, complied with the order and did not retain their leftover samples.[15] Without providing any details on the designated organizations or information on how to obtain such designation, Communication No. 3 also stipulated that organizations and individuals "shall not release information about the results of the pathogenic testing or experimental activities." Papers and results must be vetted and approved by the commissioning department before publication.

The Management of Pathogen Verification and Diagnostic Test Kit Development

With the January 3 "gag order" in place, it is unsurprising that the NHC also imposed a news blackout while launching an official program for the detection and verification of the pathogen responsible for the viral PUE cases in Wuhan. Although commercial laboratories and the WIV had already made much progress in identifying the novel coronavirus, the NHC leadership could not accept such results as official. Some NHC leaders still remembered well the humiliation of the China CDC laboratory mis-identifying the pathogen for SARS in 2003.[16] Taking advantage of the four sets of bronchoalveolar lavage (BAL) samples that Dr. Zhang Dingyu and his team at Wuhan Jinyintan Hospital had prepared, on January 1–2, 2020, Minister Ma Xiaowei's NHC epidemic response leading group arranged for four state laboratories, including the WIV, to investigate the Wuhan samples in parallel (see Table 6.1).[17] All four of the laboratories had researchers who had done research on coronaviruses; all but the WIV participated in the identification and verification of the H7N9 avian influenza virus in 2013.

The China CDC, with the blessing of the NHC, "coordinated four organizations [laboratories] to carry out the genomic sequencing of the coronavirus and isolate the virus."[18] Academician Xu Jianguo from the China CDC was appointed to lead an expert panel (NHC Pathogen Detection Results Evaluation Expert Panel) to evaluate the laboratory pathogen identification results and the diagnostic test kits to be developed. Since Xu publicly stated that there was no human-to-human transmission, it made sense that he and others felt they could afford to take a few more days to follow through on the official pathogen

Table 6.1 Laboratories in the NHC Pathogen Detection/Verification Initiative

The National Institute of Viral Disease Control and Prevention of the China CDC
The Institute of Pathogen Biology of the Chinese Academy of Medical Sciences
Wuhan Institute of Virology of the Chinese Academy of Sciences
The Academy of Military Medical Sciences of the People's Liberation Army Academy of Military Sciences

detection and verification process rather than push for action based on the fastest results from the laboratories, which the WIV had already produced.

Teams at the four laboratories went into emergency response mode and worked continuously 24 hours a day. With its head start, the WIV team led by Shi Zhengli had already identified a novel coronavirus on December 31, 2019. As the NHC program proceeded, the WIV team obtained the whole genome of the novel coronavirus on January 2, 2020, and isolated the live novel coronavirus (SARS-CoV-2) on January 5.[19] On January 7, the WIV team confirmed through experimentation and PCR (polymerase chain reaction) analysis that a novel coronavirus was the cause of the disease and proceeded to carry out studies of the virus using animal models.[20]

The Institute for Viral Disease Control and Prevention (IVDC) team at the China CDC obtained the whole genome of the novel coronavirus at 11 PM on January 3, 2020, and isolated the virus strain on January 6.[21] The IVDC team observed the novel coronavirus with electron microscopy the next day and submitted the transmission electron microscopic image of the novel coronavirus to the NHC on January 8.[22] The other two laboratories were also successful in sequencing the virus. All four laboratories had come up with whole-genome sequences for the novel coronavirus by January 4, 2020, and offered their analyses.

Even before the virus verification process was completed, the four laboratories had begun to lead or contribute to the development of diagnostics, vaccines, and therapeutics. The China CDC IVDC laboratory developed its high-specificity and high-sensitivity PCR test reagent (test kit) on January 4, 2020.[23] Also noteworthy was the decision, on January 5, 2020, by the leadership of Sinopharm (China National Pharmaceutical Group Corp.) to begin development of an inactivated virus vaccine for the disease (COVID-19) in partnership with the WIV. The WIV provided both the isolated virus strain and a biosafety lab space for ensuring vaccine development by Wuhan Institute of Biological Products Co., a Sinopharm subsidiary.[24] At the Chinese Academy of Medical Sciences, a team led by Jiang Jiandong began screening for potential therapeutic drugs on January 6 and settled on azvudine as a promising therapeutic drug on January 29, 2020.[25]

On January 8, the NHC Expert Panel chaired by Xu Jianguo met to assess the laboratory results. The group concluded that the novel coronavirus as identified by the laboratories was the etiological agent causing the outbreak in Wuhan. The announcement of this conclusion came out the following day in the form of a bland Xinhua News Agency interview with Xu Jianguo.

Much consideration appears to have gone into how to communicate the conclusion that the expert panel had reached and to clear the release the previous day and overnight. Even if we leave aside the even earlier discoveries of the commercial laboratories, a week had elapsed since the WIV team first obtained its own full genome of the novel coronavirus. In comparison, during the SARS epidemic in 2003, research teams at laboratories worldwide made announcements of their findings in real time.

Referring to components of Koch's postulates for determining the causes of diseases, Xu Jianguo stated that the expert panel concluded that the pathogen of the viral pneumonia in Wuhan was a novel coronavirus (then named "2019-nCoV"). He revealed that, as of January 7, a total of 15 cases of novel coronavirus infections, out of a total 59 reported, had been confirmed using the nucleic acid testing method. He stated plainly that "further scientific research is needed to gain a better understanding of the virus" and made no mention of the alarm that researchers in different laboratories, including that of his former postdoctoral fellow Zhang Yongzhen, had raised (see the following section).[26] Instead, in an interview with *Science* a day later, Xu placed his bet with the public statements coming out of Wuhan, albeit with recognition that his own assessment depended on these public statements being reliable: "No new patients have appeared, as far as I understand. It's good news. People fear something like the SARS of 2003, but this is a different disease. The outbreak is limited."[27] In retrospect, Xu's remark was a striking indication of how far removed he had become from the scenes of patients seeking treatment in fever clinics in Wuhan.

With this relaxed attitude, Xu Jianguo and an expert panel, under the auspices of the NHC, presided over a blind test and evaluation of five PCR nucleic acid test kits for the novel coronavirus on January 10. The Hubei Provincial CDC laboratory served as the validation laboratory. The three submitting laboratories were the WIV, the IVDC/China CDC, and the Institute of Pathogen Biology of the Chinese Academy of Medical Sciences.[28] The IVDC submitted three of the five entries and handily won the "blind test." In fact, the IVDC had also formulated the "Guidelines for Laboratory Testing of Novel Coronavirus," which included the specific probes and primer sequences used for testing and listed the IVDC as the designated entity for authoritative diagnostic testing of samples.[29] Even some members of the China CDC complained to me that the process and the standards for the evaluation of the test kits were designed to favor the IVDC's entries.[30]

Following the January 10 validation and evaluation of the test kits, the NHC designated the IVDC 2019-nCov (novel coronavirus) nucleic acid test reagent as the reagent used for testing in labs of the China CDC and provincial/municipal CDCs.[31] The IVDC worked out deals with three companies in Shanghai to manufacture and supply the 2019n-CoV (SARS-CoV-2) test kits to the Chinese CDC system nationwide. Each of the three companies paid one million yuan, presumably to the IVDC/China CDC, for early access to information and the right to sell to the Chinese CDCs across the country.[32]

Had the Wuhan outbreak been quickly contained, this contracting for test kits in an emergency would not have attracted much attention because the firms involved had to incur investment costs for a situation that might not have worked out. However, as the outbreak spiraled out of control, the decision by the IVDC/China CDC to contract the diagnostic test kits business to three small players in nucleic acid diagnostic test kits invited scrutiny. This was because at least two of the three firms had clear personal and previous sponsorship ties to the China CDC community.[33]

Warnings from a Wuhan University Laboratory and the Zhang Yongzhen Team in Shanghai

Despite the January 3 NHC gag order, at least two non-commercial laboratory teams managed to obtain genomic sequences of the novel coronavirus from Wuhan patient samples in early January. One team was located at the Wuhan University State Key Laboratory of Virology (WUSKLV). This team investigated two BAL samples from Wuhan University Zhongnan Hospital and successfully obtained the whole genome of the novel coronavirus on January 7, 2020. Notably, one of the two samples came from a 21-year-old female who had no direct exposure to the Huanan market. She was infected after a vendor from the Huanan market visited her at home.[34]

Although the WUSKLV team was not part of the NHC-organized pathogen detection initiative, it provided "instant progress reports" to the China CDC starting on January 3, 2020, and submitted a written report once it had the whole genome on January 7, 2020.[35] The WUSKLV team noted that the SARS-like coronavirus was "grouped within the notorious CoV clade (i.e. SARS like) with history of cross-virus transmission to humans and [has been] demonstrated to have strong zoonotic potential."[36] In other words, based on their analysis of the genome, the WUSKLV team concluded that the novel coronavirus they were studying was likely to be infectious to humans.

The other team was led by Zhang Yongzhen, a former postdoctoral fellow and collaborator of academician Xu Jianguo. The unique contributions of Zhang's team, in offering advice to the Chinese government and sharing the genomic sequence with the international community, merit recognition. In this context, it is intriguing to examine how Zhang, even though based in Shanghai, managed to establish research collaboration networks that enabled him and his team to play a crucial role in investigating the novel coronavirus in early January 2020.

Zhang Yongzhen: The Dark Horse of Shanghai

Zhang Yongzhen earned his doctorate in 1998 at the Kunming Institute of Zoology of the Chinese Academy of Sciences, subsequently securing a postdoctoral position with Xu Jianguo at what later became the Institute for Communicable Disease Control and Prevention (ICDC) of the China CDC. After completing his postdoctoral work, Zhang remained at the ICDC and, for the first decade or so, focused on rabies and hemorrhagic fever with renal syndrome, which were important but relatively routine research subjects at the ICDC.

While the ICDC primarily concentrates on bacterial pathogens, Zhang increasingly shifted his focus to viruses. In the early 2000s, his geographical journey from peripheral institutions—animal science at Shihezi University in Xinjiang and South China Agricultural University in Guangzhou, zoology at the Kunming Institute of Zoology in Yunnan—to Beijing culminated in his pioneering work on the genomic structure of the Jingmen tick virus and the discovery of an evolutionary link between unsegmented and segmented viruses.[37] Since then, Zhang has honed his research on the diversity and evolution of viruses, and he has also collaborated with clinicians to identify the causative agents of undiagnosed diseases.[38] Specifically, he has pursued a research program on the RNA virosphere, underpinned by robust social and organizational skills, including intellectual partnerships in China and abroad. This is exemplified by a 2016 *Nature* article, titled "Redefining the Invertebrate RNA Virosphere," for which Zhang is the corresponding author. The article reports the discovery of 1,445 RNA viruses, some named after ancient Chinese states, and offers valuable insights into the dynamics of virus ecology and evolution, characterized by "host switching and co-divergence," resulting in frequent cross-species transmissions.[39] Both Xu Jianguo, his mentor, and Edward C. Holmes of the University of Sydney are co-authors. With the 2016 *Nature* article, Zhang was honored with the inaugural National Innovation Ahead Award.[40] Gao Fu, then a deputy director general of the China CDC, was the other winner. Zhang's achievements were even more impressive considering he was at the ICDC, which was increasingly overshadowed by the IVDC within the China CDC.

Around that time, Zhu Tongyu became director of the Shanghai Public Health Clinical Center (SPHCC) and sought to move the SPHCC away from the traditional infectious diseases hospital model by attracting top-notch personnel with strengths in fundamental research and in combining research with clinical practice.[41] Zhang Yongzhen has mainly worked at the SPHCC (and Fudan University) since 2018 but retained his appointment with the ICDC through 2020.

Like others in the virological community, Zhang was captivated by information on the viral pneumonia outbreak in Wuhan early on, particularly because his colleagues from the China CDC were participating in the emergency response effort in Wuhan and Beijing. He remembered that Zhu Tongyu, Eddie Holmes, and others asked him on January 1, 2020, if he was working on the so-called PUE that had emerged in Wuhan. He smiled at Director Zhu, noting wryly that he "hardly had a chance at this type of good opportunity." "New and sudden infectious diseases are generally good for publishing high-impact articles," he explained, "and everyone wants to seize [the chance to work on them]."[42]

However, Zhang had maintained ongoing relationships with the Wuhan Municipal CDC. According to Dr. Zhao Su, the chief physician of respiratory medicine at the Wuhan Central Hospital (WCH), the WCH served as a sentinel hospital for a collaborative project between the SPHCC and the Wuhan CDC, called "Major Natural Sources of Epidemic Viruses in China." Periodically, scientists at the Wuhan CDC would courier samples collected at the WCH to the SPHCC for high-throughput genomic sequencing and bioinformatics analysis.

On the afternoon of December 30, 2019, a senior staff member from the Wuhan CDC, likely Tian Junhua or Yu Bin (both of whom had collaborated with Zhang Yongzhen on a published study), picked up a BAL sample from the WCH.[43] The sample belonged to a 41-year-old male patient surnamed Chen. Patient Chen worked at the Huanan Seafood Market and began developing symptoms such as fever, cough, and shortness of breath around December 20, 2019. He was admitted to WCH Houhu Branch on December 26, and the BAL sample was taken on December 30.

Tian sent the BAL sample, along with other specimens, to Zhang Yongzhen's team in Shanghai on January 2, 2020. If he had known the urgency of the situation, he would not have waited 3 days to dispatch the sample. It is reasonable to suspect that some of the communication Zhang had with Tian at the beginning of 2020 concerned the unusual pneumonia outbreak in Wuhan and that a patient sample from WCH was part of the shipment of samples originating from Wuhan. Zhang later mentioned that it was by chance that his team received the patient sample that would ultimately test positive for the novel coronavirus.[44]

The Wuhan shipment arrived at the SPHCC around 1:30 PM on January 3, 2020. Song Zhigang, head of the Biosafety Level 3 (BSL-3) Lab at the SPHCC, and his colleagues processed the BAL sample in the BSL-3 Lab.[45] As with Vision Medicals and other labs, high-throughput sequencing was employed for RNA sequencing to obtain the reads. Working around the clock, Zhang's team managed to assemble the whole genome of the SARS-like coronavirus and map it by approximately 7 AM on January 5, 2020.[46]

Zhang then contacted Dr. Zhao Su in Wuhan to discuss the patient's clinical symptoms.[47] Putting the genomic information on the SARS-like coronavirus together with the patient's clinical manifestations (severe respiratory infections), Zhang drew upon his experience researching viruses and infectious diseases to conclude that the illness "must be more severe than avian influenza."[48] This comparison with avian influenza is significant because the SPHCC had been well known for its role in detecting the H7N9 avian influenza in 2013.

Even though the official news from Wuhan was reassuring, Zhang did not hesitate to act on his own intuition and assessment. He quickly drafted a short report of his findings and recommendations and met with Director Zhu Tongyu and his colleagues to brief them at 8 AM. He also made calls with his contacts at the NHC to report on his team's findings and assessments; one name he mentioned was He Qinghua (贺青华), a deputy director general in the Department of Disease Prevention and Control of the NHC.[49] He found sympathetic ears at the NHC and was encouraged to submit a written report.

Motivated by the significance and urgency of Zhang Yongzhen's findings, the leadership of the SPHCC, notably Director Zhu Tongyu, agreed to submit a report to the NHC directly (with a copy for the Shanghai Municipal Health Commission) in the name of the SPHCC. This decision was unusual from a bureaucratic perspective. Had Zhang Yongzhen been at a typical municipal hospital, the hospital administration could have submitted a report of his findings to the district or municipal CDC and perhaps the municipal health commission, but the report might not be passed on to the NHC immediately. However, the SPHCC leadership drew confidence from their past experience; as one informant observed, the SPHCC won major accolades, including a National Science & Technology Progress Special Prize and significant government support, for being the first to identify and report human H7N9 avian influenza cases in 2013.[50] In a later interview, Lu Hongzhou, party secretary and deputy director of the SPHCC, proudly noted that the report to the NHC bore the official stamp of the SPHCC.[51]

The SPHCC report to the NHC opens by noting that Professor Zhang Yongzhen's team was in collaboration with the WCH and the Wuhan CDC, which implied that the Wuhan CDC was informed of the results. It says that, on January 5, 2020, the Zhang team detected a SARS-like coronavirus in the sample of a Wuhan patient. The whole genomic sequence of this novel coronavirus—named "Wuhan-Hu-1 coronavirus"—was obtained and found to be 89.11% similar to SARS-like coronaviruses. The patient had worked at the Huanan Seafood Market in Wuhan and was critically ill. Based on the clinical features of this patient and others, the report suggested,

> the unexplained febrile pneumonia outbreak at Wuhan's Huanan Seafood Market may be caused by the novel coronavirus Wuhan-Hu-1. Because this virus is homologous with the coronavirus that caused the SARS epidemic, it may be transmissible via the respiratory tract. It is recommended that appropriate prevention and control measures be taken in public places and that antiviral treatment be utilized in clinical treatment.

In other words, Zhang Yongzhen and the SPHCC leadership concluded that the novel coronavirus Wuhan-Hu-1 was infectious from human to human. He later explained that he "thought it was more infectious than the flu virus."[52]

Based on bureaucratic protocol, the NHC personnel would have shared the SPHCC report with the ministerial leadership and most likely with the China CDC leadership (including academician Xu Jianguo, who was leading the official pathogen detection effort). It was also most likely that Zhang directly communicated with members of the China CDC leadership, including Xu Jianguo, Zhang's former supervisor and collaborator. However, Xu's published interviews on January 4 and January 9 did not indicate a sense of alarm. (On January 8, ahead of a lecture he was to give in Wuhan the following day, Zhang Yongzhen met with Dr. Zhao Su of the WCH and Dr. Yu Bin of the Wuhan CDC and others and further exchanged views on the disease[53].)

Zhang's tireless advocacy went further after he felt that the SPHCC report had barely created an echo in the bureaucratic machinery, as so often happens with submittals in the bureaucratic system. Driven by his sense of crisis, Zhang submitted another report, presumably to someone higher up in the Chinese hierarchy or with special access to it, to warn of the dangers of the novel coronavirus.[54] He has declined to reveal further details about this additional action.

Information Control and the Deliberate Speed of Genome Release

As noted earlier and will be elaborated further in Chapter 7, Xu Jianguo was lulled by the apparent calm in Wuhan. So was Gao Fu, the China CDC director general. Gao or his associate began negotiating with the Global Initiative on Sharing All Influenza Data (GISAID), a global data depository for sharing genomic data of influenza viruses and coronaviruses, for a curated release of the novel coronavirus genome as early as January 8, 2020.[55] However, in keeping with the official process for pathogen validation, the three non-military state laboratories designated by the NHC to submit genomes to GISAID were told to release the genomes "at the same time."[56]

On January 12, 2020, the three laboratories released five genomes of the novel coronavirus on GISAID. While Zhang Yongzhen, through Eddie Holmes, released his team's "novel 2019 coronavirus genome" on Virological.org on January 10, 2020 (January 11 Beijing time),[57] the Chinese government white paper declared January 12 as the official genome release date.[58]

According to Gao Fu, the China CDC coordinated the curated release with GISAID to ensure submission quality. However, it was clear that the deliberate process and speed were due to Gao and his colleagues not feeling a strong sense of great urgency. In a 2021 interview, Gao Fu recalled that "we would not share results we were not 100% sure of." He then expressed regret: "If [I] had known [the outbreak] would turn into such a pandemic, why seek the curation, won't a straightforward release have done the job? Hindsight is 20/20."[59] As Mike Ryan, the executive director of the World Health Organization's (WHO's) Health Emergencies Program, emphasized in spring 2020: "Perfection is the enemy of the good when it comes to emergency management."[60]

Discussion and Conclusion

Following China's failure to identify the causative agent for the SARS epidemic, Chinese policymakers and experts in disease prevention and control were keenly aware of the need to invest in research and detection capabilities. In a 2011 co-authored article, Feng Zijian, then head of the emergency response office (Emergency Operations Center) at the China CDC, emphasized the need for China to continue building capacities for detecting emerging infectious diseases through pathogen-based surveillance.[61] Over the next decade, China drew on the global genomic revolution and invested heavily in government-funded laboratories and numerous commercial diagnostic laboratories. These investments have steadily increased China's diagnostic and detection capabilities and enabled China to effectively respond to a variety of infectious diseases, most notably the H7N9 outbreak, fostering optimism in China's ability to handle emerging diseases.[62]

In late December 2019 and early 2020, a combination of commercial and government laboratories swiftly identified and verified the SARS-CoV-2 novel coronavirus. As discussed in previous chapters, commercial diagnostic laboratories played unique and pivotal roles in the initial detection of the novel coronavirus and of COVID-19, although they have hardly received a mention in the official history of China's response to the outbreak in Wuhan. Leading state laboratories were quickly mobilized to join in a multi-lab effort to verify the pathogen and engage in research and development activities.

The discipline and secrecy surrounding the pathogen detection and verification process allowed authorities to mitigate institutional and personal rivalries among major state laboratories. It took approximately 10 days from the initial announcement of the outbreak on December 31, 2019, to the official announcement of virus identification on January 9, 2020. In contrast, it took several months to identify and confirm the SARS coronavirus in 2003 and over 20 days to identify the H7N9 avian influenza in 2013. If the novel coronavirus (SARS-CoV-2) had turned out to be limited in transmissibility, as was incorrectly assumed, China's health policymakers would have received accolades for their tightly managed process of virus identification and verification.[63]

Yet, the effective handling of an outbreak requires far more than accuracy and speed in pathogen detection and verification. At the same time it orchestrated the pathogen verification initiative, the NHC, in the name of biosafety, imposed strict restrictions and control on laboratories that substantively and adversely affected the handling of the outbreak.

First, the most immediate impact of the stringent controls on disclosure of epidemic information by the laboratories was the failure to promote engaged discussion among specialists and share information with the public. While the pathogen verification project was in process, the Chinese public health system maintained an organized posture of ignorance. There was no effort to communicate to the public what was already known about the coronavirus, let alone the alarms raised by scientists and medical professionals. For example, the WIV, a laboratory with a higher biosafety rating than the China CDC laboratory, had sequenced the whole genome of the novel coronavirus by January 2, 2020; but the WIV was not permitted to announce its achievement immediately. In another revealing moment, the IVDC leadership of the China CDC convened an all-staff meeting on January 19, 2020, and relayed a set of guidelines from the NHC leadership: "Politics first, safety second, science third."[64]

The inability of the laboratories to immediately share their findings in January 2020 was in stark contrast to the situation during the SARS crisis and other infectious disease outbreaks. During the SARS crisis of 2003, scientists of research laboratories in Hong Kong, Atlanta, and Rotterdam vied with those in Guangzhou and Beijing to search for the pathogen causing SARS. As they made discoveries, they also made nearly real-time public announcements of their findings. The flourish of releases both offered valuable scientific information and stimulated public discussion about the virus of concern. In contrast, all state laboratories, not to mention the commercial laboratories being sidelined, were studious in maintaining public silence under the spell of the January 3 NHC gag order, effectively depriving the global health community of these important voices.

WHO officials, eager for case details and genomic information, put on the front of praising China for reaching the conclusion on the etiological agent. In private, they were deeply frustrated with the amount of information China provided.[65] The WHO had to wait until the Chinese government had completed the verification and validation process and still further for the disclosure of the genome. International organizations rarely have leverage when dealing with superpowers. The WHO can try to cajole, but it cannot dictate and must wait.

Second, by curbing the autonomy of the scientific community in the dissemination of their scientific findings, the NHC January 3 order also dimmed the level of alert that the public could have received of the risk from the novel coronavirus. Instead, the Chinese system kept using the lingo of the so-called PUE or pneumonia of uncertain etiology through January 9, until the identification of the novel coronavirus was officially declared complete. Even then, the official statement through academician Xu Jianguo failed to convey any of the concerns about the novel coronavirus, especially in view of the strong warning from Professor Zhang Yongzhen, Xu's former postdoctoral fellow and collaborator. The NHC authorized the WMHC to refer to the so-called viral PUE as pneumonia caused by the novel coronavirus on January 11–12 but continued to leave the disease in legal limbo as an infectious disease.

Since we know that Chinese state laboratories had assembled multiple whole genomic sequences of the novel coronavirus between January 2 and January 7, 2020, one could imagine Chinese laboratories such as the WIV announcing their assembly of the whole genome on January 2 or 3, thus sending a powerful message to the public, especially the people of Wuhan, that the novel coronavirus had been identified and that they—most especially the medical staff—needed to take serious precautions. If the other laboratories, including the Zhang Yongzhen team, had been allowed to make their own announcements, the effect of the WIV announcement would have been reinforced and the public would have received significant warning.[66]

Third, if laboratories had been permitted to announce their findings in real time, the subsequent wave of announcements and awareness of multiple cases infected by the same novel coronavirus would likely have sparked public discussion on human-to-human transmission. This would have led to a more in-depth examination of the epidemiological information on early patients, especially if such announcements were supported by more open press reporting. As Peter Daszak, president of EcoHealth Alliance who had collaborated with researchers at the WIV, noted on January 9, 2020, "I don't understand how you can get so many cases without human-to-human transmission. . . . This is something I have a red flag on."[67]

Lastly, the NHC's restrictions on laboratories significantly reduced testing capacity when it was most needed, limiting the identification of new patients with novel coronavirus infections in the first 2 weeks of January 2020. As the NHC January 3 "gag order" was disseminated, hospitals such as the WCH could no longer rely on third-party commercial diagnostic labs. Instead, they had to submit patient samples for suspected cases to the CDCs for diagnosis and verification.[68] But the ability of the CDCs to conduct such tests was hardly available before mid-January 2020 and painfully limited immediately afterward. Considering the critical roles played by commercial diagnostic labs, such as BGI and Vision Medicals, in detecting the virus and the extremely limited testing capacity through the Chinese CDC system during early January, the January 3 "gag order" and other control measures effectively hindered the identification of new cases and of community spread.

7

The China CDC, the Huanan Seafood Market, and Epidemiological Tunnel Vision

In the challenging domains of field epidemiology and public health emergencies, decision makers are often required to make swift and complex decisions amid incomplete information and uncertainties. The *Field Epidemiology Manual* also notes that initial decisions may need to be modified as new information emerges through further investigation.[1] As the eminent epidemiologist Patricia Happ Buffler famously noted, "The work of epidemiology is related to unanswered questions, but also to unquestioned answers."[2]

In retrospect, it is evident that there were a rapidly growing number of so-called viral pneumonia of uncertain etiology (VPUE) cases that had no connection to the Huanan Seafood Market in the early weeks of the Wuhan outbreak. It is now also certain that many such cases were indications not only of the novel coronavirus circulating beyond the market but also of its person-to-person transmission, regardless of whether the original virus came from animal sources within the Huanan market or if the market simply played an amplifying role after an intermediary host had carried the virus into it. A crucial question arises: why did it take approximately 2 weeks for the National Health Commission (NHC) to modify the case definition requiring exposure to the Huanan market for cases of VPUE/novel coronavirus infections, as will be detailed in Chapter 10, when the number of such infections without Huanan market exposure was multiplying in Wuhan-area hospitals during the first half of January 2020?

Feng Zijian, the deputy director general of the China CDC who rushed to Wuhan on December 31, 2019, later defended the focus on the Huanan market exposure, citing the need to "determine if this is an independent and new disease, or if [it was one of the] other diseases that suddenly showed up as clusters during this season."[3] Without elaborating on why determining the disease required the fixation on Huanan market exposure, Feng admitted that it was necessary to broaden the scope of the epidemiological search to include cases without exposure to the Huanan market in due course.[4] However, Feng and the China CDC did not address why it took so long for the China CDC and, by extension, the NHC leadership to review the early January 2020 data from the Wuhan outbreak and recognize and act on their significance for human-to-human transmission of the novel coronavirus.

In fact, following the New Year's Eve meeting, a good number of NHC officials and staff, which later became known as the NHC front-line working group, along with a China Centers for Disease Control and Prevention (China CDC) emergency response team, were stationed in Wuhan. Amid the information clampdowns, the implementation of the inclusion–exclusion criteria, discussed in Chapter 8, kept the number of confirmed cases down and diminished the sense of urgency about the outbreak for public health leaders who relied on the case numbers from Wuhan to assess outbreak severity. Equally remarkably, Feng revealed that the China CDC leadership did not review the pre–January 3 novel coronavirus case data from Wuhan until nearly 3 weeks later. Feng's revelation came in response to the public uproar following the publication of two articles in *The Lancet* and the *New England Journal of Medicine* (*NEJM*) by Chinese researchers showing that a significant portion of the cases had no connections with the Huanan market.[5] The findings shocked the Chinese public not because they conclusively proved human-to-human transmission, which was already public knowledge by the time of publication, but because the case data supporting such a conclusion were for the period of December 2019 through January 2, 2020. It is important to note that data on the first 40-plus cases were accessible to the China CDC leadership much earlier.

The response gap by the China CDC leadership led directly to deficiencies by the China CDC and the NHC in making timely adjustments to epidemic response measures, such as updating the case definition. It thus contributed to the prolonged delay in ascertaining human-to-human transmission of the novel coronavirus. Given the China CDC's often-touted capabilities and the amount of manpower devoted to the Wuhan outbreak, the considerable delay by the China CDC leadership in reviewing and acting on early case data from the beginning of January 2020 is both astounding and puzzling. It raises issues of cognition, leadership, and coordination within the China CDC, the preeminent institution responsible for providing expertise on disease prevention, control, and health emergency response. Thus, the China's CDC's response delay holds an important key to understanding the challenges China faced in responding to the Wuhan outbreak and why the novel coronavirus spread unimpeded in Wuhan and beyond for much of January 2020.

Drawing on speeches and interviews of China CDC leaders, this chapter examines the causes of the significant cognitive and response gap displayed by the China CDC leadership and by extension the health authorities while the number of suspected VPUE cases in Wuhan-area hospitals increased rapidly without official recognition. It posits that the China CDC's failure to act was likely due to an inadequacy in epidemiological imagination, which refers to the inability to seriously consider and explore alternative scenarios for the initial outbreak.[6] During the first 2–3 weeks of January 2020, China CDC director general Gao Fu, his colleagues, and, by extension, China's national health leaders adopted and applied a rigid set of cognitive priors regarding the severe acute respiratory syndrome (SARS)–like novel coronavirus. Enthralled by this cognitive framework, Gao and others harbored strong assumptions about the behavior of the novel coronavirus, its potential for person-to-person transmission, and the appropriate prevention and control measures based on their experience with SARS. Within the political-administrative context of fragmented authoritarianism, this cognitive framework and the introduction and enforcement of the inclusion–exclusion criteria—discussed in the following chapter—were mutually constitutive. This led to the downplaying and even dismissal of cases that suggested human-to-human transmission in early January 2020.

What Gao Fu and Others Thought of Human-to-Human Transmission Early On

As previously discussed, China CDC director general Gao Fu analyzed the genomic sequence of the novel coronavirus on December 31, 2019. There is little doubt that Gao and others at the China CDC were aware of the potential threat posed by the novel coronavirus. However, they also played a part in the official deployment of ambiguous language with the public.

The Wuhan Municipal Health Commission (WMHC) updates and Wuhan CDC director Li Gang's interview on January 5–6, 2020, were made with the approval and guidance of the NHC. They were later criticized for downplaying the outbreak's severity. Given the substantial amount of information available to health leaders and experts in early January 2020, it is now clear that the official statements employed coded language. When the WMHC update mentioned that "some patients are operators in the Wuhan Huanan Seafood City (Huanan Seafood Market)," we can now interpret it as indicating that not all patients had a (and thus some had no) connection to the Huanan market.

The updates and interview of January 5–6 also stated that "No clear evidence of human-to-human transmission has been found." At the time, the public interpreted this statement to mean there was "no . . . evidence of human-to-human transmission." But did they genuinely mean what the public understood them to mean?

According to Gao Fu's extensive interview with *Caijing Magazine* on the first anniversary of the Wuhan outbreak, it turns out that the public's understanding was not what the China CDC and NHC intended. I have quoted the relevant question and answer by Gao Fu in their entirety here:

> *Caijing*: It was finally made clear to the public on January 20, 2020 that the novel coronavirus was transmissible from human to human, what was done before that date?
>
> Gao Fu: On January 6, 2020, Wuhan CDC Director Li Gang said to the public, there was at present "no clear evidence of human-to-human transmission." Please note that this statement indicates that there *was* human-to-human transmission, but it was not obvious. At the beginning of January, we reached our assessment on this issue that [we] absolutely couldn't say that there was no human-to-human transmission at that time. We were constantly looking for evidence [of human-to-human transmission].
>
> At the beginning of January, this judgment [of human-to-human transmission] was definitely there, no need to doubt [it]. But [from asking] whether or not to communicate to the public, to announcing it to the public on [January] 20th, there was a process, so I hope everyone can understand (italics added; words in brackets are added for clarification).[7]

Gao Fu was thus quite candid in stating that he and others believed there was human-to-human transmission as of early January 2020. However, the WMHC, Dr. Li Gang, as well as the China CDC were limited in what they could say publicly. When Gao pleaded that there was a process and he hoped "everyone can understand," he was also conveying to the public that it was beyond the China CDC's control what could be said publicly and thus implicitly absolving themselves the blame for the failure to inform the public that he and his colleagues thought there was human-to-human transmission. Although he did not specify those constraints, we can recall that China CDC staff were explicitly told by the NHC leadership to put "politics first, safety second, science third."

The China CDC Activation of Emergency Response (Level II) and Xi's "Requirements"

By January 5–6, 2020, the China CDC leadership had the updated number of cases from Wuhan that had more than doubled from December 31, 2019. They also received additional findings from laboratory analyses on the novel coronavirus. These developments, combined with their prior understanding of the dangers associated with the SARS and Middle East respiratory syndrome (MERS) coronaviruses, led the China CDC leadership to activate its emergency response at Level II. Level II (of three levels) necessitates significant involvement of the China CDC Public Health Emergency Center staff and participation from more than two China CDC institutes or departments beyond normal operations.[8]

Although this emergency response activation was a somewhat delayed acknowledgment of the extent of China CDC activities in Wuhan and Beijing since the end of December 2019, it sent a strong signal within the China CDC of how the China CDC leadership assessed the severity of the situation. It was also well timed. January 6 marked the first day of the 2-day National Health Work Conference, and the China CDC activation of the emergency response helped to garner the national health leadership's attention to the Wuhan outbreak.[9] While the official news release on the health work conference at the time did not mention the unusual pneumonia outbreak in Wuhan, other official sources confirm that the NHC briefed conference participants about the outbreak in Wuhan and called for strengthening monitoring, analysis, assessment, and prompt epidemic response.[10] However, individuals familiar with the conference proceedings noted that the briefing at the conference did not convey a strong sense of urgency.

As the health leadership reported to the national leadership on the outbreak, the measures taken in Wuhan, as well as the assessment and recommendations of the NHC and China CDC, they had the attention of national leaders. On January 7, 2020, General Secretary Xi Jinping chaired an annual meeting of the Politburo Standing Committee (PBSC) to hear reports from the leaders of the National People's Congress, the State Council, and other state institutions.[11] Xi personally disclosed a month later that, at some point during the January 7 PBSC meeting, he "made requirements on the prevention and control of the novel coronavirus pneumonia outbreak."[12]

The specifics of Xi's "requirements" have not been made public, but Xi's later speeches and comments suggest that he wanted the outbreak to be brought under control while he reminded the relevant authorities to be mindful of the overall sociopolitical environment and social stability. Neither at the

National Health Work Conference nor in Xi's instructions of January 7 was there a sense of great urgency. As the following chapter will detail, the NHC then dispatched another expert team, including senior members of the China CDC, to visit Wuhan. It was not until January 15 that the China CDC discreetly activated its highest level of emergency response (Level I).

When Did the China CDC Confirm Human-to-Human Transmission? Or, Were They Actively Searching for It?

Gao Fu's earlier answer to the *Caijing* reporter's question about actions taken before January 20 did not specifically address what the China CDC did between January 7 and January 20. Since *The Lancet* and *NEJM* articles utilized data from before January 2 to demonstrate significant human-to-human transmission of the novel coronavirus, relevant follow-up questions would involve when the China CDC obtained the data on the first 40-plus cases, how these data were used, and when the China CDC specialists and leadership conclusively determined the existence of human-to-human transmission. It is important to note that the clinicians who published in *The Lancet* conducted their own epidemiological investigations.

Recall that Li Qun, Feng Zijian's colleague and successor as the director of the China CDC Public Health Emergency Center, traveled to Wuhan on December 31, 2019, and led the development of guidelines for surveillance, contact tracing, and management of close contacts with infected patients. On January 15, 2020, Li Qun, speaking on China Central Television from Wuhan, said, "We have made meticulous investigation, careful screening, and prudent assessment of each patient's exposure and contact situation."[13] Three groups of Li Qun's colleagues carried out epidemiological investigations on 89 (novel coronavirus-infected) patients being treated at Jinyintan Hospital earlier.[14]

Under the title of a national, provincial, and municipal joint investigation team, Li Qun and his colleagues published their findings in the English-language *China CDC Weekly* on January 31, 2020. The report utilized data as of January 19, 2020, and was submitted on January 20 and accepted the next day. This suggests that the findings of this investigation were available to the China CDC leadership and national health leadership on January 20, if not earlier. The following excerpt from this report is of particular interest:

> The epidemiological investigation of 198 confirmed cases [as of January 19, 2020] revealed that 22% of patients had direct exposure to the Huanan Seafood Wholesale

> Market before illness onset; 32% of patients had contact with patients with fever or respiratory symptoms; and 51% of cases had neither visited the Huanan Seafood Wholesale Market nor had contact with similar patients before their illness onset.[15]

The January 20 report referred to confirmed cases with no history of exposure to the Huanan market, exported cases in other countries and other provinces, and healthcare worker infections as evidence for human-to-human transmission. It suggested that community transmission was "taking place in Wuhan" and stated that "further spread is almost certain." It recommended implementing measures like exit screening to prevent or reduce transmission.[16]

Surprisingly, in his rare interview representing the China CDC during the public uproar, Feng Zijian did not mention or claim credit for the January 20 report led by Li Qun. Instead, he stated that "this inference [of human-to-human transmission] was made when [we] received the data [for the *NEJM* article] on January 23 and saw that there were some cases without a history of exposure to the Huanan Seafood Market."[17] This *NEJM* article, "Early Transmission Dynamics in Wuhan, China, of Novel Coronavirus-Infected Pneumonia," revealed that only 26, or 55%, of 47 patients before January 1, 2020, had a history of exposure to the Huanan Seafood Market. In other words, 45% of the 47 cases had no exposure to the Huanan market.[18] Feng is the primary investigator for the *NEJM* article and Li Qun of the China CDC was first author, joined by Guan Xuhua of the Hubei provincial CDC. Ben Cowling, a co-author based at the University of Hong Kong confirmed that the analysis for the article was completed on January 26, 2020, and then provided to the China CDC.[19]

Feng's revelation in his interview is shocking for at least two reasons. First, it implied that Feng and his senior China CDC colleagues did *not* obtain and review the early case data and associated analyses—even if they only concerned patients with novel coronavirus infections at Jinyintan Hospital—until January 23, 2020. Comparing Feng's statement with the January 20 report led by Li Qun and comments by Xu Jianguo and Zeng Guang raises questions about internal communication and coordination among senior China CDC leaders during this major health emergency.

Second, as part of its standard operating procedures during a major health emergency response, it was expected that the China CDC leadership and expert staff would have conducted ongoing and repeated review of the case data and relevant information. There was a widely perceived failure of the China CDC to ensure that timely epidemiological investigations were carried out and that basic facts and data on the outbreak were readily available.[20] In an interview with *Science*, Gao Fu admitted that the delay in recognizing "clear evidence of human-to-human transmission" was because "detailed epidemiological data were not available yet."[21]

Since China CDC leaders such as Gao Fu had thought that the SARS-like novel coronavirus was likely transmissible from human to human and since the data on cases from December 2019 through January 2, 2020, were so clear-cut on the issue of human-to-human transmission, it is baffling and hard to believe that the China CDC leadership did not review the cases through January 2 until January 19 (study led by Li Qun) or January 23 (interview with Feng Zijian). Thus, the question remains, why were such epidemiological data not available earlier when the China CDC had an emergency response team based in Wuhan and was directly involved in epidemiological investigations?

In his interview representing the China CDC, Feng Zijian attributed the delay to the unavailability of diagnostic tests for the novel coronavirus.[22] However, this explanation is unconvincing. First, two rounds of testing on the early cases were carried out, on January 6 and January 10, 2020; and the results of these tests formed the basis of the WMHC announcement of January 11. Second, even if diagnostic test kits were not yet available, the NHC and the China CDC leadership, if they had felt a great sense of urgency, could have mobilized the China CDC laboratory or the Wuhan Institute of Virology (WIV), among others, to help with testing when the number of cases was relatively small. Such testing capability was evidently available because the China CDC laboratory was testing a large number of environmental samples at the time.

It is notable that Feng Zijian was the only member who served on both the first and second NHC expert teams. As China CDC deputy director general, he was in a unique position to play a coordinating and leadership role. However, the information that has emerged about the visit of the second team (January 8–16) to Wuhan paints an unflattering picture of the support and coordination that were available and for which the China CDC and NHC leadership could have done something even if they were on the turf of Wuhan/Hubei. A member from the second team lamented that the team members received little background information about the investigations by the first expert team and those of Hubei and Wuhan: "we did not get to see a formal report, including how the disease came about, how it was identified, what investigations had been carried out, what the findings were, and which cases were found in the beginning. . . . We got to know none of these."[23]

When this same team member became interested in the possibility of human-to-human transmission among the two family clusters in the early cases, he "went to ask an expert in the [China] CDC system [perhaps Feng

Zijian?], and the answer he got was, there was no way to determine [whether the clusters were caused by] person-to-person transmission."[24]

Strikingly, the second team members were present in the conference room at Jinyintan Hospital on January 13, 2020, when the WMHC hosted infectious disease specialists from Taiwan, Hong Kong, and Macau in what was billed as a "professional exchange" organized by the NHC. An NHC official and leaders from the Hubei and Wuhan health commissions attended the session. Among the non-mainland visitors were Dr. Chuang Yin-Ching, an epidemiologist who led the Communicable Disease Control Medical Network in the Taiwan CDC. During the session, the chair and local presenter presented the non-mainland visitors with images of the computed tomographic (CT) scans used for diagnoses. While he stated that 28 out of the 41 confirmed cases were associated with the Huanan Seafood Market, he also gave the official line that there was no evidence of human-to-human transmission.[25] The use of these numbers shows that epidemiological data on the early cases were already available and in use in Wuhan at that time.

Dr. Chuang Yin-Ching and other non-mainland visitors did not take the interpretation offered by mainland officials and experts for granted. During the presentation, they asked why 13 infections could not be traced to the Huanan market. As the presenter did not have a satisfactory answer, they focused on a family cluster and asked probing questions about how the wife, who had not recently been to the Huanan market due to limited mobility, could have been infected directly from the market.[26] Under relentless questioning, the NHC official present was apparently persuaded of at least the possibility of limited human-to-human transmission. He stood up and physically stopped the presenter from continuing to repeat the no human-to-human transmission line: "why do [you] give an old conclusion? Now the conclusion is that limited human-to-human transmission cannot be excluded."[27] This became the new official line from Wuhan on January 14, 2020.

Dr. Chuang was surprised at the paucity of epidemiological information available and the problems in monitoring close contacts.[28] According to the Taiwan visitors, their hosts appeared to believe in their own rhetoric and didn't realize how bad the situation had already become. They even tried to persuade Dr. Chuang and his colleague to go sightseeing, an offer they declined.[29] Instead, the Taiwan visitors returned from their field trip to Wuhan convinced that the outbreak was much worse than officially presented in Wuhan.[30] On January 16, 2020, the Taiwan CDC issued a level II travel alert for Wuhan. In their news conference, Dr. Chuang referred to the family cluster and the fact that 30% of the 41 confirmed cases in Wuhan had no direct exposure to the Huanan Seafood Market.[31]

The Taiwan CDC also explicitly spelled out that "limited human-to-human transmission generally means that people within one meter of an infected person for about 10 minutes could contract a disease," thus putting members of the same household and medical professionals caring for or treating infected patients at higher risk.[32] What was not generally recognized then or now was that Chinese epidemiologists' understanding of limited human-to-human transmission was heavily influenced by their experiences with N7N9 and H5N1 avian influenzas. Feng Zijian was the director of the China CDC Health Emergency Center in 2013, when the concept of limited human-to-human transmission was used. According to Feng, limited human-to-human transmission when used in 2013 meant that "there is generally no multigenerational transmission, at most, there are two generations of patients, but not three generations and more."[33]

Bringing in these different understandings of "limited human-to-human transmission" helps us understand why Taiwan health policymakers reacted vigorously to the outbreak in Wuhan, while their counterparts on the mainland were still quite relaxed. This contrast suggests that the delay by the China CDC (and by extension the NHC) in examining the early January 2020 case data for evidence of human-to-human transmission was fundamentally due not to a lack of data or lack of capacity to collect and analyze the data but to rather a lack of willingness or sense of urgency to pursue such actions. In other words, an explanation for the action or inaction of the China CDC needs to be sought in the cognitive framework of the China CDC leadership, which in turn shaped the responses of the national health leadership.

The "Zoonosis in the Huanan Seafood Market" Thesis and Its Epidemiological and Policy Implications

A review of the interviews and speeches of Gao Fu and his colleagues suggests that their belief in the zoonosis-in-the-Huanan-market thesis, combined with and reinforced by the clinician–epidemiologist/virologist divide, led them to underestimate the potential for viral spread. This contributed to a slower pursuit of empirical evidence for human-to-human transmission in the first half of January 2020.

The shutdown of the Huanan Seafood Market on January 1, 2020, was a pivotal moment. Accompanied by reports of illegal wildlife sales in the market, the market's closure solidified the belief that the outbreak, caused by the SARS-like coronavirus, began with an animal-to-human zoonotic transmission at this location. For officials and the public who remembered the link between SARS and civets in 2003–2004, this appeared logical and consistent.

As the China CDC director general and an academician, Gao Fu, a virologist specializing in emerging and zoonotic infectious diseases, was not physically present at the New Year's Eve meeting in Wuhan. However, since he had analyzed the genomic sequence of the novel coronavirus before the meeting, his input carried significant weight with Liang Wannian and others. For Gao, the idea that the Huanan market was the site of the zoonotic jump was both scientifically interesting and epidemiologically important. Identifying the source of the infection could help cut off that source and eliminate it, similar to the culling of civets and chickens in response to past SARS and avian influenza outbreaks. In the words of (William) Liu Jun of the China CDC, a close associate of Gao Fu who led the origins tracing effort in Wuhan, "finding this intermediate host is critical for us" because it would help "cut off the chains of transmission from the intermediate host to humans."[34]

In early January 2020, Gao directed much of his own focus and the resources of the China CDC toward sampling at the Huanan market and sequencing collected samples for clues about the source of the novel coronavirus. Despite his stature as an academician and the China CDC director general, he personally traveled to Wuhan in early January 2020 to join the China CDC virus origins tracing team, collecting samples and epidemiological information in and around the Huanan market.[35]

The assumption of zoonosis—that the novel coronavirus originated from an animal-to-human transmission at the Huanan Seafood Market—provided Gao Fu and China's public health leaders with the conceptual framework for seeking and interpreting evidence as they made decisions within the China CDC and offered policy recommendations to the NHC during this period. Although Gao avoided the public spotlight before January 20, 2020, he became the most prominent authority and public advocate for the zoonotic origin at the Huanan market thesis through April 2020. On January 20, 2020, in his first public appearance during the outbreak, Gao briefly introduced the topic to the public:

> This novel coronavirus is the seventh [coronavirus]. In the past we encountered six [coronaviruses], including SARS-CoV. They all came from mammals, some wildlife, through an intermediate host, and then infected humans. This was the consistent pattern in the past. . . . Based on the characteristics [of this novel coronavirus], and its similarity [to other coronaviruses], we hypothesized that wildlife played a very critical role in [its spread to humans].[36]

Thus, Gao explained to reporters why he and other experts inferred the origin of the coronavirus in the Huanan Seafood Market, adding, erroneously, that "all patients at the earliest stage were related to the Huanan Seafood Market."[37] Three days later, on the day of the Wuhan lockdown, Gao Fu confidently addressed the national audience on China Central Television about the importance of the Huanan market and the China CDC's work there:

> After this epidemic started, we quickly identified the [outbreak] source at the Huanan Seafood Market, where illegal wildlife was on sale. We discovered the virus's genome in stalls selling illegal wildlife, which should be conclusive evidence that the virus originated from wildlife. Unfortunately, we still face limitations now because the market was hastily shut down. We haven't pinpointed the exact wild animal [that was the virus's intermediate host], but *it's only a matter of time* (emphasis added).[38]

Subsequently, the question of how the novel coronavirus SARS-CoV-2 arrived at the Huanan market in Wuhan—whether it was carried by one or more animals as an intermediate host or by a human who might have become infected with the virus elsewhere—has become one of the most hotly debated issues ever in science and public health.[39] Initially, Gao Fu believed that the bamboo rat (竹鼠), raised on specialty farms, was the intermediate host for the novel coronavirus.[40] Based on samples collected in the Huanan Seafood Market between January and March 2020, which by definition could not fully represent the situation between November and December 2019, the China CDC team, led by William Liu Jun, Gao Fu and Wu Guizhen, reported detecting live SARS-CoV-2 viruses in environmental samples, as well as the presence of at least 18 species of animals. Although some of the mammalian animals could be susceptible to SARS-CoV-2, the China CDC team emphasized in the published version of their study in 2023 that they did not detect the SARS-CoV-2 virus in the animal samples.[41] In contrast, scientists outside of China have relied on data of early human cases and genomic diversity to argue in favor of the Huanan market as the pandemic epicenter and likely site of the initial zoonotic spillover.[42]

The Strength of Gao Fu's Belief in the Huanan Market Zoonosis Theory

The belief in zoonosis in the Huanan market seemed to have had a powerful influence on Gao Fu and his colleagues in early 2020. Even though some scientists began to question the validity of the Huanan market zoonosis theory at the end of January 2020, Gao Fu remained committed to it for several more months.[43] In April 2020, Gao gave a high-profile interview on CGTN in English. When discussing the earliest cases presented at the New Year's Eve meeting, he matter-of-factly referred to all the initial cases in Wuhan as being connected to the Huanan Seafood Market: "In that market, from the very beginning, all the clusters and all . . ."; when he realized he had misspoken, particularly because he was a co-author of the January 2020 *NEJM* article, he corrected himself mid-sentence, ". . . most, let's say, 'all' is not a good word. If you go back, from the very beginning, we thought it's 'all', but now it's 'most'. Most of the cases, they're from that market."[44]

In a surprising turn, Gao then questioned the reliability of the information on the case that had no Huanan market exposure history and suggested that the absence of Huanan market exposure for that case should be discounted:

> You realize, all these patients, they have some connections [to that market]. Of course, even from the very beginning, you have one, or two, some cases . . . they have no, I call it, no evidence to have a direct connection with that market. Pay attention to the word I am using, 'evidence.' . . . I remember one of the patients, from [December] 27th, no clue [of connection]. But you talk to the patient, when you do this investigation, it looks like there might be some clue, he or she might have some connections [with the Huanan market].[45]

Studies of decision-making have found that decision makers with strong statistical training—with its emphasis on null hypothesis significance testing—may be more inclined to interpret evidence dichotomously rather than continuously and, as a result, "either disregard evidence that fails to attain statistical significance or undervalue it relative to evidence that attains statistical significance."[46] Gao Fu's discussion of the case, made 3 months after the public confirmation of human-to-human transmission of the novel coronavirus, aligns well with such an interpretive mindset. That Gao would publicly dismiss the significance of a December 27 case months after the novel coronavirus had been known to transmit easily among humans raises questions about how dismissive he must have been of the case and of other evidence that did not align with his mindset at the end of December 2019 or early January 2020.

After April 2020, Gao Fu publicly moved away from the Huanan market zoonosis thesis. In May 2020, he speculated that the Huanan market might not have been the source of the coronavirus's initial infection in humans: "At first, we conjectured the [Huanan] Seafood Market might be [the source of the virus], but now it looks like the seafood market itself was likely a victim, since the virus existed beforehand."[47] To date, the zoonosis-in-the-Huanan-market thesis remains a matter of intense debate among virologists and epidemiologists interested in tracing the origins of SARS-CoV-2. Efforts of surveillance of SARS-CoV-2 in wild animals have returned negative results in China.[48] Researchers at the Chinese Academy of Medical Sciences, the WIV, as well as a team led by Zhang Yongzhen of the Shanghai Public Health Clinical Center also sampled bats native to Wuhan or the wider Hubei Province but have not found a bat-borne coronavirus closely related to SARS-CoV-2.[49]

As far as our current review is concerned, it was the Huanan market zoonosis theory, as stated by Gao Fu in early 2020, that dominated the discourse and provided the conceptual framework for health emergency decision-making in China in the weeks and months following the December 31, 2019, New Year's Eve meeting. This theory became a powerful rallying cry for policy action and prompted the National People's Congress Standing Committee to issue the "Decision on a Complete Ban of Illegal Wildlife Trade and the Elimination of the Unhealthy Habit of Indiscriminate Wild Animal Meat Consumption for the Protection of Human Life and Health" on February 24, 2020.[50]

Gao Fu's Three Stages of Zoonosis and Implications for Understanding Human-to-Human Transmission

In his CGTN interview, Gao referred to the December 2019 cases specifically, suggesting that he and colleagues had carefully reviewed these cases and that they likely also took a similar attitude toward the early January cases with no connection to the Huanan market, such as those uncovered by the clinicians at Wuhan University Zhongnan Hospital. The initial certainty about the zoonosis-in-the-Huanan-market thesis by Gao Fu and others made it difficult to entertain alternatives, especially because this belief was also embodied in the inclusion–exclusion criteria that prevented the submission of cases lacking Huanan market exposure.

Gao and his colleagues' embrace of the zoonosis-in-the-Huanan-market thesis carried important implications for understanding how the novel coronavirus might behave in humans and thus what prevention measures should be adopted. Drawing on analogies to the SARS outbreak in Guangdong, MERS in the Middle East, and China's experiences with H7N9 and other avian influenza outbreaks, Gao Fu spoke on various occasions of three likely stages in the zoonotic process. "At the earliest stage *all patients* were related to the Huanan Seafood Market," he said on January 20, 2020. "It was very clear, [the coronavirus first] jumped from animals to humans, it had adaptive mutation, there was [then] *limited* human-to-human transmission" (italics added).[51] The third stage of the zoonosis process would involve "efficient human-to-human transmission" of the coronavirus.[52]

Within this framework of zoonotic stages, the identification of one or more cases of human-to-human transmission appeared less concerning. In fact, when Dr. Anthony Fauci of the US National Institute of Allergy and Infectious Diseases first heard that all those unusual pneumonia patients in Wuhan had become infected by animals in the Huanan market, his reaction was that the transmission would likely not be efficient initially.[53] Within this conceptual framework, one could understand why the China CDC leaders thought the novel coronavirus could transmit from human to human early on and yet did not panic upon learning that some cases did not have an obvious history of exposure to the Huanan market. During a press conference on January 20, 2020, China CDC chief epidemiologist Zeng Guang revealed that he had suspected that the pneumonia outbreak in Wuhan was infectious from the start, saying he "would be surprised if this disease did not transmit from human to human."[54] Both Gao Fu and Feng Zijian also said later that they suspected that the novel coronavirus could be transmitted from human to human early on.[55] In April 2020, Gao Fu reminisced as follows:

> We already suspected there might be human-to-human transmission or person-to-person transmission. And, more importantly, based on the knowledge, based on the understanding of other coronaviruses we know, there *must be* human-to-human transmission. The only thing is whether or not it is *very serious*. . . . Or, if there is human-to-human transmission, is it limited human-to-human transmission or is it really very efficient? (italics added)[56]

As late as January 20, 2020, both Gao and Zeng still thought the novel coronavirus was in the limited human-to-human transmission phase, meaning that the transmission had yet to become efficient. Zeng Guang also noted that, "looking at the whole country, it has not been found that imported cases led to further infections." He called for preventing second-generation case transmission and to "certainly not allow the emergence of a third generation." "The situation can be completely reversed if measures are taken now," Zeng stated.[57]

Both Gao and Zeng also sought to reassure the public and to galvanize action. Gao Fu appealed to the public to "believe in science." He vowed that, based on a scientific understanding of the novel coronavirus, "we will prevent and control [the outbreak] scientifically, and handle the situation scientifically, so everyone, please don't panic." While calling for strengthening prevention and control actions, Zeng appealed to the public to "believe in us, the China CDC can quickly gain control [of the outbreak]."[58]

The Coronavirus Zoonosis Framework and China CDC Actions

With the China CDC leadership's firm belief in zoonosis within the Huanan market from animal to humans, as well as Gao Fu's personal research interests, it was logical for the China CDC to work with local CDCs and make substantial efforts to collect samples from the Huanan Seafood Market. They aimed to test the samples for insights into the virus's origin even when testing capacity was extremely limited.

Simultaneously, the authorities, through the WMHC but advised by the China CDC and approved by the NHC, adopted what Feng Zijian called a "conservative, and certainly cautious" stance in disclosing information about the novel coronavirus's transmissibility.[59] Some believe this conservatism arose from concerns about the potential political repercussions of their judgments and recommendations.[60] Such an interpretation makes sense in the context of China's preoccupation with stability maintenance. Given our understanding of the cognitive framework that informed the decisions of China's health leadership, this caution also aligned with their understanding of the novel coronavirus's behavior, an understanding that proved to be tragically incorrect.

As a technocrat navigating China's intricate and perilous political landscape, Gao Fu emphasized his role as a scientist, in line with the China CDC's primary function as a research and advisory organization for the NHC. He often used the analogy of a scientist as a detective "trying to figure out the suspect." "From the very beginning," Gao said, "I don't think any scientist would be in a position to say there was no human-to-human transmission . . . you're looking for evidence."[61]

However, Gao's critics accused him of prioritizing scientific accuracy over an effective response to the Wuhan outbreak. Much of the public's initial outrage was directed at the China CDC and Gao—and by extension the national health leadership—for failing to recognize and even misleading the public about the contagiousness of the novel coronavirus outbreak in Wuhan. As mentioned earlier, Gao also insisted on the disclosure of the novel coronavirus genomes as a complete package, sacrificing speed in the process.

From December 31, 2019, to January 19, 2020, the outgoing Gao Fu did not make a single public statement on the Wuhan outbreak as the China CDC director general.[62] Instead, he chose to provide assessments to the NHC and national leadership through internal channels, avoiding tying himself to public statements that downplayed the novel coronavirus's threat. This also meant that he was publicly silent about the virus's dangers during these critical weeks. After the Wuhan lockdown was lifted in spring 2020, Gao addressed the earlier public uproar about his role, stating in English that he "never said there was no human-to-human transmission in public. Never, ever."[63]

In the absence of public discussions, the China CDC leadership's discounting of cases unrelated to the Huanan market might have been counterbalanced if the leadership included epidemiologists advocating for alternative scenarios. Unfortunately, this was not the case. Feng Zijian, a deputy director general and the leading epidemiologist within the China CDC leadership, shared Gao's perspective. Zeng Guang, the China CDC chief epidemiologist, was absent from Wuhan on December 31, 2019, and did not arrive in the city until January 9, 2020. His brief visit exemplified the China CDC's leadership challenges as a conglomerate of multiple centers. In the meantime, with the inclusion–exclusion criteria requiring Huanan market exposure history and a strong assumption that the outbreak was still in the initial phase of a SARS-like zoonotic event with inefficient transmission, members of the Hubei and Wuhan CDCs, alongside China CDC members, concentrated their epidemiological efforts in Wuhan during the first 3 weeks on patients connected to the Huanan market and their close contacts.[64]

Despite official statements that the disease in the Wuhan outbreak was not SARS, experts and policymakers agreed that the symptoms of the novel coronavirus infections resembled those of SARS. As previously mentioned, clinicians initially reported that the symptoms of patients at Jinyintan Hospital were strikingly similar to those of SARS.[65] In his first anniversary interview, Gao Fu reiterated that everyone initially thought the novel coronavirus was similar to the SARS and MERS coronaviruses.[66]

The SARS coronavirus was believed to have relatively "low transmissibility" and predominantly symptomatic transmission, with peak infectiousness occurring after the onset of clinical symptoms.[67] As Zeng Guang summarized, "Mild and asymptomatic infections are virtually absent. We confirmed that the SARS virus is not contagious during the incubation period, i.e., a SARS patient in contact with the outside world won't pass the virus to others if the patient does not develop symptoms."[68] Consequently, the SARS epidemic was contained in late April 2003 with basic public health measures like isolating and quarantining patients and their close contacts, along with mass mobilization that forced most people to stay at home and sharply reduce social contact.[69]

Keeping the SARS containment experience in mind and operating under the assumption that the novel coronavirus had limited transmissibility, Chinese health leadership adopted much of the SARS containment strategy in Wuhan in early January 2020. This strategy involved isolating and quarantining symptomatic patients and their close contacts. The big difference between the first half of January 2020 and late April 2003 was the lack of public involvement and mobilization. Since the WMHC had already coordinated with the Wuhan municipal CDC and major hospitals to transfer the first patients to Jinyintan Hospital's isolation wards and had shut down the Huanan Seafood Market, the immediate task was identifying and closely monitoring patients' close contacts.[70] These measures, along with the enforcement of the inclusion–exclusion criteria, created a false sense of security that the epidemic situation in Wuhan was under control.

Professor Linfa Wang, director of the Program in Emerging Infectious Diseases at Duke-NUS Medical School in Singapore, is a leading researcher on bat-borne viruses, especially SARS-CoV-1, and a scientific advisor at the WIV. He was closely monitoring the "explosive" situation in Wuhan in early January 2020 and attended an annual scientific retreat for scientists working on bat-borne viruses at the WIV from January 14 to 18, 2020.[71] Given the information he had on early cases and their association with the Huanan Seafood Market, Wang and his conference colleagues in Wuhan were not concerned. During an online session organized by *Science* magazine, he recalled, "When I was in Wuhan on January 14, I thought: No problem. We have done SARS. And we have all the tools right now. We can do better."[72]

The China CDC leadership, including Feng Zijian, Li Qun, and Xu Jianguo, as well as NHC and local health officials in Wuhan and Hubei, appeared to have believed they had taken the necessary steps to contain the outbreak. In fact, as noted in the exchange with visiting epidemiologists from Taiwan (see also Chapter 9), members of the second NHC expert team had access to epidemiological data showing that 13 of the 41 confirmed novel coronavirus cases at the time had no connection to the Huanan Seafood Market.[73] Since Feng Zijian was a key member of that expert team, he would have had those data; further details about the cases were within his reach if he didn't already have them. This also implies that the top China CDC leadership and others in health leadership could have had access to the same data much earlier than January 23.

Unless there is reason to accuse the China CDC leadership of willful blindness, it seems that the most plausible explanation for their failure to review the pre–January 3 data and recognize community spread is that they were influenced by a powerful cognitive framework that prevented them from seeing what was essentially right in front of them. Instead, those who spoke on behalf of the China CDC, including Xu Jianguo, Feng Zijian, Li Qun, and Zeng Guang, used their authority to reinforce the official narrative that the outbreak in Wuhan was preventable and controllable, there was no sustained human-to-human transmission, and therefore there was not much cause for concern.

Enter Zeng Guang, the China CDC Chief Epidemiologist

We have noted Zeng Guang's absence from Wuhan on December 31, 2019. During the 2003 SARS crisis, Zeng Guang was an influential player. He headed the Ministry of Health–Guangdong Provincial Health Bureau joint epidemiology team in Guangdong and later served as an advisor to the Beijing Capital SARS Command. He was known for advocating tough decisions, particularly the quarantine of the entire Peking University People's Hospital, which helped Beijing stem the scourge of SARS in 2009.

Zeng Guang officially retired from the China CDC in February 2019 but continued to hold the title of chief epidemiologist as of early January 2020.[74] Somehow the China CDC leadership neglected or failed to come up with a suitable replacement for the venerable Zeng, who no longer had to show up regularly in the office. This liminal state of appointment may explain why he was not part of the rapid response expert team that went to Wuhan on December 31, 2019, even though he was a member of the NHC health emergency advisory committee.

On the evening of January 8, 2020, Zeng Guang received an order from the NHC (rather than the China CDC) to "take the 7:15AM flight next morning to Wuhan."[75] Just as Minister Ma Xiaowei entrusted Liang Wannian to help handle the initial outbreak on December 31, 2019, the NHC leadership sought an assessment from someone with Zeng's extensive experience and prominence in the epidemiological community.[76] Zeng joined the battle at a moment's notice, stating that retired veterans should still step up when their country called.[77] However, he also explained that he was not part of the second team of experts and was not expected to be on the front lines to conduct on-site investigations as he was already retired and in his 70s. "There were lots of others doing on-site investigations," he noted.[78]

Zeng flew to Wuhan early the next morning and joined a second NHC expert team to hear briefings from local health officials and clinical experts on the *fangkong* (prevention and control) measures and treatment situation. Thus, he received an update on the outbreak situation solely from official sources in Wuhan. Zeng visited the China CDC team in Wuhan, emphasizing that controlling the outbreak, rather than publishing academic papers, was the priority.[79] He returned to Beijing the same day without joining the hospital visits and seeing patients already on ventilators.

Zeng later regretted his limited use of the internet and social media, which hampered his access to valuable information.[80] He did not know until January 29, 2020, that the eight so-called rumormongers punished in Wuhan in early January were doctors. He also did not learn Dr. Zhang Jixian's name until much later and did not speak with her during his January 9 visit. The lack of access to alternative sources of information may have predisposed him to limit his visit and trust the information from the official briefing. Although he later lamented the limited access he and other experts had in Wuhan/Hubei, it was no surprise that he echoed the official mis-assessment of the outbreak at the time:

> The severity of this disease was found to be similar to that of seasonal viral pneumonia. At that time, hospitals [in Wuhan] had isolated the patients, and no second-generation cases emerged during the quarantine process. The person-to-person transmissibility of the virus had not been demonstrated at that time. Consequently, we had the impression at the time that the disease's infectivity was not strong.[81]

In another interview, Zeng cited the clinicians to defend himself: "My impression was that [this disease] wasn't very severe. That's also the assessment of the clinicians. That view reflected the actual situation."[82] While he brought this benign assessment back to Beijing, he recommended strengthening the quarantine of suspected cases and close contacts.[83] In a later interview, Zeng pointed out that stallholders and other workers at the Huanan market were all close contacts and should have been quarantined immediately and tested when possible.[84]

Zeng's self-justifying explanation for his role made sense for him, particularly because a large contingent from the China CDC and a second NHC-organized expert team were already in Wuhan when he was there. However, the highly limited involvement of the China CDC chief epidemiologist in the early days of what would become the COVID-19 pandemic raises important questions about the nature of Zeng's appointment in the China CDC and the China CDC leadership's responsibility for having a chief epidemiologist who should be playing a full-time, hands-on role at such a critical juncture. It is a legitimate question to ask how much difference might have been made to the course of the pandemic if the China CDC chief epidemiologist had been actively and deeply involved on the front lines in Wuhan from December 31,

2019, with the visit of the first expert team, rather than dashing in and out of Wuhan more than a week later.

Conclusion

In hindsight, despite Gao Fu's claim that they were constantly looking for evidence of human-to-human transmission, it is remarkable that the NHC and China CDC leadership, having contributed to and abetted an environment of secrecy and information hoarding, did not give serious attention to evidence indicating that the novel coronavirus was already circulating and spreading outside the Huanan Seafood Market until it was too late. How did the China CDC leadership have human-to-human transmission in their view "from quite early on" and yet fail to identify such transmission until after Dr. Zhong Nanshan from Guangdong went to Wuhan and then made his public announcement? The answer, I suggest, lies not in the lack of testing capabilities or the unavailability of epidemiological data but in the mindset of the China CDC leadership in a political-administrative environment of fragmented authoritarianism that made it difficult for key decision makers to consider abnormal information and alternative ideas.

The evidence considered in this chapter suggests that a major cause for the delays in China's January response to the Wuhan outbreak was a failure of epidemiological imagination and intellectual leadership. The China CDC leadership, comprised of some of China's leading virologists and epidemiologists such as Gao Fu and Feng Zijian, adopted a cognitive framework centered on the novel coronavirus having had its zoonotic jump to humans in the Huanan market. According to this view, the coronavirus would likely go through stages before it could transmit efficiently from human to human.

This framework lent support to the enforcement of the inclusion–exclusion criteria that required Huanan market exposure (as detailed in Chapter 8). However, the strict implementation of the criteria and additional measures to suppress case reporting in turn thwarted the identification of new cases among those who had no exposure to the market. The absence of new cases served to reinforce the initial belief in the zoonosis-centered framework. This cognitive framework had a circular and self-reinforcing character until it could no longer be sustained. It thus helped to produce and sustain the epidemiological tunnel vision and contributed to the considerable delay in mobilizing the public to respond to the outbreak.

8

Fragmented Authoritarianism, Inclusion–Exclusion Criteria, and Suppression of Case Submissions

The New Year's Eve meeting focused on the Huanan Seafood Market as the source of infections. The Hubei/Wuhan authorities cracked down on health workers who shared information about the outbreak. The national health authority restricted the number of laboratories authorized to carry out testing of patient samples and gagged laboratory scientists. In this political-regulatory environment, the first week of January 2020 became a pivotal turning point for handling the outbreak, just the wrong kind. Since it is now common knowledge that COVID-19 is among the most infectious diseases the world has ever known, what prevented the identification of new cases after January 5, when there was a growing number of patients with the so-called VPUE symptoms in hospitals in the greater Wuhan area?

In this chapter, I first provide an overview of the officially announced number of viral pneumonia of uncertain etiology (VPUE)/novel coronavirus cases in the first 3 weeks of January 2020. In the first week of January 2020, front-line clinicians and hospital administrators in Wuhan reported more VPUE cases, including cases that lacked exposure to the Huanan Seafood Market. Some of them also warned that the VPUE caused by the severe acute respiratory syndrome (SARS)–like coronavirus was contagious. Had these warnings been heeded, there could have been a real chance for containing the outbreak before it spiraled out of control. Yet in an epic failure, the reports and warnings in early January were ignored. Instead, for much of this period the number of confirmed cases was fixed at 41.

The rest of the chapter presents two major factors that made it extremely difficult for clinicians and hospital administrators to submit new VPUE cases in Wuhan. One was the introduction and implementation of the inclusion–exclusion criteria, instead of the Diagnosis and Treatment Protocol developed by clinicians, that made exposure to the Huanan market a necessary condition for classifying a case as a so-called VPUE case and later, beginning on January 12, a case of pneumonia caused by novel coronavirus infection. The other was the strong motivation on the part of the political and health leadership in Hubei/Wuhan to create a pleasant environment for the "two sessions" meetings held in Wuhan over the January 6–17 period. In the political administrative context of fragmented authoritarianism, submission of VPUE/novel coronavirus cases became the casualty.

The Official Case Numbers and the "Two Sessions" Political Season

As I discuss later, major hospitals in Wuhan reported a growing number of suspected VPUE cases, including cases with no exposure history of the Huanan Seafood Market in early January. Following investigations by the local Centers of Disease Control and Prevention (CDC) team and review by the Wuhan Municipal Health Commission (WMHC), the number of cases, according to the WMHC, rose from 27 as of December 31, 2019, to 44 on January 3 and 59 on January 5, 2020. Table 8.1 presents the officially announced VPUE and, beginning on January 10, novel coronavirus cases over the December 31, 2019–January 20, 2020, period.

As the WMHC released these figures, it also informed the public that "the *fangkong* [prevention and control] work is progressing in an orderly manner." The increase in case numbers resulted from a citywide effort to screen for VPUE cases. All identified patients were being quarantined and treated; 163 close contacts were under medical observation. The tracing of close contacts continued. The Huanan Seafood Market had been shut down and disinfected. Besides "proactively carrying out epidemiological investigation," national and provincial efforts to carry out confirmation of the pathogen and search for the source of the pathogen were underway.[1] Nonetheless, the WMHC update of January 5 reminded residents to "maintain indoor air circulation, avoid going to closed, poorly ventilated public places and crowded locations, and wear a mask if necessary."[2] The January 5 update was followed by a question-and-answer (Q&A) with Li Gang, director of the Wuhan Municipal CDC. Although he indicated that the case numbers might increase slightly, Dr. Li Gang reassured the public that the *fangkong* measures Wuhan had adopted "have effectively reduced the risk of infection to the public."[3]

In light of Dr. Li Gang's Q&A, one would have expected additional updates from the WMHC. However, the WMHC did not release its next update until 6 days later. In fact, January 6 marked the start of the political "two sessions" season in Wuhan. The annual plenary sessions of the people's congresses

Table 8.1 Officially Announced Number of Viral PUE–Novel Coronavirus Cases, December 31, 2019–January 20, 2020

Data date	Data release date	Confirmed	Critical/serious	Under observation
2019-12-31	2019-12-31	27	7	
2020-01-03	2020-01-03	44	11	121
2020-01-05	2020-01-05	59	7	163
2020-01-10	2020-01-11	41	7	739[a]
2020-01-11	2020-01-12	41	7	717
2020-01-12	2020-01-13	41	6	687
2020-01-13	2020-01-14	41	6	576
2020-01-14	2020-01-15	41	6	313
2020-01-15	2020-01-16	41	5	119
2020-01-16	2020-01-18	45	5	95
2020-01-17	2020-01-19	62	8	82
2020-01-18	2020-01-20			
2020-01-19	2020-01-20	198	44	90
2020-01-20	2020-01-21	258	63	249

[a]Including 419 medical staff.

Source: Wuhan Municipal Health Commission.

and political consultative conferences for Wuhan municipality (January 6–10) and Hubei Province (January 11–17) were held in Wuhan from January 6 to January 17, concluding on the morning of January 17 with a final plenary meeting of the Hubei Provincial People's Congress. During the "two sessions" period, the Hubei/Wuhan press under the direction of the party propaganda department specialized in publishing news to foster an atmosphere of harmony and prosperity.[4] Reports about the two sessions and on the achievements of Wuhan/Hubei dominated the front pages of *Hubei Daily* and *Changjiang (Yangtze) Daily*. News that reflected badly on the provincial and subprovincial authorities was avoided.

The release of WMHC updates about the Wuhan outbreak paralleled the course of the "two sessions" season. As noted earlier, the WMHC announced 59 VPUE cases on January 5 right before the two sessions season started. It then went quiet for 6 days when the Wuhan "two sessions" were being held. One delegate to the Wuhan Municipal People's Congress suggested postponing the Wuhan municipal "two sessions," but he was ignored.[5] Hardly any attendee at the Wuhan municipal "two sessions" wore a facemask as the leadership wanted business as usual.

The WMHC resumed issuing updates on January 11, coinciding with the start of the provincial "two sessions" and the beginning of the peak Lunar New Year travel season. It stated that as of January 10, 41 patients were confirmed for novel coronavirus infections with nucleic acid testing, resulting in a decrease in the number of official cases. The WMHC then provided daily updates, but the number of confirmed novel coronavirus cases remained fixed at 41 for January 11, 12, 13, 14, and 15. The official number of confirmed cases rose to 45 for January 16, but this was not announced until January 18, the day after the Hubei provincial "two sessions" concluded. Over the same period, the number of people officially under observation for possible infection declined sharply. These numbers created a public atmosphere suggesting that the outbreak was being contained.

The announcements by authorities during the "two sessions" period were just as reassuring as the trend in official case numbers. On January 11, the WMHC stated that epidemiological investigations by national, provincial, and municipal experts "have not found any newly infected patients after January 3, 2020" and "have not found clear evidence of human-to-human transmission."[6] On January 15, the WMHC stated the following in a Q&A from January 14 on its website: "No clear evidence of human-to-human transmission has been found; limited human-to-human transmission cannot be ruled out, but the risk of sustained human-to-human transmission is low."[7] The National Health Commission (NHC), which had approved these announcements, also provided the same information to the World Health Organization (WHO). The WHO in turn shared it with the rest of the world. As later became widely known, this reference to the low risk of "sustained human-to-human transmission" could not have been more incorrect.

The officially announced case numbers, along with the official statements and explanations, gave the public and even leading experts at the China CDC the strong impression that the outbreak in Wuhan was being contained. The day after the China CDC activated Level II emergency response (January 6), the China CDC's "Summary of Daily Intelligence Meeting on Key Infectious Diseases and Public Health Emergencies," which is distributed to the NHC and all province-level CDCs, noted that there were no domestic infectious disease outbreaks or public health emergencies of particular concern.[8] The reality, as the world discovered later, was precisely the opposite.

Clinical Diagnostic Criteria and Case Reporting from Hospitals

A long-standing challenge since the SARS crisis has been the coordination and integration of clinical and disease prevention and control approaches to epidemic outbreaks. During SARS, clinicians and epidemiologists worked together and collaborated to formulate a pragmatic case definition and diagnosis criteria in Guangdong. However, the fissures between these two groups were already apparent during the New Year's Eve meeting in Wuhan. These fissures became even more pronounced in early January 2020 in the form of separate approaches to case definition.

The Clinical VPUE Case Definition

As mentioned in Chapter 4, clinical experts led by Cao Bin and Li Xingwang, working with experts from Hubei/Wuhan, developed the "Diagnosis and Treatment Protocol for Viral Pneumonia of Unknown Etiology" on January 3, 2020. In contrast to the case definition in the Joint Investigation Team report from December 30, 2019, the clinicians drew on their clinical observations. They pointed to the possibility of family clusters in their epidemiological discussion. They noted that most admitted cases had a history of exposure to the Huanan Seafood Market, but this left the door open to cases that might not have been exposed to the market. Their use of the term "viral" PUE to refer to the disease of concern indicated their awareness that the VPUE was caused by a novel coronavirus, pending official confirmation and announcement.

Following the 2007 Ministry of Health protocol for PUE surveillance and investigation, as well as their own epidemiological understanding of the outbreak when no standard diagnostic test was available, the clinical experts introduced a case definition that was not exclusively focused on individuals with a history of exposure to the Huanan Seafood Market. The clinicians' case definition for the Wuhan outbreak includes a checklist of four items: (1) fever, (2) having the imaging characteristics of pneumonia (computed tomographic [CT] scan), (3) low or normal total white blood cell (leukocyte) count or low lymphocyte count early in the illness, (4) no improvement or progressive worsening symptoms after 3 days of standard antimicrobial drug treatment.

A patient was identified as a case of VPUE if they had a history of exposure to the Huanan Seafood Market and presented the symptoms contained in the first three items of the checklist. If the patient did not have a history of exposure to the market but had exposure to confirmed VPUE patients, the same diagnosis applied. Even if the patient had neither exposure to the market nor exposure to confirmed VPUE patients, they would still be diagnosed as a VPUE case if they satisfied all four checklist items and could not be diagnosed with another type of pneumonia.

By making the VPUE diagnosis in Wuhan open to symptomatic individuals without exposure to the Huanan Seafood Market and confirmed cases, the VPUE Diagnosis and Treatment Protocol formulated by clinical experts clearly took into account the possibility that the SARS-like coronavirus transmitted from human to human. In the absence of easily available diagnostic tests, application of the clinical case definition for VPUE diagnosis would likely have resulted in the identification of some false-positive cases. Given the need to strengthen surveillance and identify possible community spread of a dangerous virus about which much remained to be known, this seemed to be a reasonable price to pay.

A useful comparison to the clinicians' case definition was the approach taken in Hong Kong. Drawing on the lessons of SARS, the Hong Kong government acted early and decisively. It activated, with immediate effect, the "serious" level of its Preparedness and Response Plan for Novel Infectious Disease of Public Health Significance on January 3, 2020.[9] Meanwhile, the Hong Kong Center for Health Protection strengthened temperature surveillance at ports of entry and broadened the scope of surveillance. Individuals with fever and acute respiratory or pneumonia symptoms who had visited Wuhan within 14 days before disease onset were to be immediately referred to public hospitals for isolation, treatment, and testing.[10] Professor Yuen Kwok-yung, chair of Infectious Diseases at the University of Hong Kong, was a member of a four-person expert team that advised the Hong Kong leadership on their response. According to Dr. Yuen, it was necessary to make the criteria for suspected cases as broad as possible, i.e., to cast the net wide, to avoid missing any cases, even if this approach invited public pressure.[11]

Growing Number of Suspected VPUE Cases in Wuhan Hospitals

In contrast to the trend shown in the official number of cases, clinicians and hospital administrators in Wuhan encountered a growing number of patients in early January that they believed should be identified as VPUE cases, in accordance with the Diagnosis and Treatment Protocol. They were particularly alarmed by cases with no exposure to the Huanan Seafood Market and recognized that the so-called VPUE was spreading in the population. In this subsection, I draw on information from some hospitals to convey the situation faced by clinicians and hospital administrators in early January 2020.

As the most prestigious hospital in Wuhan, Tongji Hospital took the lead among comprehensive hospitals in implementing proactive measures to respond to the so-called VPUE outbreak. However, as I will report below, the cases encountered at Zhongnan Hospital, located quite far from the Huanan market, were of special importance as we examine how the Chinese health system responded to the outbreak in early January.[12] In the meantime, hospitals close to the Huanan Seafood Market area, the epicenter of the initial outbreak, experienced much greater increases in the number of VPUE patients. These included Hankou Hospital, Wuhan Red Cross Society Hospital, Wuhan Central Hospital (WCH), and Hubei Provincial Hospital of Integrated Chinese and Westsern Medicine (Hubei Integrated Medicine Hospital). It should be borne in mind that Wuhan has many more hospitals than can be described here. For instance, Wuhan No. 5 Hospital, affiliated with Jianghan University, set up a dedicated fever clinic on January 2 and admitted several suspected patients, including a family cluster, on January 6, 2020.[13]

Tongji Hospital Took the Lead

Of the four most prominent 3A (tier 1) research and teaching hospitals in Wuhan, Tongji Medical College of Huazhong University of Science and Technology (HUST) and the Wuhan University Medical School each boasts two of them. HUST has the more historic Tongji and Union Hospitals on the side of the Yangtze River where the Huanan Seafood Market was located; Wuhan University has People's (Renmin) and Zhongnan Hospitals on the other side. Each of these four hospitals played major roles in the early response to the outbreak.

Among the four top hospitals, Tongji and Union Hospitals saw more early cases in December 2019 and early January 2020 because of their relative proximity to the Huanan market and strong reputation in respiratory medicine. Under Dr. Zhao Jianping's leadership, Tongji had already identified 12 cases in the Respiratory Ward alone by December 28, 2019, and these 12 cases were transferred to Jinyintan Hospital in the year-end emergency response. According to Wu Jing, the Tongji Hospital party secretary, the hospital leadership convened a special meeting on December 31, 2019, to develop reporting criteria and clarify suspected patient–contact relationships for the so-called VPUE.[14] Thus, Tongji clinical leaders who were at the New Year's Eve meeting, especially Dr. Zhao Jianping, had additional information from the hospital.

Recognizing that the fever clinic on the Tongji Hospital main campus was inadequate for the growing number of VPUE patients seeking treatment, President Wang Wei made a critical decision to convert an old building for internal medicine outpatients into an expanded fever clinic.[15] The hospital leadership also mobilized staff for the clinic from respiratory medicine, emergency critical care medicine, and the infection section to form working teams on January 5–6, 2020.[16] Around this time, Dr. Lu Jun in emergency medicine began to show symptoms of the so-called VPUE from infection with the novel coronavirus. Dr. Zhao and his colleagues of an ad hoc expert team provided care to Dr. Lu Jun and reported the case of medical staff infection to the health commission.[17] Because Tongji Hospital is directly under the provincial health commission, it is quite likely that this information went to the provincial health leadership.

Wuhan Red Cross Society Hospital

The Wuhan Red Cross Society Hospital, less than a mile away from the Huanan Seafood Market, was the closest comprehensive hospital to that location. Dr. Fan Zhongjie, head of Respiratory Medicine there, was accustomed to seeing patients with the flu from the Huanan market each winter. In retrospect, Dr. Fan saw the first COVID-19 patient, a wholesaler at the Huanan market, on December 17, 2019. Later, when he had three patients with similar symptoms, he suspected that they had the same viral pneumonia and reported it to the hospital leadership. On December 27, 2019, Wuhan Red Cross Society Hospital was one of at least four Wuhan-area hospitals that reported unusual PUE cases to the local CDCs and health bureaus/commissions.[18]

Dr. Fan and his colleagues also took precautions to avoid infections.[19] At the end of December 2019, when the 30-bed respiratory ward was getting full, Dr. Fan reported to the hospital leadership. They converted the medical examination center into a new 30-bed respiratory ward on January 5, 2020, which was also filled in 2 days.[20]

The Red Cross Society Hospital submitted another batch of 10 suspected cases of the so-called PUE on January 5, 2020; and, according to the hospital, these cases were included in the 59 cases announced by the WMHC.[21] Dr. Fan and other staff also learned that some of the so-called PUE patients had no exposure to the Huanan market, and they thought the official rhetoric "there is no clear evidence of human-to-human transmission" seemed obviously incorrect.[22]

WCH Houhu Branch

Located within easy walking distance of the Huanan Seafood Market, the WCH (Houhu Branch) was in the center of the viral storm in late December 2019 and early January 2020. A doctor in the Emergency Section of the hospital began to live in a hotel near the WCH starting on January 3, 2020, in order to avoid passing on the infection to family members. For this clinician and his colleagues, the so-called VPUE was evidently contagious. "All you need to do is go to the fever clinic site and ask two random patients, and you'll quickly conclude that this is an infectious disease and can be passed from person to person, without the need for in-depth investigation."[23]

This doctor recalled that he and his colleagues saw a steady stream of several dozen patients each day before January 8, 2020. Beginning on January 9, however, the number of patients with fever and VPUE symptoms "began to double [each day], increasing exponentially." It would reach more than 800 a day at one point.[24] The WMHC January 11 statement saying that there was no human-to-human transmission was greeted with disbelief and consternation by WCH doctors who treated patients with VPUE symptoms. "There were so many outpatients coming to the Emergency Section, entire families with the same illness. At that point, there were already health workers infected at the Wuhan Central Hospital."[25]

Wuhan Pulmonary Hospital

The Wuhan Pulmonary Hospital, a dedicated infectious disease hospital, was made a "reserve designated hospital" early on and had good communication with the WMHC. Dr. Du Ronghui, chief of Respiratory Medicine, recalled that five or six patients showed up at the fever clinic on January 3, 2020. Dr. Du and her colleagues were struck that the patients "were remarkably similar [in their radiological images], as if [they were] the same person."[26] In an early February interview, Dr. Du pointed to the ground glass opacities on patients' CT scan images and explained that the images for these patients differed from those for typical pneumonia cases.[27]

Dr. Du and the hospital leadership were alarmed by these cases. They raised the level of protection to Level III, the highest, by January 6 and made a dedicated fever clinic available for receiving a growing number of outpatients with similar symptoms but no history of exposure to the Huanan Seafood Market. Medical staff in the fever clinic and isolation wards were required to wear full protective suits and N95 facemasks as a precautionary move against infection, even though health authorities had not warned of human-to-human transmission.[28] In consequence, Wuhan Pulmonary Hospital did well in protecting its own medical and support staff.

Wuhan University Zhongnan Hospital

Similar to other major hospitals in Wuhan, the Wuhan University Zhongnan Hospital Medical Affairs Department received emergency notices from the

WMHC on the afternoon of December 30, 2019. In accordance with WMHC regulations, the Zhongnan Hospital leadership, including Vice President Yuan Yufeng and Dr. Pan Zhiyue, director of the Medical Affairs Department, directed the Emergency Center and the Respiratory Medicine Section to screen for the so-called PUE patients.

On the following morning, the Respiratory Medicine Section identified two suspected PUE cases. Both patients exhibited fever, cough, and ground glass opacities in their chest CT scans. Patient 1, a 39-year-old male admitted on December 25, worked as a fish vendor at the Huanan Seafood Market. Patient 2, a 21-year-old female admitted on December 22, did not have direct exposure to the Huanan market but had been visited at home by a vendor at that market.[29]

Upon identifying these cases, the Zhongnan Hospital leadership promptly initiated an emergency response. Vice President Yuan Yufeng led an ad hoc PUE prevention and control working team, devising a multi-pronged emergency response strategy that included quarantining suspected cases, screening for similar cases throughout the hospital, providing protective equipment for front-line staff, and opening a dedicated fever clinic. The team also reported the cases to the Wuchang District CDC and the District Health Bureau (Medical Administration Section).[30]

Under the leadership of Dr. Cheng Zhenshun, chief of Respiratory Medicine, staff in the Respiratory Section took and sent bronchoalveolar lavage samples of the two patients to BGI (Wuhan) for high-throughput genomic sequencing on January 1, 2020.[31] The following day, Cheng learned that BGI had identified a novel coronavirus in the samples that was approximately 80% similar to the SARS coronavirus. Intriguingly, Dr. Li Yirong, chief of Zhongnan Hospital's own laboratory, and his team found that the two samples tested positive using SARS test kits.[32] "I immediately realized that the situation was not good," Dr. Cheng recalled.[33]

Zhongnan Hospital reported the two patients' diagnostic results to the Wuchang District CDC and the WMHC. On the afternoon of January 2, 2020, a team of three from the Wuhan Municipal CDC, dispatched by the WMHC, arrived to investigate. The two patients were subsequently transferred to Jinyintan Hospital.[34] As reported in Chapter 6, the Zhongnan Hospital laboratory staff collaborated with a research team at the Wuhan University State Key Laboratory of Virology to investigate the novel coronavirus. This team sequenced two whole genomes of the novel coronavirus and provided the results to the China CDC.

On January 3, 2020, three more suspected cases, forming a family cluster, were identified at Zhongnan based on clinical symptoms. The cluster consisted of a 92-year-old father and his son and daughter-in-law. The father, hospitalized in the neurology ward, was the first to exhibit symptoms. All three tested positive using the SARS test kits at the Zhongnan Hospital lab. None of them had visited the Huanan Seafood Market.

Zhongnan Hospital president Wang Xinghuan was alarmed. During the SARS crisis, Dr. Wang was a section chief in the Guangdong People's Hospital, where a chief nurse in his section died from SARS—a painful memory he has carried since.[35] With the identification of the family cluster, Dr. Wang and his colleagues realized they were facing a more severe outbreak than health officials had indicated. "Most importantly," Dr. Wang said, the three patients had "no epidemiological history of association with the Huanan Seafood Market. We therefore concluded that this disease is definitely transmissible from human to human."[36]

Determined not to take chances, Wang directed Zhongnan Hospital to initiate "war-time general mobilization" and adopt "SARS-class" prevention and control measures to address the outbreak.[37] On January 4, the fever clinic was relocated and expanded to reduce the chances of cross-infection. Staffing for the clinic was increased to more than 20 experienced physicians to handle the growing number of outpatients visiting the fever clinic.

Armed with their own evidence regarding the novel coronavirus and its infectivity, the 12 members of the Zhongnan Hospital leadership convened for their weekly meeting on the morning of Monday January 6, 2020. They unanimously approved President Wang Xinghuan's proposal to activate SARS-class infection control and treatment measures throughout the hospital.[38] Both the intensive care unit (ICU) in the Emergency Center and the ICU in Critical Care Medicine created separate sections with 16 beds each for treating patients suspected of being infected with the novel coronavirus.

In the meantime, the Medical Affairs Department staff at Zhongnan Hospital reported the first five cases, including the family cluster with no connection to the Huanan Seafood Market, to the Wuchang District Health Bureau and the district CDC. Staff at the District Health Bureau promptly arranged specialist consultations for the patients, while district CDC staff collected swab samples from the patients, conducted epidemiological reviews, and sent the samples to the Wuhan municipal CDC laboratory for investigation.[39]

The Mystery of the WMHC Inclusion–Exclusion Criteria (Case Definition)

If the Chinese public health system had been receptive to reports about an increasing number of cases unrelated to the Huanan market and heeded front-line clinicians' warnings about the VPUE's contagious nature, it would have been evident that the so-called VPUE was spreading in the community in early January. In consequence, confirmation and disclosure of human-to-human transmission of the novel coronavirus would have likely occurred well before January 20, 2020.

As of early January 2020, the various components of China's health system seemed to operate in harmony. Both the NHC and the China CDC publicly affirmed that they provided guidance to provincial and municipal health commissions or CDCs. In Wuhan, the epicenter of the outbreak, the WMHC displayed its deference to provincial and national authorities. On January 3, the WMHC announced that the national and Hubei provincial health commissions were paying significant attention to the outbreak and had dispatched work and expert teams to Wuhan to offer guidance on handling the outbreak.[40]

Within this hierarchical political-administrative context, the WMHC intensified its emergency response. To avoid alarming the public, the WMHC discreetly established the WMHC Command for Responding to Pneumonia of Uncertain Etiology (PUE) and brought the Wuhan municipal health system—including the WMHC, district health bureaus and CDCs, and municipal hospitals—into "war-time status." A significant concern of this response was not the medical or infectious disease risk but controlling the behavior of hospital administrators and medical staff. In the evening, leaders of municipal hospitals, such as WCH, held emergency meetings with hospital leadership, including department heads, to follow up on implementing the WMHC's directive. According to minutes reported by a *Caixin* reporting team, WCH leadership emphasized the importance of strict discipline, prioritizing "politics, discipline, and science" in that sequence. Department heads were instructed to "keep a close eye on their own staff, strictly enforce confidentiality protocols, and require medical personnel not to disclose confidential information in public or discuss patients' medical conditions using text and images that could be retained as evidence."[41]

Meanwhile, instead of simply adopting the case definition found in the Diagnosis and Treatment Protocol created by clinicians, the WMHC discreetly but assertively introduced the more restrictive "Inclusion–Exclusion Criteria for Viral Pneumonia of Uncertain Etiology " for managing the outbreak through the Chinese disease prevention and control system.[42] Borrowing terms from the 2007 health ministry (NHC) protocol for PUE monitoring and screening, the inclusion–exclusion criteria specify that a viral PUE case must exhibit *all* four clinical manifestations, including

a. Fever ≥38°C
b. Lung imaging characteristic of pneumonia
c. Normal or lower than normal white blood cell count in the early phase of the disease or lower than normal lymphocyte count
d. Lack of improvement or deterioration following 3 days of standardized antimicrobial treatment[43]

Additionally, the patient must have a direct or indirect link to the Huanan Seafood Market in terms of epidemiological history: (a) being a long-term trader or hired hand and working staff; (b) having worked for 3 hours or more in processing, selling, slaughtering, handling, and moving at the Huanan market within 2 weeks of disease onset; (c) having been in contact with poultry or wildlife at the Huanan market within 2 weeks of disease onset; and (d) having lived or studied with or having accompanied those who satisfied the case definition, including medical staff, without effective protective measures.

Patients who met the inclusion criteria, based on both clinical symptoms and epidemiological history, were to be tested to exclude a range of viral and bacterial diseases, including influenza, adenovirus, mycoplasma, and chlamydia pneumonia. The final remaining patients were then considered suspected PUE cases, pending laboratory confirmation (of novel coronavirus infections) by a government-authorized laboratory.

The Inclusion–Exclusion Criteria, Ascertainment Bias, and the China CDC

Epidemiological practitioners are trained to identify and mitigate various biases in studying and managing disease outbreaks.[44] Many of these biases are related to systematic distortions in measurement, known as "ascertainment bias." By requiring exposure to the Huanan market as a necessary condition for confirming a VPUE case in early January 2020, the inclusion–exclusion criteria introduced a major ascertainment bias by excluding symptomatic individuals without a Huanan market exposure history from being considered as VPUE cases. Enforcing the inclusion–exclusion criteria rather than the case definition found in the Diagnosis and Treatment Protocol thus contributed substantially to the delay in recognizing the spread of novel coronavirus infections among people with no exposure to the Huanan market in Wuhan.

When this glaring bias and associated failure became public knowledge, much of the public's anger was directed at the WMHC. However, the WMHC had consistently stated that it had support from national and provincial authorities. Dr. Zhang Dingyu, president of Jinyintan Hospital (which directly reports to the WMHC), acknowledged that the guidelines at the time made exposure to the Huanan market "a requirement and condition for diagnosis."[45] Meanwhile, the China CDC disclosed that its staff collaborated with those from the Hubei and Wuhan CDCs on epidemiological investigations, as well as data management and analysis. Li Qun, director of the China CDC's Public Health Emergency Center, led the development of the protocol for VPUE emergency surveillance and epidemiological investigations. China CDC staff, in three groups, investigated 89 patients being treated at Jinyintan Hospital.[46] In summary, based on publicly available information, the China CDC leadership and experts, within the cognitive framework reviewed in Chapter 7, were directly involved in designing and executing the epidemiological investigations with the inherent bias. The enforcement of the inclusion–exclusion criteria, by hindering the identification of VPUE cases lacking in Huanan market exposure, further reinforced the existing cognitive framework.

While acknowledging the need to expand testing and gradually search for cases with similar pneumonia characteristics but without a history of exposure to the Huanan market, Feng Zijian of the China CDC defended the choices made in early January: "Failing to prioritize exposure history at the outset can result in many misclassifications, as it is called in epidemiology."[47] "Misclassification bias" refers to a type of systematic error by which an individual is assigned to a different category from the one to which they should be assigned.[48] In the interview, Feng, who had participated in a training program in infectious disease surveillance and health emergency management at the U.S. CDC a decade earlier, said "misclassification" in English first before explaining it in Chinese.

According to Feng, if the epidemiological investigations had included individuals without Huanan market exposure, many individuals with symptoms not necessarily caused by the novel coronavirus infection would have been included.[49] Feng's reasoning was that there was not yet a diagnostic test available, and as a result, "it is impossible to classify the cases because there are also many influenza and adenovirus infections during this season."[50] However, this argument by Feng is questionable at best. On the one hand, as mentioned earlier, Hong Kong adopted broader case screening criteria with the explicit goal of trying not to miss suspected cases. On the other hand, the WMHC statement on January 5 clearly stated that diagnostic tests were to be conducted to rule out influenza, avian influenza, adenovirus, SARS, and Middle East respiratory syndrome, among others.[51] Meanwhile, Feng neglected to mention that by excluding symptomatic individuals without exposure to the Huanan market, the inclusion–exclusion criteria introduced a far more detrimental form of misclassification from the perspective of infectious disease prevention and control.

The Inclusion–Exclusion Criteria in Practice

On January 4, 2020, the WMHC conducted a training session for doctors and infection control specialists in Wuhan.[52] A white-covered handbook containing 10 documents was distributed to participants. The first two documents in this handbook were the Diagnosis and Treatment Protocol and the WMHC inclusion–exclusion criteria.[53] The handbook stated that hospital administration should convene experts to examine a suspected PUE case within 12 hours and report the suspected PUE case to the local CDC of the disease prevention and control system using the infectious disease report card for submitting infectious disease cases.[54]

The WMHC promoted the adoption of the more restrictive inclusion–exclusion criteria discreetly through hospital leaders, particularly in major municipal hospitals directly under WMHC leadership. In one top-grade hospital, hospital administrators communicated the inclusion–exclusion criteria to department leaders and doctors in face-to-face meetings, as well as by phone or voice message, prohibiting written messaging.[55] In another hospital, department heads were required to participate in a training session on the so-called VPUE, informally referred to as "viral lung" disease by the practitioners to avoid association with SARS or coronavirus. The participants were required to keep the training materials confidential and were explicitly told that those who took and leaked photos of the materials would be held responsible.[56] In orally conveying these instructions, emphasis was on exposure to the Huanan Seafood Market as a necessary condition for considering a patient for further testing as a suspected VPUE case.

The WMHC Command for Responding to PUE oversaw and managed the transfer of so-called VPUE patients to Wuhan Jinyintan Hospital for quarantine and treatment. With strict application of the inclusion–exclusion criteria, however, only patients with a history of exposure to the Huanan Seafood Market were given permission for transfer to Jinyintan Hospital. Patients with similar clinical symptoms but no history of exposure to the Huanan market were excluded and remained in the general hospitals.[57]

According to a doctor at the WCH, the WMHC Command instructed the WCH to transfer seven patients to the Jinyintan Hospital between December 29, 2019, and January 2, 2020. "The Command gave notices and sent ambulances to transfer [the patients]." "They only transferred those [patients] with an exposure history to the Seafood Market, including those we had almost cured . . . but they didn't want any [patient] without a history of contact with Seafood Market."[58]

As epidemiological investigations being conducted focused on n-cov (novel coronavirus)–infected patients in Jinyintan Hospital, the selective transfer of so-called PUE patients by exposure to the Huanan market evidently decreased the chance of uncovering the viral spread among patients with no exposure to the Huanan market. Meanwhile, the general hospitals, such as the Wuhan Red Cross Society Hospital, the WCH, and the Wuhan University Zhongnan Hospital, all had to expand the number of wards dedicated to patients with the unusual pneumonia symptoms in early January 2020. In hindsight, it is evident that many patients who were denied transfer to Jinyintan Hospital were also infected by the novel coronavirus, and some of them became sources for new chains of infection transmission.

At that time, the epidemiological team from the China CDC was in Wuhan. Besides sampling from the Huanan market, team members conducted investigations on 89 patients at Jinyintan Hospital. They focused their attention on individuals who had worked at the Huanan market and the clinics nearby.[59] In hindsight, this approach resembled the proverbial story of searching for lost keys only under the streetlights. This was because the implementation of the more restrictive WMHC criteria was directly connected to the screening of patients as suspected cases of the so-called viral PUEs and whether such cases could be reported to the local CDC or health bureau/commission and become available for further review and examination by the China CDC. The obstacles to case submission are examined in the next section.

Fragmented Authoritarianism and the Politics of Case Submission: Delays, Obstacles, and Outright Deletion

In the first half of January 2020, doctors in Wuhan hospitals treated a growing number of patients with the clinical manifestations typical of the so-called viral PUE but without any direct or indirect link to the Huanan market. They also struggled to have their reports of these cases as suspected VPUE cases accepted by the government health administration. Instead, case submission became a casualty of the politics of fragmented authoritarianism.

Firstly, control over case submission through the national disease reporting system remained a contentious issue despite the seeming unison of the national–provincial–municipal health authorities. In early January, the NHC vice-ministerial emergency work team stationed in Wuhan asked the WMHC leadership to report the so-called VPUE cases through the national disease direct report system.[60] In theory, doctors and hospital administrators in Wuhan should have been able to report suspected VPUE cases directly to the information system for specialists at CDCs of the district, municipal, provincial, and national levels to see and respond to. In practice, hardly any such reporting of the so-called VPUE cases materialized on the national disease direct report system in the first half of January 2020. According to the China CDC's daily surveillance report, only Jinyintan Hospital reported, on January 4, 2020, a backlog of 19 clinically diagnosed PUE cases.[61]

Confirming this development, Feng Zijian, deputy director general of the China CDC, acknowledged that case reporting from Wuhan "ceased coming afterward, for some unknown reason."[62] By alluding to "some unknown reason," Feng seemed not only to recognize the significance of this issue but also to deflect responsibility away from the China CDC. Interviews conducted during the Wuhan lockdown period provide intriguing insights into the role of provincial and municipal health authorities in obstructing case submissions.

Since WCH made use of case report cards to submit suspected cases to the local CDC, the focus of bureaucratic obstructions was centered on delaying the submission of the report cards. However, the situation inside the hospital was different. As the number of unusual pneumonia cases increased, clinicians felt obligated to file reports in accordance with the Law on Infectious Disease Prevention and Treatment and were concerned about being held responsible for failing to report. Procedurally, they could have used the electronic medical record system to inform the Public Health Section of the hospital of the cases; staff in the Public Health Section could then use the information supplied by the clinicians to make direct reports into the national disease reporting system. Yet, according to an emergency room doctor at the WCH Houhu Branch, "with this [disease] it's different. From the beginning [we were] told not to talk about it."[63] When clinicians checked with the Public Health Section for guidance about reporting suspected cases, they were told to wait. Another doctor expressed frustration that, when suspected cases were not being reported, the patients concerned were not treated as being infectious; allowing these patients to roam around enabled further spread of the disease.[64]

As will be noted below, there was at least one exception to the lack of case submission on the national disease reporting system, and that exception revealed that the provincial health administration was actively engaged in making such reporting disappear from the system during the "two sessions" period. Information on suspected PUE cases submitted from Wuhan hospitals remained within Wuhan.

Secondly, in medical practice, clinicians typically exercise some discretion, whether in clinical diagnosis or prescription writing. Dr. Zhao Zigang, deputy director of the Emergency Center of the Wuhan University Zhongnan Hospital, explains that "policy standards tend to be rigorous, but the people who implement them are flexible."[65] However, during the outbreak in Wuhan, doctors found it difficult to have cases accepted as VPUE/suspected novel coronavirus cases even when the patients exhibited the required clinical symptoms stated in the Diagnosis and Treatment Protocol. One doctor at the Wuhan Youfu Hospital complained that the criteria for officially diagnosing a VPUE case "were so strict, not a single patient [at the Youfu Hospital] met them" due to the Huanan market exposure condition strictly enforced by the WMHC.[66]

Thirdly, the inclusion–exclusion criteria and the Diagnosis and Treatment Protocol seemed to pit disease prevention (the CDC system) against clinicians. The Hubei provincial and Wuhan municipal health authorities were not neutral arbiters. A *Caixin* report reveals that when members of the NHC and Hubei provincial expert teams, likely leading clinical experts, saw the inclusion–exclusion criteria, they "were outraged. [They] demanded that the Wuhan Municipal Health Commission recall the Handbook [containing the inclusion–exclusion criteria]."[67] In response, the WMHC quickly printed a replacement green-covered handbook without the "criteria." However, this gesture was only a tactical move to avoid confrontation with national and provincial medical experts. In practice, the WMHC staff continued to enforce the same more restrictive inclusion–exclusion criteria, emphasizing Huanan market exposure, to determine whether a patient should be classified as a VPUE case for transfer to Jinyintan Hospital for centralized treatment.

As noted earlier, Wuhan-based hospitals treated more and more patients with VPUE/n-cov symptoms in the first 2 weeks of January. The WMHC and the Wuhan CDC, backed by provincial interests, acted as gatekeeper to enforce the restrictive criteria for identifying and transferring VPUE/n-cov cases. Consequently, doctors and hospital administrators in Wuhan struggled to have cases accepted when the patients lacked Huanan market exposure history. Wuhan Pulmonary Hospital and WCH, along with Jinyintan Hospital, are among the 13 hospitals with a direct report relationship to the

WMHC; and they adhered to the more restrictive criteria. Wuhan Pulmonary Hospital designated three floors of its Renji Building for patients with VPUE symptoms on January 6. The 102 beds on these floors were quickly filled, and the total number of such patients reached 380 by January 18. President Peng Peng observed that the patients couldn't meet the criteria for VPUE diagnosis, despite exhibiting "typical clinical manifestations" of the condition.[68]

In the rest of this section, I examine the experiences of WCH and Wuhan University Zhongnan Hospital to provide further insight into how VPUE case reporting was constrained and suppressed in January 2020, especially during the "two sessions" period. The WCH directly reports to the WMHC, while the Wuhan University Zhongnan Hospital has a higher administrative ranking and directly reports to the Hubei provincial health commission. Various other hospitals faced similar situations.

Suppression of Case Reports from the WCH

As one of the first hospitals to report unusual pneumonia cases, WCH had identified seven pneumonia patients with connections to the Huanan Seafood Market as of December 29, 2019. Dr. He Xiaoman and Dr. Yin Wei of WCH's Public Health Section communicated with officers from the Wuhan Municipal CDC and the Jianghan District CDC regarding these cases. That evening, staff from both CDCs visited WCH to collect patient samples and investigate. When Dr. Yin inquired about submitting reports on the cases, Wang Wenyong, chief of the Infection Prevention Section at the Jianghan District CDC, told Dr. Yin on January 3, 2020 to wait for further notice before filing reports.[69] On January 4, WCH hospital administrators received the restrictive inclusion–exclusion criteria instead of authorization to submit cases.

As the number of suspected cases increased, Dr. Yin filed nine PUE report cards (cases) on January 8, four more on January 9, and another on January 10, totaling 14 cases in 3 days.[70] When the WMHC started referring to pneumonia caused by novel coronavirus infections on January 11, the WCH's Medical Affairs Department contacted the Jianghan District Health Bureau about a suspected case requiring review and testing. They were instructed to contact the district CDC about sampling and epidemiological investigation. However, the director of the Jianghan District CDC said that they could not proceed without instruction from the District Health Bureau.[71] Apparently under pressure from superior levels of administration, neither the District Health Bureau nor the district CDC was willing to proceed. It was later discovered that Hu Ziwei, an emergency ward nurse, was clinically diagnosed as having VPUE symptoms on January 11. After Dr. Ai Fen, the director of Emergency Medicine, promptly informed the Medical Affairs director, WCH hospital leadership demanded that the reference to viral pneumonia be removed from Hu Ziwei's medical record.[72]

The following day, the reason for the impasse at the district level became apparent. Xu Jian, director of the Supervision Division of the Hubei Provincial Health Commission (HPHC), visited WCH Houhu Branch and provided instructions on case submission: "Infectious disease report card submission requires prudence. Submit a case report card only after joint provincial and municipal ascertainment."[73] Within Wuhan's medical community, Xu and his colleagues were known to have conveyed a "new spirit [from the HPHC] for submitting novel coronavirus cases."[74] At a time when novel coronavirus cases were increasing rapidly in hospitals, hospital leaders were told not to submit cases until authorized by provincial and municipal CDCs/health commissions. By thus controlling case submission, the provincial and municipal health administrations effectively halted the case reporting process for VPUE cases.

On January 13, Wu Fengbo, director of WMHC's Disease Prevention and Control Division, reiterated the need for caution in submitting PUE cases at WCH. He explained that suspected PUE cases should undergo extensive testing and reviews within the hospital before being brought to the district level for consultation and sample collection, followed by testing at the district, municipal, and provincial levels. If the causes of unexplained pneumonia cases remained unknown after this process, cases could be formally submitted as PUE cases with approval from the HPHC.[75] Wu's explanation outlined a lengthy process with several steps, including testing requirements outside of hospitals' control. Once again, the health leadership in Hubei and Wuhan appeared determined to use complex submission procedures to minimize the number of PUE cases filed.

On the same day, the Infection Prevention Section chief of the Jianghan District CDC instructed Dr. Yin at WCH to change the cause of disease for the PUE cases filed on January 10 to "other," meaning not due to novel coronavirus infection. When Dr. Yin asked about the January 11 case review request, staff at the Jianghan District Health Bureau told Dr. Yin to wait for further instruction.[76]

The Frustration of Wuhan University Zhongnan Hospital

Armed with independent information on novel coronavirus infections and higher administrative ranking, the Wuhan University Zhongnan Hospital adopted a more aggressive approach in communicating with health administrations and reporting suspected cases. As a result, the challenges faced by Zhongnan Hospital in reporting these cases highlighted the barriers to identifying and submitting new cases during the "two sessions" period.

When Wuhan University Zhongnan Hospital identified its first five patients in early January 2020, Dr. Pan Zhenyu of the Medical Affairs Department sought guidance from the WMHC on reporting the suspected cases through the direct reporting system. He did not receive a response. The reporting issue was put aside since the WMHC and local CDCs had already investigated the cases.

After the Zhongnan Hospital Emergency Department admitted a patient from the city of Huanggang with severe symptoms on January 6, 2020, the Zhongnan Hospital leaders decided to report the case instead of waiting for administrative instructions. The patient was from another city, was critically ill, and had been denied admission by other hospitals. Consequently, there was a high likelihood that the so-called VPUE infections had spread to other cities. Dr. Peng Zhiyong, the chief of Critical Care Medicine who made the decision to admit the patient, emphasized the importance of reporting the case.[77]

Since the local CDCs had become unresponsive, Zhongnan Hospital's Medical Affairs Department used the national disease reporting system to submit reports of two VPUE cases on January 9, 2020. The system indicated a successful submission.[78] This meant that different levels of health administrations and CDCs, including the China CDC, should have been able to view the cases submitted by Zhongnan Hospital.

The online case submission by Zhongnan Hospital and likely one other institution was crucial for neighboring Huanggang city. Staff at Huanggang Central Hospital had seen patients with unusual pneumonia symptoms since early January and sought help, unsuccessfully, from the Huanggang municipal CDC.[79] When Huanggang health leadership learned through the online disease reporting system about three patients from Huanggang being treated in Wuhan for the so-called VPUE, they quickly launched epidemiological investigations of the cases. Two patients (Mr. Hu, a poultry seller, and Mr. Du, a delivery truck driver) were connected to the Huanggang Central Produce Market and often traveled to the Huanan Seafood Market in Wuhan. This prompted Huanggang municipal leadership to disinfect the Huanggang Central Produce Market and other markets on January 12. By that time, Huanggang Central Hospital was already handling a significant number of patients with suspected novel coronavirus infections.[80]

While Huanggang benefited from the information submitted through the online disease reporting system, it turned out that the cases Zhongnan

Hospital had submitted were deleted from the system shortly afterward and were not recorded in the China CDC daily surveillance reports. Zhongnan Hospital "definitely did not delete" the submissions. The Wuhan district and municipal levels lacked the authority to make such deletions.[81] Thus, it is almost certain that the HPHC intercepted the submissions and removed them from the online reporting system, an action they had the authority to take.

Faced with difficulties in submitting cases using the national disease reporting system, staff at Zhongnan Hospital nevertheless attempted to report directly to the district and municipal health commissions as they dealt with the rapid increase in the number of suspected cases. However, they knew that the cases did not meet the Huanan market exposure requirement of the inclusion–exclusion criteria. To circumvent this requirement, Zhongnan Hospital's leadership assembled a team of clinical experts, led by Dr. Cheng Zhenshun and Dr. Yang Jiong from the hospital's Pulmonary and Critical Care Medicine department, to evaluate cases for submission. Based on clinical symptoms, including chest CT scans, this expert team selected 21 suspected novel coronavirus cases, which the Zhongnan Hospital Public Health Section submitted on January 11. Anticipating objections based on the inclusion–exclusion criteria, Dr. Pan Zhenyu added a special note explaining that the cases were chosen based on "hospital testing," likely referring to tests conducted by the Zhongnan Hospital laboratory using SARS test kits it had recently purchased. On the following day, the WMHC sent a team of three specialists to Zhongnan Hospital to follow up on the cases. While the specialists acknowledged that patients displayed symptoms resembling those of novel coronavirus infections, they emphasized that the inclusion–exclusion criteria required a history of exposure to the Huanan market.[82] This meant that none of the 21 patients could be transferred to designated hospitals for treatment.

During this period, the number of patients with VPUE/n-cov symptoms at Zhongnan Hospital increased rapidly, from 5 on January 8 to 45 on January 12, 55 on January 13, and 62 on January 14. Concerned about the government's inadequate response, Dr. Wang Xinghuan, the Zhongnan Hospital president, arranged an urgent meeting with a provincial leader, likely vice governor Yang Yunyan, on January 14. Drawing on lessons from the SARS crisis, Dr. Wang urgently warned,

> I have carefully examined the patients' CT scans; they definitely have novel coronavirus pneumonia. The number of such patients is growing, and the hospital is running out of beds to accommodate them. The relevant department [WMHC] currently claims that this disease is preventable and controllable, with no clear evidence of human-to-human transmission found. I believe this assessment must be incorrect. If action is not taken, the situation will become dire.[83]

This meeting prompted the HPHC to send a team from its Department of Medical Administration to Zhongnan Hospital that afternoon. In an unusual move that signaled their displeasure with the number of suspected cases that Zhongnan Hospital intended to report, the HPDC team donned protective suits to inspect the wards and verify the count of suspected patients. That evening, the WMHC sent its own team to follow up. Comprising one bureau official and four specialists, the WMHC team reviewed each of the suspected cases against the inclusion–exclusion criteria.[84] According to Dr. Peng Zhiyong, these specialists acknowledged that the patients exhibited clinical symptoms reminiscent of SARS. However, they insisted on adherence to the Huanan Seafood Market exposure requirement.[85] "They first excluded cases without a history of exposure to the Huanan Seafood Market, then carefully reviewed other items, finding one reason or another for not meeting [the WMHC criteria], and thus forcefully eliminated the majority of the suspected cases," recounted Dr. Zhao Yan, vice president and chief of Emergency Medicine at Zhongnan Hospital.[86]

Thus, the Hubei and Wuhan Health Commissions were able to whittle down the number of suspected novel coronavirus cases at Wuhan University Zhongnan Hospital, if only for a few days. In fact, all of the first 40 suspected cases identified by the Zhongnan Hospital clinical expert team tested positive for the novel coronavirus later on when nucleic acid testing became available.[87]

Conclusion

How did the health establishment in Hubei and Wuhan fail to recognize the growing numbers of patients with novel coronavirus infections in the first half of January? The truth is, they did not. Instead, they kept the number of confirmed novel coronavirus cases at 41 due to a combination of factors.

Firstly, the adoption of the inclusion–exclusion criteria and the requirement of exposure to the Huanan market as a necessary condition for VPUE/n-cov case diagnosis played a role. By excluding symptomatic patients without exposure to the Huanan market, the implementation of the inclusion–exclusion criteria introduced a significant ascertainment bias in the initial handling of the outbreak. With strict application of the inclusion–exclusion criteria, the official number of new VPUE/n-cov cases associated with the Huanan market dropped to zero after January 3, 2020. This created an illusion for scientists and health policymakers at the China CDC and the NHC that the outbreak had been contained, which in turn dulled the official response across multiple dimensions. By the time the NHC working team had organized experts to produce an updated diagnosis and treatment protocol accounting for community spread, it was already too late.

In Wuhan, the strict enforcement of the inclusion–exclusion criteria and related measures showed the features of fragmented authoritarianism at work as the health leadership of Hubei/Wuhan sought to create a pleasant environment for the "two sessions" during the January 6–17 period. Even though front-line clinicians and hospital administrators quickly recognized the rapidly growing number of suspected VPUE cases and, in some instances, conducted tests to detect the novel coronavirus and concluded that the virus was contagious, the political-administrative apparatus in Wuhan and Hubei utilized the inclusion–exclusion criteria to hinder VPUE case submissions. When clinicians and hospital administrators persisted in submitting new VPUE cases, the experiences of WCH and Zhongnan Hospital show that the health leadership of Hubei/Wuhan were determined to slow down case submissions for the duration of the "two sessions" season. They used various internal mechanisms to prevent cases from being submitted, and in one instance the provincial health authorities actively intercepted and removed submissions made through the online reporting system.

From the outset, the health leadership in Wuhan prioritized politics and discipline over scientific evidence. As time progressed, the initial dominance of the disease prevention establishment in implementing the inclusion–exclusion criteria became increasingly influenced by provincial and municipal political considerations associated with the "two sessions" season. When Dr. Wang Xinghuan, the president of Zhongnan Hospital, persisted in warning of the novel coronavirus's potential dangers, he encountered repeated criticism in Hubei/Wuhan for "failing to adopt the appropriate political stance."[88]

In a more open organizational and information environment, the built-in ascertainment bias centered on exposure to the Huanan Seafood Market could have been corrected quickly as front-line clinicians encountered and reported cases that contradicted the faulty premises and when such cases were tested. However, due to the controls and prohibitions imposed on health workers, hospitals, laboratories, and the media, as well as tenacious efforts by the Hubei/Wuhan health leadership to keep cases from being reported, the original ascertainment bias developed into an organized silence in Wuhan.

Reflecting on human-made disasters, Diane Vaughan observed, "there is nothing so deadly in a crisis as the sound of silence."[89] As late as January 19, 2020, Dr. Li Gang of the Wuhan CDC still asserted that "the risk of sustained human-to-human transmission is low."[90]

9

The Wall of Silence Surrounding Health Worker Infections

Following Xi's January 7 "requirements" and the official conclusion on January 8 that a severe acute respiratory syndrome (SARS)–like novel coronavirus was the pathogen causing the viral pneumonia of uncertain etiology (VPUE) in Wuhan, the National Health Commission (NHC) leadership stepped up efforts to respond to the novel coronavirus outbreak. These efforts included dispatching a second NHC-organized expert team, along with Zeng Guang, to Wuhan; engaging in international communication and exchange with the US Centers for Disease Control and Prevention (CDC) and the World Health Organization (WHO); disclosing the novel coronavirus genome internationally; and hosting visits of experts from Taiwan, Hong Kong, and Macau. Simultaneously, while continuing to collaborate with the Hubei/Wuhan authorities on public messaging that downplayed the risk from the novel coronavirus, the NHC also reinforced its own working team in Wuhan, which had been led by a vice minister. Key mid-level officials and staff in the NHC relocated to Wuhan and would play critical roles in the following weeks and months. By January 15, the NHC had orchestrated the updating of a 63-page set of prevention and control documents for handling the novel coronavirus pneumonia outbreak. Most of these efforts were conducted covertly as the country entered the busy Lunar New Year holiday travel season.

Whereas the previous chapter explored the difficulties clinicians and hospital leaders in Wuhan encountered in reporting suspected VPUE/novel coronavirus cases, this chapter focuses on the January 8–16 visit by the second NHC national expert team to assess the severity of the outbreak in Wuhan. In Chinese public memory, this expert team's January 10 interview helped the authorities downplay the severity of the outbreak by stating that it was "preventable and controllable."[1] In reality, after the authorities acknowledged the possibility of limited human-to-human transmission, the team's mission shifted to verifying rumors of healthcare worker infections.

This chapter first introduces the second NHC expert team and describes the mounting pressures in Wuhan's major hospitals, particularly Jinyintan

Hospital. While members of the expert team were initially welcomed when their views aligned with the official discourse, they soon encountered resistance when they urged local authorities to release data on the number of suspected cases. Connecting the data on medical staff infections with the official rhetoric reveals that Wuhan/Hubei authorities, including Wuhan party secretary Ma Guoqiang, received crucial alerts about the severity of the outbreak around January 11–12, 2020. Particularly important was the growth in the number of health worker infections. However, within the confines of fragmented authoritarianism, Hubei/Wuhan authorities used political discipline, heightened emphasis on stability, and fear of sanctions against hospital infections to erect a wall of silence surrounding health worker infections. Despite their persistent efforts to verify rumors of such infections, the second expert team failed to obtain confirmations of health worker infections with the novel coronavirus.

The NHC and the Organization of the Second Expert Team

The members of the second NHC expert team, like the first, were once again composed of public health and clinical experts from Beijing-based organizations. They were selected from the NHC advisory committees for health emergency response and respiratory diseases.[2] All of them had experience dealing with SARS in 2003 (Table 9.1).

The two public health specialists on the team had both headed the emergency response office (center) in the China CDC previously. Feng Zijian, the only member who was part of both the first and second teams, served as a key

Table 9.1 The Second NHC Expert Team to Wuhan, January 8–16, 2020

Feng Zijian, deputy director general and former director of the China CDC Public Health Emergency Center, China CDC
Yang Weizhong, vice president, Chinese Preventive Medicine Association; former deputy director general, and former director, Office of Disease Control and Emergency Response, China CDC
Dr. Gao Zhancheng, director of Respiratory Medicine, Peking University People's Hospital
Dr. Jiang Rongmeng, director of the Second Section of Infectious Diseases, Beijing Ditan Hospital (affiliated with Capital Medical University; arrival January 9)
Dr. Wang Guangfa, director of Pulmonary and Critical Care Medicine, Peking University First Hospital

link between the rest of the China CDC leadership, the China CDC emergency team in Wuhan, the NHC working team in Wuhan, and other NHC officials. Yang Weizhong, Feng's predecessor at the China CDC, had led the development of the national disease reporting and surveillance system in the early 2000s and was the Chinese co-leader of the China–WHO H7N9 Joint Mission Team.

The clinicians Gao Zhancheng and Wang Guangfa were leading respiratory specialists in their respective hospitals affiliated with Peking University. Jiang Rongmeng had had extensive domestic and international field experience dealing with infectious diseases outbreaks, such as avian flu, Ebola, and plague. He was an expert contributor to multiple infectious disease diagnosis and treatment protocols.[3]

When the NHC staff organized this second group of experts for Wuhan, it also sent additional staff to join the NHC working team in Wuhan, as did the China CDC. After the initial alarm and urgency in responding to the outbreak, the level of urgency had decreased significantly. The team of experts was there to learn and to offer advice, particularly to help update the Diagnostic and Treatment Protocol. Upon their arrival in Wuhan, the team members were specifically instructed by an NHC official that "[under the principle of] territorial management, the locals are in charge, and [you] experts are here to provide assistance."[4]

The Mounting Pressure in Jinyintan Hospital

As the second expert team began its mission in Wuhan, one of the first stops was Jinyintan Hospital. Initially, most of the so-called VPUE patients were transferred to Jinyintan Hospital for treatment. As a result, the hospital, which usually maintains a small staff, quickly required reinforcements. With the coordination of the Hubei Provincial Health Commission (HPHC) and the Wuhan Municipal Health Commission (WMHC), an expert team of at least 26 members, led by Dr. Zhao Jianping and Dr. Huang Chaolin, provided treatment. They were joined by Cao Bin and Li Xingwang from the first NHC expert team. With such support, Zhang Dingyu, the hospital president, initially thought that the epidemic situation was manageable and life would return to normal by late January 2020.[5]

However, Zhang soon felt the weight of the situation. "By January 3–5," he recalled, "there were already 70–80 patients [in Jinyintan] and quite a few were critical care patients, some were already in a dying state [on extracorporeal membrane oxygenation]. So we knew this was very serious."[6] As with the enforcement of the inclusion–exclusion criteria or the January 10 efforts to test and verify cases, the authorities preferred figures that made the outbreak appear less severe whenever possible. Officially, the first death from novel coronavirus infections—Mr. Zeng—occurred on January 9.[7] In fact, Mr. Zeng was preceded by a 67-year-old male patient on January 7 (some sources also use January 6). This patient was, like Mr. Zeng, transferred to Jinyintan Hospital the night of December 31, 2019, and on ventilation. He had the clinical symptoms but did not receive nucleic acid testing. A panel of five experts agreed that the deceased died of pneumonia but could not be certain he had died of novel coronavirus infection. In consequence, this case was not counted as a death from novel coronavirus infection.[8]

Especially misleading was the official number of confirmed novel coronavirus cases. Following extra-strict testing rules that required each confirmed case to have tested positive using two different test kits, the WMHC announced that there were 41 confirmed novel coronavirus cases in Wuhan as of January 10. But that double-testing scheme ruled out many cases that tested negative on one or both diagnostic tests. In fact, according to Dr. Zhao Jianping, Jinyintan Hospital alone had five non–intensive care unit (ICU) wards full of novel coronavirus pneumonia patients on January 10; each ward had more than 40 patients.[9] Many more cases were kept away from Jinyintan Hospital and not even counted as suspected cases because of the Huanan market exposure requirement in the inclusion–exclusion criteria.

In the ensuing days and weeks, the gravity of the situation at Jinyintan Hospital became crystal clear to all involved. According to an investigative report by *Southern Weekend*, the ICU of Jinyintan Hospital took in nine so-called PUE patients between December 31, 2019, and January 8, 2020. Not a single one of these patients survived.[10] Dr. Zhong Qiang in Emergency Care at Tongji Hospital led a team of five to join Dr. Wu Wenjuan's ICU team on S7 in Jinyintan Hospital beginning on January 11.[11] On his first tour to check on the patients in the ICU, Zhong was struck by the fact that "many critically ill patients were already on ventilators."[12]

With a large number of patients requiring intensive care even in non-ICU wards, the Jinyintan Hospital administration faced a major staffing crisis. While efforts were made to bring in doctors and nursing staff from other hospitals, more than 50 of the medical orderlies, about half of the total for the hospital, quit between January 12 and 15.[13] In Chinese hospitals, medical orderlies perform a variety of essential non-medical tasks of patient care.

On January 13, 2020, President Zhang Dingyu activated the hospital's full mobilization mode. Bowing before his colleagues, he announced that all staff must report to work and that all time off for weekends, holidays, and vacations was canceled. Administrative and other non-medical staff were enlisted to help with various tasks in the patient wards, such as delivering meals to patients.[14] Zhang declared, "We are already in the eye of the storm, and we must not back down now! All we have to do, all we can do, is to save the patients, protect our people, protect our city!"[15]

In this context, the NHC working team in Wuhan also brought in reinforcements from Beijing. Among the new faces was Li Dachuan, director of the Medical Management Division in the NHC Medical Administration Department. Li went to Wuhan on January 12 at a time when there was a growing number of patients in severe conditions and a strong need to improve treatment. According to the NHC, Li Dachuan helped arrange for the transfer of patients to designated hospitals. After making visits and speaking with physicians, he assisted in the decision by Jinyintan Hospital to open three new wards for treating patients with novel coronavirus pneumonia and having the Wuhan Tongji and Union Hospitals and Wuhan University People's Hospital each assume responsibility for one ward in mid-January.[16]

Expert Team Members and Their Challenging Quest for Infection Information

When the second team of experts began its visit in Wuhan, it was presented with the same information as Zeng Guang and similarly persuaded that the outbreak situation was manageable. Dr. Wang Guangfa of the Peking University First Hospital stated on the evening of January 10, 2020, that the illness, which became known officially the next day as "pneumonia caused by the novel coronavirus," was less severe than SARS and the outbreak was "preventable and controllable."[17]

As of January 10, 2020, the second team appeared to have a good working relationship with the Wuhan/Hubei authorities. Before the WMHC announcement on January 11, the team met with the leadership of the HPHC and the WMHC. During the meeting, they discussed the 41 laboratory-confirmed cases. While the official testing program suggested that the outbreak was limited, there was significant discussion and debate regarding the number of cases, the criteria for confirmed cases, and what information should be shared with the public. At one point, the conversation with Zhang Jin, the party secretary of the HPHC, became tense. The team urged the Wuhan/Hubei authorities "to report truthfully." Zhang Jin did not address the implied criticism directly but disarmed the team by asking, "You suspect me of underreporting, don't you?"[18]

A major reason for the prolonged discussion and tense exchange was the existence of a list of over 100 suspected cases that had not been laboratory-tested.[19] When the meeting concluded, the expert team members believed they had secured an agreement with the authorities to disclose both the confirmed and suspected case numbers to the public. Disclosing suspected case numbers had been a well-received practice during the SARS outbreak in late spring 2003. "We all agreed to it before we left the meeting," recalled a team member.[20]

However, to their dismay, the WMHC did not disclose the number of suspected cases, as the team thought they had agreed upon, during the second expert team's stay in Wuhan. The expert team was sharply reminded of its limited influence. "What happened behind the scenes, I just don't get it," lamented a team member.[21]

As noted in Chapter 7, under persistent questioning from non-mainland visiting epidemiologists, an NHC official was persuaded that "limited human-to-human transmission cannot be excluded." This official stance was included in the WMHC question-and-answer (Q&A) of January 14, 2020, in the form of doublespeak that characterized official communications during this period. The Q&A also mentioned a husband–wife cluster, noting that the wife denied any history of exposure to the Huanan Seafood Market.[22] In hindsight, this Q&A was an indirect admission that there were cases of human-to-human transmission, given that authorities had received multiple reports of suspected cases of human-to-human transmission in early January.

Meanwhile, as mentioned below, the team members heard rumors that some healthcare workers had become infected with the novel coronavirus. Medical staff, especially doctors, wore facemasks and had relatively brief exposure to patients. As a result, cases of healthcare worker infections could be seen as indications of serious infectivity, providing powerful evidence for a more vigorous response. Consequently, the second expert team was particularly interested in inquiring about medical staff infections with the novel coronavirus during its hospital visits.

However, the second team had not received an affirmative answer to the question of healthcare worker infections by the time it left Wuhan. In one instance, the team was able to contact a doctor believed to have been infected with the novel coronavirus, but the doctor denied being infected. In fact, during the time of the second expert team's visit to Wuhan, there was a growing number of medical staff infections. The failure of the second expert team to confirm the existence of such cases offers a unique perspective on the power of vested interests at work in Wuhan/Hubei.

The Trend in Medical Staff Infections, January 1–18, 2020

According to a presentation slide from the China CDC in early February 2020, 13 hospitals in Hubei Province, including all of Wuhan's nationally renowned hospitals, reported at least 15 confirmed COVID-19 infections among medical staff each.[23] Table 9.2 lists the Wuhan-area hospitals. I have organized the list by the earliest disease-onset dates up to January 15, 2020, the final full day of the second expert team's stay in Wuhan.

While the dates of disease onset do not correspond to the dates of confirmation, the information from the China CDC presentation slide serves as a valuable indicator. Two major studies, one by the China CDC Epidemiology Team and another by Zheng, Wang, Zhou, et al., include more systematic official data on confirmed healthcare worker infections in January 2020.[24] I have excerpted the number of confirmed healthcare worker cases by date for the period of January 1–18, 2020 (Table 9.3).

WMHC Reticence on Medical Staff Infections

Many of these healthcare worker cases were initially diagnosed based on clinical symptoms and lung infections observed in computed tomographic (CT) scan images. Case confirmation through laboratory-based diagnostic testing was significantly delayed. However, as we have noted, the availability

Table 9.2 Known Medical Staff Infections in Wuhan Hospitals by Date of Disease Onset (as of Early February 2020)

Wuhan Municipal First Hospital, 2019-12-27
Hubei Provincial Hospital of Integrated Chinese and Western, 2020-01-01
Wuhan Red Cross Society Hospital, 2020-01-5
Wuhan Tongji Hospital, 2020-01-5
Wuhan University People's Hospital, 2020-01-10
Wuhan University Zhongnan Hospital, 2020-01-10
Wuhan Union Hospital, 2020-01-11
Hubei Provincial No. 3 People's Hospital, 2020-01-13
Wuhan Municipal No. 4 Hospital, 2020-01-14
Wuhan Municipal No. 3 Hospital, 2020-01-15
Wuhan Central Hospital, 2020-01-20

Source: China CDC presentation.

Table 9.3 Number of Lab-Confirmed Healthcare Worker COVID Cases in Wuhan, January 1–18, 2020

Date in January 2020	Number of healthcare worker cases	Date in January 2020	Number of healthcare worker cases
1	0	10	8
2	0	11	13
3	0	12	9
4	4	13	15
5	0	14	11
6	1	15	16
7	1	16	20
8	3	17	37
9	1	18	29

of laboratory testing capacity was primarily influenced by political and regulatory considerations when the number of cases was relatively small. Some leading hospitals in Wuhan managed to deploy limited laboratory testing capacity or utilize university-based research laboratories.

As Dr. Zhao Jianping of Tongji Hospital pointed out, the date of January 10, 2020, marked a significant turning point in Wuhan's epidemic situation regarding new symptomatic cases. According to the data in Table 9.3, the same was true for the number of healthcare worker infections. Even with the Huanan market exposure requirement of the inclusion–exclusion criteria, the number of healthcare workers exhibiting clinical symptoms was enough to raise concern among hospital administrators about in-hospital infections.

Health commission officials in Hubei and Wuhan possessed significantly more information about healthcare worker infections than they disclosed at the time. However, a subtle yet critical shift occurred in the WMHC updates, which largely went unnoticed. Up until January 11, 2020, the WMHC consistently stated that no medical staff had been identified as infected with VPUE or novel coronavirus pneumonia. Beginning on January 12 (data for January 11) and continuing through January 20, 2020, the WMHC updates no longer addressed the issue of medical staff infections.

It was not until 9 days later that the WMHC's silence on medical staff infections was recognized for what it truly was: the WMHC leadership had confirmation of cases of medical staff infections by January 11 at the latest, most likely following the round of diagnostic testing conducted on January 10, 2020.[25] As I shall relate in Chapter 10, Wuhan party secretary Ma Guoqiang publicly expressed regret for not having implemented decisive containment measures around January 12, 2020. On January 21, 2020, the WMHC finally disclosed on its Weibo social media account that 15 medical staff had been diagnosed with pneumonia caused by novel coronavirus infections, with one in critical condition.[26] This number, not surprisingly, was a significant understatement, as can be inferred from Table 9.3.

The Second Expert Team and the Management of Its Hospital Visits

The second NHC expert team members, however, were not given access to the information on healthcare worker infections that the provincial–municipal health leadership possessed at the time. Instead, the expert team received attention and care of a different kind from local authorities who viewed them as experts "coming from above." Representatives of the same interests that hindered the submission of suspected cases also selected the hospitals for site visits and briefed hospital administrators ahead of the team visits. They carefully chose the hospitals that the experts were taken to on closely chaperoned visits and limited the amount and type of information offered to the experts. It is a classic game that anyone familiar with inspections in China would recognize. What the hosts for the visiting experts did not realize was the magnitude of the stakes, not only for Wuhan but also for the entire world.

The second expert team visited six of Wuhan's major hospitals: Jinyintan Hospital, the center of treatment for patients infected with the novel coronavirus and the site of presentations and exchanges for other visitors, such as those from Taiwan and Hong Kong; Wuhan Pulmonary Hospital; Wuhan University People's Hospital (aka Hubei General Hospital); Wuhan Municipal No. 1 Hospital; Wuhan Union Hospital; and Wuhan Tongji Hospital.

In addition to the specialized Jinyintan and Pulmonary Hospitals, which were already designated for treating patients with novel coronavirus pneumonia, four other top hospitals with strong ties to the WMHC (Municipal No. 1 Hospital) and the HPHC (People's, Tongji, and Union) were included. Notably, both Tongji and Union are affiliated with the Huazhong University of Science and Technology (HUST) Tongji Medical School. It is worth noting that Ma Guoqiang (Wuhan party secretary), Zhang Jin and Liu Yingzi (party secretary and director general of HPHC, respectively), and Jiao Yahui (deputy director general of the NHC Department of Medical Administration) are all alumni of HUST/HUST Tongji Medical School.

Among the major hospitals not listed on the second NHC expert team itinerary, three are particularly noteworthy. The Wuhan Central Hospital, situated near the outbreak's epicenter, had fallen out of favor with Wuhan/Hubei health leadership due to doctors who shared outbreak information in late December 2019. The absence of the Hubei Provincial Hospital of Integrated Chinese and Western Medicine and Wuhan University Zhongnan Hospital from the itinerary is also of special interest.

Dr. Zhang Jixian and the Hubei Provincial Hospital of Integrated Chinese and Western Medicine

At the Hubei Provincial Hospital of Integrated Chinese and Western Medicine, located close to the outbreak's epicenter, Dr. Zhang Jixian played a crucial role in drawing the HPHC's and WMHC's attention to the VPUE cases. After the first group of patients was transferred to Jinyintan Hospital on December 29, 2019, new patients with similar symptoms continued to arrive at Dr. Zhang's respiratory section.[27] She was skeptical of the initial WMHC releases that dismissed the possibility of human-to-human transmission. When the WMHC enforced the inclusion–exclusion criteria, Dr. Zhang advocated for broadening the criteria to include screening of patients with clinical symptoms but no Huanan market exposure.[28] By the time the second expert team conducted hospital visits, the Radiology Section of Dr. Zhang's hospital had identified at least two medical staff members—one in respiratory medicine (January 6) and the other in neurology (January 11)—who exhibited ground glass opacities on their CT scans that were characteristic of patients with novel coronavirus infection in the lungs.[29]

Considering her significant role and expertise and the proximity of her hospital to the Huanan Seafood Market, Dr. Zhang Jixian would have been an ideal candidate for expert interviews. Unlike many other doctors in Wuhan who were intimidated by official injunctions, Dr. Zhang appeared irrepressible. However, it seemed as if the Hubei and Wuhan health authorities decided to keep Dr. Zhang out of sight during this period. None of the expert teams met or interviewed Dr. Zhang during their visits to Wuhan.[30] China CDC chief epidemiologist Zeng Guang did not learn of Dr. Zhang's name until long after his visit to Wuhan.[31]

If Dr. Zhang had been given the opportunity to meet with the visiting expert teams, she would likely have highlighted the increasing number of patients with similar clinical symptoms at her hospital. She would also likely have mentioned the first cluster of family members she had seen on December 26–27, 2019, a family cluster that had no connection to the Huanan market.[32]

When "people who lived near the Huanan Seafood Market had such symptoms, you say they are not [infected from other people]. That's impossible," she emphasized.[33] When later asked how she felt about authorities downplaying the risk of human-to-human transmission, Dr. Zhang responded, "Very anxious, extremely anxious, that is not the average anxious. The official line was that there was no human-to-human transmission, but that's really not the same as what I saw. How can one not be worried and anxious!"[34]

The Wuhan University Zhongnan Hospital

Wuhan University Zhongnan Hospital was the first to recognize the novel coronavirus's contagious nature at the hospital level and implemented strong preventive measures within the hospital. The Zhongnan Hospital leadership persistently attempted to alert and persuade provincial and municipal health leaders, including Vice Governor Yang Yanyun, about the outbreak's severity.[35] To emphasize the seriousness of their recommendations, the Zhongnan Hospital leadership invoked the joint party and administrative leadership conference mechanism to formally submit three reports and analyses on the prevention and control of novel coronavirus pneumonia to the provincial party leadership.[36] This left little doubt that the Zhongnan Hospital leadership wanted the Hubei and Wuhan leaders to understand the gravity of the situation and respond accordingly.

Had the second NHC expert team visited Zhongnan Hospital, it would likely have received an honest assessment. The Zhongnan Hospital leadership began holding daily meetings on epidemic response starting January 6, 2020, fostering an open atmosphere for sharing and assessing epidemic information. President Wang Xinghuan was forthright and risked his hospital presidency to speak the truth. Colleagues like ICU chief Peng Zhiyong were also unafraid to express their opinions. Dr. Yang Jiong, chief of Pulmonary and Critical Care Medicine, recalled, "If they had come to ask me, I would have certainly told them that the [outbreak] situation was very serious and there were already medical staff members who had become infected."[37]

The exclusion of three major hospitals that were known for their outspoken physicians and health administrators regarding the outbreak suggests a systematic effort to put on the itinerary hospitals that would adhere to the official stance of the Hubei/Wuhan provincial–municipal health leadership. For the hospitals selected for the expert team's itinerary, the Hubei–Wuhan health leadership contacted the hospital leaders to prepare for the NHC experts' visits. In response, most hospital leaders, following years of campaigns to enhance party leadership and promote political discipline, instinctively prioritized political considerations and confidentiality. At each hospital, senior WMHC staff and administrators, including a president or vice president and the Medical Affairs director, escorted the expert team members during their visits to the hospital complexes. In particular, the handlers and local experts that the expert team encountered were tight-lipped about the specifics of healthcare worker infections.

The Wall of Silence Surrounding Healthcare Worker Infections

The issue of nosocomial, or in-hospital, infections, particularly those involving medical staff, is a complex and sensitive topic for hospital administrators and doctors in China. Nosocomial infections play a significant role in the assessment and certification of hospitals, particularly comprehensive hospitals.[38] According to the Administrative Methods for Hospital Infection (2006), a strict responsibility system exists for nosocomial infections, complete with detailed regulations on reporting and response measures. If a hospital outbreak has five or more cases, causes a patient death, or injures three or more people, the outbreak must be reported to the NHC within 24 hours after a provincial investigation. Those responsible for the outbreak may face severe punishment, including demotion or even loss of professional licenses.[39]

In April 2019, following the deaths of five infants due to echovirus 11 at the Shunde Hospital of the Southern University of Medical Sciences, the Guangdong Provincial Health Commission revoked the hospital's 3A status and imposed sanctions on the hospital and the "responsible persons" of the municipal and district health commissions. In response to the Shunde incident, the NHC's Department of Medical Administration directed provincial health administrations to strengthen oversight of hospital infection prevention and control and to conduct reviews.[40] The HPHC, for example, adhered to the NHC directive by urging hospitals to prevent and control in-hospital infection.[41]

Because the NHC has given heightened attention to nosocomial infections, these infections are considered a significant threat to the reputation of hospitals, particularly highly rated ones. Following the loss of Shunde Hospital's 3A status, health commission officials, hospital administrators, and key medical staff got a strong reminder of the importance of focusing on in-hospital infection prevention and control.

There is a saying in regulation, "What gets measured, gets managed," which applies to both banking and hospital administration.[42] When the stakes are especially high and organizations such as health commissions and hospitals have much discretion and little public scrutiny, the leaders of these organizations have a strong temptation to not reveal problems such as serious in-hospital infections unless they must.

Looking back, members of the second expert team encountered a wall of silence regarding medical staff infections, maintained by health commission officials, hospital administrators, and doctors. Fears of sanctions against hospital infections, emphasis on political discipline, and repeated reminders to keep secrets following the crackdown on doctors in early January 2020 contributed to this silence. In such an environment, it would be unwise for hospital administrators and doctors in selected hospitals in Wuhan to disclose medical staff infections to visiting experts sent by the NHC. In response to the subsequent public outrage over their apparent failure to uncover medical staff infections, Dr. Wang Guangfa recalled, "The information we obtained at that time was 'NO.' Based on the materials we had [received], there were certainly no medical staff infections."[43]

During visits to fever clinics in five different hospitals (Jinyintan Hospital only accepted transfer patients), members of the second NHC expert team repeatedly inquired about medical staff infections. They were consistently told "there were none." They also pursued other leads: "When we heard there might be medical staff infected [with the coronavirus] at certain places, we made phone call after phone call to check, but in the end, we were told the information [we received] was not true."[44]

The Case of Dr. Lu Jun of Wuhan Tongji Hospital

Tongji Hospital is the primary institution of Dr. Zhao Jianping, leader of the Hubei provincial medical expert team. Dr. Zhao's respiratory section played a significant role in reporting initial cases and in preventing staff infections with the novel coronavirus beginning in late December 2019. In early January 2020, Tongji Hospital leadership followed the recommendation of Infection Section specialists to take decisive action against the so-called VPUE outbreak. They revived SARS procedures and mandated staff to wear N95 facemasks.[45] Therefore, when members of the second NHC expert team visited, they were not surprised to learn that Tongji had performed well. According to a member of the second team, "We visited Tongji Hospital after January 10, and the response we received at that time was that no medical staff had been infected."[46]

However, members of the second team also observed that doctors in Tongji's Respiratory and Emergency Sections seemed to have taken excessive protective measures. They not only wore N95 facemasks but also donned protective suits and goggles while making rounds to check on patients in the wards. One team member wondered if the Tongji doctors were overreacting since official rhetoric had only mentioned the possibility of limited human-to-human transmission.[47]

Approximately a week later, it was revealed that there had already been medical staff infections at Tongji Hospital when the expert team visited. The case of Dr. Lu Jun, a 31-year-old emergency medicine doctor, received enormous attention. Firstly, Lu Jun was diagnosed several days before the second expert team's visit and is known as the earliest laboratory-confirmed case of medical staff infection with the novel coronavirus. Secondly, Lu became critically ill and experienced respiratory failure. To dispel rumors of his death, Dr. Lu Jun later shared short video clips of himself recovering, garnering considerable sympathy and attention.[48] His resilience, survival, and recovery served as an inspiration for the infected, particularly front-line healthcare workers, during China's darkest weeks of the epidemic. However, Dr. Lu's case also indicated an organized effort to conceal his situation from the expert team.

Dr. Lu Jun worked the night shift on January 2, 2020. He saw approximately 30 patients, mostly feverish, that night and personally took pharyngeal swabs from over 10 patients for diagnostic tests. Some of these patients later tested positive for the novel coronavirus. Despite wearing an N95 facemask for protection, he became infected and developed a fever on the evening of January 5. He had never visited the Huanan Seafood Market.[49]

By January 7, Lu Jun's infection had spread to both lungs. He was placed in an isolation ward the previous day, making his case known to the hospital administration. In a later interview, Dr. Lu believed that he was infected with both influenza B and the novel coronavirus as of January 7. According to the Red Cross Society of China, with information from Tongji Hospital, Dr. Lu Jun's novel coronavirus infection was diagnosed on January 7, 2020, and later confirmed by nucleic acid testing.[50]

As Dr. Lu Jun's condition worsened, he was admitted to the respiratory ward of Tongji Hospital on January 10 and given supplemental oxygen, followed by ventilation.[51] He was in critical condition when transferred to Jinyintan Hospital on the evening of January 17.[52] The transfer to Jinyintan Hospital signified that Dr. Lu Jun's coronavirus infection was confirmed by a nucleic acid diagnostic test and arranged through the WMHC.

This overview of Dr. Lu Jun's treatment history in January reveals that his situation was well within the purview of his hospital section and the Tongji

Hospital administration. After Lu Jun began experiencing symptoms, medical staff at the Tongji Hospital fever clinic quickly elevated protection to Level II. This also prompted Dr. Zhao Jianping to establish a pulmonary and critical care medicine expert team within the hospital and implement stronger infection control measures.[53] As the leader of the Hubei provincial expert team for treatment of the so-called VPUE, Dr. Zhao led Dr. Lu Jun's treatment. Tongji Hospital's official commendation of Dr. Zhao Jianping also praised him for being vigilant about the possibility of human-to-human transmission from the beginning, saying that he "provided the most detailed, objective, and timely situation updates and suggestions to higher authorities," presumably the HPHC.[54]

Since Dr. Lu Jun's case had received significant attention in the respiratory and emergency medicine sections at Tongji Hospital, it is evident that leading physicians and hospital administrators of Tongji Hospital concealed Dr. Lu Jun's case from members of the second NHC expert team during its visit to Tongji Hospital and on other occasions when they interacted. When asked about the concealment later, Dr. Lu Jun deflected the question, saying, "we were all victims."[55]

The Union Hospital Cluster of Healthcare Worker Infections

Another destination on the second NHC expert team's itinerary was Union Hospital, which began providing outpatients with 24-hour access to a fever clinic in early January 2020, under the leadership of Dr. Yuan Li. The number of patients seen at the clinic quickly grew from around 50 on its first day to over 500 by January 10, 2020. Dr. Yuan recognized that "the situation was not right and that the epidemic was serious."[56]

Amid the rapidly increasing infections, Patient ZH underwent neurosurgery on January 7, 2020, at Union Hospital. The medical team did not take extra precautions because Patient ZH had no history of exposure to the Huanan market and was not considered an infection risk. However, Patient ZH developed a fever on January 11. Based on clinical symptoms, CT scan results, and diagnostic tests for various pathogens (as a test kit for the novel coronavirus was not yet available), Patient ZH was considered a suspected case of novel coronavirus pneumonia.

Suddenly, in the words of Dr. Zhao Hongxiang, chief of Neurosurgery, his section was plunged into "the darkest moment."[57] Medical staff who had participated in Patient ZH's operation began exhibiting fever and other symptoms on January 12. Due to Patient ZH's stay in four different wards before and after surgery, many individuals were exposed to him and considered close contacts.

The infection of Patient ZH raised alarm at Union Hospital. At the time, the novel coronavirus testing protocol was managed at the provincial level. Dr. Zhao Hongxiang and Union Hospital leadership acted quickly, given the circumstances, to secure testing for Patient ZH. On January 15, Patient ZH was confirmed to have contracted the novel coronavirus and was immediately transferred to Jinyintan Hospital.[58] This indicated that the Hubei provincial CDC, the HPHC, and the WMHC were not only informed but also directly involved in addressing the infection situation at Union Hospital.

News of staff infections at Union Hospital and other hospitals spread rapidly within the wider Wuhan medical community. Dr. Tong Jun, a professor at Tongji Medical School and chief physician at the Wuhan Mental Health Center, recalled her shock on January 15 upon learning of such infections and hearing that Jinyintan Hospital was full.[59] A passerby at Wuhan Central Hospital heard that several medical staff members at Union Hospital had been infected with novel coronavirus pneumonia around this time.[60]

Mr. Q, a diagnostic test manufacturer's salesperson, learned on January 15, 2020, from a former colleague that several Union Hospital doctors had contracted the unusual pneumonia; one of them was in serious condition and on a ventilator. He was also informed that Jinyintan Hospital staff had been infected even earlier. Mr. Q went to Union Hospital the following morning to investigate the situation. He was struck that staff of the Infection Section wore protective suits. He described the scene as "a sight [he] had never seen in his ten-plus years in Wuhan."[61] Mr. Q's intelligence proved valuable for his company, which later developed its own diagnostic test kits for the novel coronavirus.

For Dr. Zhao Hongxiang of the Union Hospital, the crisis in his section was far from over. Even though the medical staff exposed to Patient ZH displayed symptoms such as fever and ground glass opacities on their CT scans, they were not quarantined due to the absence of diagnostic testing for novel coronavirus infection. "The longer this situation persisted, the more people would get infected," Dr. Zhao observed.[62] For several more days, Dr. Zhao and the Union Hospital leadership struggled to secure testing for medical staff members at a time when such testing was incredibly challenging to arrange.[63]

Conclusion

In attempting to understand the challenges faced by the second NHC expert team in pushing for better information disclosure and verifying cases of medical staff infections, we gain a particularly sharp insight into the political and institutional dynamics of epidemic information manipulation and concealment during the weeks leading up to the Wuhan lockdown.

During the second expert team's visit to Wuhan, there were multiple cases and clusters of medical staff infections caused by the novel coronavirus. Even with the limited information that has become publicly available, it is evident that the health and political leadership in Wuhan and Hubei had more substantial information about the outbreak's risks at that time. However, within the confines of party-state dominance and fragmented authoritarianism, the intricate web of political and organizational interests that hindered the reporting of suspected cases also prevented local officials, hospital administrators, medical experts, and even infected doctors from confirming medical staff infections to the external expert team members.

While even passersby on the streets in Wuhan heard of medical staff infections, the authorities in Hubei/Wuhan were nonetheless able to maintain a wall of silence around medical staff infections. As an anonymous member of the second expert team stated, they "didn't tell us the real situation." In an apparent reference to Zhang Jin, party secretary of the HPHC, this team member added, "From what we now know of the real situation, [he] was lying [to us]."[64] Many days after the Wuhan lockdown, a member of the second expert team received a phone call from a doctor in Wuhan. The doctor "admitted that he did not tell the truth to the expert team at the time [of their visit]. [He was] clearly infected with the virus but did not admit that he was."[65] All available evidence implies that the doctor infected with the virus was likely pressured to conceal his condition from members of the second expert team.

During an impassioned online discussion on a forum of HUST alumni, one speaker noted that HUST alumni were among the most influential groups in health and politics in the city of Wuhan and Hubei Province. The speaker then asked, "Didn't they know the virus could be spread from person to person when staff of an entire department had fallen sick? Why didn't they tell the truth?" He subsequently answered, "They didn't dare!"[66]

The repercussions of obstructing and concealing information about epidemic infections are universally understood. As Dr. Wang Chen, the president of Peking Union Medical College and the Chinese Academy of Medical Sciences, succinctly stated, "The key to handling infectious diseases lies in maintaining openness and transparency, rather than adopting an ostrich-like approach. An abscess left untreated can escalate into sepsis."[67] Regrettably, despite the worsening crisis, the emergency response to the novel coronavirus outbreak remained veiled in secrecy through January 19, 2020.

10 Conducting Public Health Emergency Response in Stealth

In retrospect, the time frame during which the second National Health Commission (NHC) expert team visited Wuhan (January 8–16) presented another crucial opportunity for authorities to implement more robust public health emergency measures. While members of the second expert team independently attempted to verify cases of medical staff infections, cases of novel coronavirus infections were identified not only outside Wuhan/Hubei but also outside China. After an overview of the national and provincial environment, this chapter turns to the emergence of new cases beyond Wuhan's borders, specifically in Beijing, Guangdong, and Thailand. These cases spurred the NHC leadership to advocate for stronger prevention and control (*fangkong*) measures. However, contrary to the China Centers for Disease Control and Prevention's (China CDC's) later assertions, neither the NHC nor the Wuhan/Hubei authorities were willing or able to execute a proactive public strategy to tackle the outbreak during this critical period of rapid virus transmission from Wuhan.

Adhering to the principle of avoiding social panic, the Hubei/Wuhan authorities continued to emphasize the low risk of sustained human-to-human transmission, striving to maintain normalcy in Wuhan. The NHC adopted a cautious "hope for the best, but monitor, wait and see" approach. They convened a confidential national meeting of provincial health commission leaders to enhance surveillance and issued the first edition of the NHC *fangkong* documents on novel coronavirus pneumonia. This edition expanded the case definition beyond those exposed to the Huanan market.

Within 3 days after distributing the first-edition *fangkong* documents, the NHC received significant new information on the further spread of the novel coronavirus, including compelling evidence of human-to-human transmission in a familial cluster in Shenzhen, Guangdong. This revelation prompted the NHC to further update the *fangkong* documents, acknowledging the coronavirus's continued propagation. Regaining its *fangkong* focus and invigorated, the NHC leadership assembled a third expert group, spearheaded by the esteemed 83-year-old Dr. Zhong Nanshan, to embark on an emergency visit to Wuhan.

Novel Coronavirus Cases outside Hubei and Changing Perceptions of the Epidemic Situation

In previous discussions, I emphasized the strong motivation of political leaders to create the "right" atmosphere during the "two sessions" season for both Wuhan and Hubei. As the Lunar New Year (January 25, 2020) approached, coinciding with the peak holiday travel period, the national leadership participated in a series of high-profile meetings to conclude a busy year. Unless absolutely necessary, national and local officials, including those from Hubei and the NHC, were reluctant to make announcements or implement measures that could disrupt the prevailing atmosphere of peace and prosperity.

Xi Jinping concluded his 6-month-long (Communist) Party Education Campaign on Aspiration and Mission with a prominent meeting on January 8, 2020. He presented the National Science and Technology Awards on January 10 and delivered the opening speech on January 13 at the plenary meeting of the Central Discipline Inspection Commission, the Communist Party's discipline and anti-corruption arm. Also on January 13, Premier Li Keqiang convened the State Council Plenary Meeting to review the draft *Government Work Report* he would present at the annual plenary session of the National People's Congress, scheduled for early March at the time. Li Keqiang emphasized that 2020 was the year for "realizing the goal of fully building a moderately prosperous society" in China and urged all localities and government departments to "strive for a successful start in economic and social development in the first quarter."[1] Furthermore, after enduring a challenging and prolonged trade war, China was finally poised to sign a Phase 1 trade agreement with the United States on January 16, 2020 (January 15 in the United States).

Amid this national atmosphere and the ongoing "two sessions" in Hubei/Wuhan, the period from January 10 to 12 emerged as a crucial turning point in understanding and managing the outbreak. After the official confirmation of the novel coronavirus, Wuhan/Hubei authorities received updates on the virus and the potential risks associated with it. On January 12, 2020, the Wuhan Municipal Health Commission (WMHC), under the NHC's guidance, finally adopted the term "pneumonia caused by novel coronavirus" to replace the previous designation of viral pneumonia of uncertain etiology (VPUE).

Simultaneously, as noted in the previous chapters, there was a significant surge in the number of fever clinic outpatients in Wuhan-area hospitals, accompanied by the emergence of medical staff infections exhibiting clinical symptoms. Adding to these developments, the identification of a new case in Thailand, along with the appearance of suspected cases in Beijing and other parts of China around the same time, prompted the health leadership to abandon their previous complacency.

The Undisclosed Novel Coronavirus Cases in Beijing and Jiangsu

During this period, suspected novel coronavirus cases were identified beyond Hubei Province within China. Individuals suspected of having the virus were isolated on January 10 in Jiangsu and on January 12 in Beijing; however, these cases were not publicly revealed until January 20 or later.[2] Remarkably, on December 31, 2019, the Jiangsu Provincial Health Commission instructed subprovincial CDCs in the province to screen PUE cases using influenza and pan-coronavirus nucleic acid test kits.[3]

The situation in Beijing, a city that experienced the devastating effects of severe acute respiratory syndrome (SARS) in 2003, was particularly concerning for public health officials. The Beijing Municipal Health Commission (BMHC) and municipal leaders closely monitored the developments in Wuhan from the outset. They also had access to valuable information through the experts who traveled to Wuhan from Beijing-area hospitals and the China CDC. For instance, both Feng Zijian and Li Qun of the China CDC were also team leaders of the Beijing Municipal Health Emergency Expert Advisory Committee.[4]

Upon the official verification of the novel coronavirus, the BMHC initiated its health emergency response plan. The commission instructed medical institutions to monitor and report patients exhibiting fever, cough, and other symptoms. It also designated three hospitals as specialized facilities for treating patients suspected of having novel coronavirus infections.[5] Qinghua Changgeng Hospital's leadership distributed PUE screening protocols on January 6 and established a novel coronavirus control leading group on January 13, 2020.[6]

Beijing Ditan Hospital, which had two doctors on the first and second NHC expert teams sent to Wuhan, was one of the designated hospitals. Its intensive care unit (ICU) was prepared when the first two suspected cases, a married couple, were transferred there on January 12, 2020.[7] The pair had attended a wedding reception in Wuhan around January 7–9 but had no exposure to the Huanan Seafood Market.[8] Three more patients, including two men who visited Wuhan briefly on January 7 and 9 and an elderly woman visiting from Wuhan, began displaying symptoms on January 13–14.[9]

Although Beijing authorities refrained from publicly announcing these cases, specific neighborhood communities in the city were discreetly alerted. For instance, Dr. Wu Hao, director of the Fangzhuang Community Health Service Center in Beijing, activated the joint control mechanism with the Fangzhuang Neighborhood Office in mid-January 2020. This put work teams in Fangzhuang on active surveillance for close contacts and suspected cases.[10]

The Wuhan Tourist Case in Thailand and World Health Organization Pressure: A Turning Point

While the official word out of Wuhan remained comforting, the national health leadership felt the pressure mounting from a source that had caused alarm in Beijing during the 2003 SARS crisis—the World Health Organization (WHO).[11] On January 8, 2020, a tourist from Wuhan was hospitalized with a fever near Bangkok. Using the genomic sequence of the novel coronavirus released by Zhang Yongzhen's team, researchers in the Thai Red Cross Emerging Infectious Diseases Health Science Center at Chulalongkorn University in Bangkok swiftly developed their own test kit. They confirmed the patient's infection with the novel coronavirus on January 12, with the result verified in the Department of Medical Science laboratory.[12]

Despite the NHC and Wuhan/Hubei health administrations' failure to update the diagnostic criteria for novel coronavirus infections, the WHO issued an interim guidance for surveillance, including a "surveillance case definition," on January 11, 2020. This guidance emphasized that the primary objective of the surveillance effort was to detect "any evidence of amplified or sustained human-to-human transmission," rather than confirming preexisting assumptions. The WHO guidance included in its case definition consideration of "history of travel to Wuhan, Hubei Province, China in the 14 days prior to symptom onset."[13]

After identifying the case of novel coronavirus infection in the traveler from Wuhan, the Thai government promptly informed the WHO, effectively breaking the testing and surveillance deadlock in China.[14] The WHO announced on January 13 that the case identified in Thailand confirmed its earlier concerns about the virus spreading beyond China. The organization also revealed that its director-general, Dr. Tedros Adhanom Ghebreyesus, had consulted with its Emergency Committee members.[15] This statement signaled an escalation in international concern for China's health leaders.[16]

China quickly conducted epidemiological investigations on the case identified in Thailand and provided the findings to the WHO.[17] A daily digest from the China CDC recorded that, according to the WHO, the patient in Thailand had no exposure to the Huanan Seafood Market but had visited another market.[18] China CDC representatives also participated in a teleconference on novel coronavirus cases as convened by the WHO diagnostics and laboratories global expert network.

As previously mentioned, several VPUE cases in Wuhan with no history of exposure to the Huanan market were reported to local CDCs in late December 2019 and early January 2020. However, their significance was largely overlooked for almost 2 weeks. Discussions about the case in Thailand, combined with inquiries from Taiwanese visitors, seemed to suddenly draw attention to the significance of cases not connected to the Huanan Seafood Market. On January 14, for example, China CDC staff participating in the daily situation assessment discussed the need to revise the risk level if the patient in Thailand had no connection to a chain of transmission in Wuhan.[19] On January 15, 2020, the China CDC raised its emergency response level to Level I, the highest, but did not inform the public.

Stalemate between NHC and Hubei/Wuhan Leadership amid Growing Outbreak Concerns

As the number of indications grew that the outbreak had not been contained and instead threatened to spread far and wide, national health leaders called for a more robust response. Minister Ma Xiaowei and others, who vividly remembered the intense international pressure during the SARS crisis, found the case in Thailand particularly alarming.

However, the reality was that Wuhan and Hubei leaders were preoccupied with the provincial "two sessions" and did not perceive the epidemic as a serious issue. Even after the conclusion of the "two sessions," Hubei Provincial Party Secretary Jiang Chaoliang continued to treat the novel coronavirus outbreak as a non-event for almost another week (until January 21).[20] In light of this, the NHC leadership sought support from the national government.

On January 13, 2020, during the State Council Plenary Meeting, Premier Li Keqiang "laid out his requirements" for the prevention and control of the epidemic outbreak in Wuhan.[21] Backed by the State Council leadership, the NHC leadership held a meeting on the same day to "deploy and guide" (部署指导),

i.e., encourage Hubei and Wuhan authorities to "further strengthen control measures."[22] Wuhan leaders were urged to "enhance temperature surveillance at ports of entry and transport hubs, and reduce crowd gatherings."[23]

It is difficult to overlook the sense of urgency in the NHC leadership's communications with the Wuhan and Hubei authorities. However, based on the information published about the following day's meeting, the NHC leadership hoped that the local authorities would take even more decisive action.

The Confidential National Teleconference on January 14 and the Initiation of Nationwide Surveillance

The emergence of cases in Thailand, Beijing, and other locations outside of Wuhan and Hubei compelled Chinese health leaders to address the novel coronavirus outbreak as both a national and an international concern. In addition to the January 13 meeting with Wuhan and Hubei authorities, the NHC leadership organized a national working teleconference on novel coronavirus pneumonia prevention and control on January 14. During the conference, Minister Ma Xiaowei addressed health commission leaders from provinces and major cities, discussing the considerable uncertainty surrounding the Wuhan situation. He emphasized that the case in Thailand signified an "important change in the epidemic prevention and control situation" and warned that "the spread of the epidemic could increase significantly, especially during the Lunar New Year travel season."[24] Ma's experience with the SARS crisis, which saw cases outside of mainland China dramatically alter the epidemic's trajectory, made him more aware than most participants of the implications of identifying Wuhan-connected novel coronavirus patients beyond China's borders.

Citing support from General Secretary Xi Jinping, Premier Li Keqiang, and Vice Premier Sun Chunlan, Minister Ma urged Hubei Province and Wuhan city to implement strict control measures, including

> focus on strengthening the control of farmers' markets; strengthen the control of individuals with fever by establishing and bolstering body temperature monitoring and fever clinic diagnosis and screening as two lines of defense; improve crowd management, reduce large public gathering activities, and advise patients with fever not to leave Wuhan; improve patient treatment, strengthen the management of close contacts, implement the most stringent measures to contain the epidemic locally, and do our utmost to prevent epidemic spread in Wuhan.[25]

The January 14 meeting marked the beginning of a national initiative urging health leaders in provinces and major cities outside Hubei to concentrate on the outbreak, activate local surveillance and detection mechanisms, and prepare to "effectively deal with possible new outbreaks promptly."[26] Minister Ma asked health leaders across the country to prioritize epidemic prevention and control in the interest of "protecting people's health, maintaining social stability, and safeguarding national public health security."[27] In essence, he advised them to be prepared but not to publicize their efforts. The national teleconference itself was convened confidentially and only disclosed weeks later when the NHC leadership sought recognition for having convened such a preparatory conference.[28]

Minister Ma Xiaowei's remarks align well with Wuhan party secretary Ma Guoqiang's admission that he regretted not intervening more decisively around January 12. Although Minister Ma advocated for the timely and transparent release of information, he simultaneously emphasized "avoiding causing panic sentiments among the public."[29] According to informed sources, Guan Xuhua from the Hubei CDC was during the conference among the last to speak to CDC officials from across the country, providing on-the-ground information. Guan, who had recognized the risks of community spread by that point, went beyond her assigned task of providing information, warning that the risks from the outbreak were real and that "many lives were at stake."[30]

The First Edition of NHC Novel Coronavirus Prevention and Control Documents and Disease Surveillance

Prior to the confidential teleconference on January 14 and immediately after, experts, particularly members of the first and second NHC expert teams, worked urgently with NHC staff support to update or create a set of prevention and control documents for novel coronavirus pneumonia.[31] The 63-page document set included the updated Diagnosis and Treatment Protocol for Novel Coronavirus Pneumonia, the Protocol for the Prevention and Control of the Novel Coronavirus Pneumonia Epidemic (covering surveillance, epidemiological investigations, management of close contacts, and laboratory testing), Requirements for Strengthening Pre-Check-in Triage and Fever Clinic Work, Procedures for Confirming the First Case of Pneumonia Caused by Novel Coronavirus Infection, and Requirements for Prevention and Control of Hospital Infections and Protection of Medical Staff. As these documents were frequently updated in the following weeks and months, this initial set of prevention and control documents for novel coronavirus pneumonia became known as the "first edition," although it was never officially released.[32]

On January 15, the day after the teleconference, the NHC provided this document set to province-level health commissions using the highest level of urgency classification, *teti* (特提), which mandates immediate attention and action within 5 hours of reception. The documents were marked "for internal working use, not to be circulated on the internet."

In line with the January 11 WHO surveillance case definition, the January 15 NHC documents revised the case definition for novel coronavirus pneumonia. In the updated definition, a patient could be considered a suspect or "observation case" for further diagnostic testing if they exhibited the previously discussed clinical symptoms and had traveled to Wuhan within 2 weeks of disease onset or had direct or indirect exposure to Wuhan markets. This revision expanded the population subject to surveillance from those who had direct exposure to the Huanan Seafood Market to the entire population of Wuhan and those who had recently visited the city. The change acknowledged that, as the case in Thailand demonstrated, the initial outbreak had spread within and beyond Wuhan. For Wuhan, this broadening of diagnostic criteria allowed for the inclusion of many more clinical cases that lacked a history of exposure to the Huanan market. Notably, the January 15 documents also required that observation or suspected cases be reported within 2 hours by medical institutions using the National Notifiable Diseases Surveillance System under the category for PUE, pending confirmation through diagnostic tests. However, this stipulation was largely disregarded in Wuhan in the following week.

The January 15 documents outlined in Annex 4 the procedures for determining the first novel coronavirus cases in provinces other than Hubei. Once a province identified a suspected case, the provincial CDC was required to obtain the coronavirus's whole genome and conduct a preliminary comparison with the whole genome of the novel coronavirus from Wuhan. If the genomes were highly similar, the China CDC would then be asked to review the case. Finally, a diagnosis expert panel organized by the NHC Leading Group would make the final determination based on laboratory test results, clinical symptoms, and epidemiological history. If the expert panel concluded that the case was a novel coronavirus pneumonia case, the NHC could then authorize the provincial health commission to publicly disclose the case.[33]

Thus, as the NHC authorized the distribution of small batches of diagnostic tests for the novel coronavirus to provincial CDCs across the country, it simultaneously established a process for case verification and disclosure that put the NHC in control of how the information would be released in the provinces. In other words, provincial health commissions could not announce their first cases without the NHC's express authorization, thereby allowing the NHC to control the pace of the public disclosures. For example, the cases in Beijing and Jiangsu were not disclosed to the public until January 20 and 23, 2020.

Maintaining Wuhan's Calm Appearance

The day following the NHC national teleconference, Minister Ma Xiaowei personally visited Wuhan to guide Hubei and Wuhan in implementing various containment measures. These included installing infrared temperature monitors at transportation hubs to screen travelers leaving Wuhan and managing and limiting mass gatherings.[34] By this time, the Hubei Provincial CDC team, led by Dr. Guan Xuhua, was already warning, through internal channels, of community transmission of the novel coronavirus outside Wuhan.[35] An informed source revealed that Dr. Guan had made an unauthorized trip to Huanggang, where she identified a family cluster demonstrating clear human-to-human transmission.

Despite the infrared thermometers at airports and other transportation hubs, there was minimal indication that the NHC national teleconference or Minister Ma's discreet visit to Wuhan significantly impacted the city.[36] Usually, there would be reports of Minister Ma Xiaowei's provincial visits, but neither Hubei nor the NHC immediately reported on this trip.[37] Wuhan and Hubei officials seemed intent on avoiding public warnings about the novel coronavirus, fearing it would cause social panic and disrupt the ongoing peak Lunar New Year travel season. Markets bustled with shoppers purchasing farm produce and other goods.

For the general public, the day's headline news on the outbreak was the statement from the WMHC question-and-answer that "the risk of sustained human-to-human transmission is low."[38] Most people overlooked the subtle warning in the WMHC statement that "limited human-to-human transmission cannot be ruled out."[39] In a January 15 interview with *News 1+1* of China Central Television, Li Qun of the China CDC (not Li Gang of the Wuhan CDC) initially echoed the official stance that the novel coronavirus's illness severity was low. However, when asked about the "low risk" assessment, he advised the public not to focus on the official wording but to take personal protective measures to prevent infection. Unfortunately, Li Qun's message about responsible behavior was overshadowed by the self-congratulatory tone of the television program lauding China's outbreak response.[40]

On January 17, 2020, the Hubei "two sessions" concluded, and Hubei provincial health leaders held a confidential video conference of health officials and experts from across the province to discuss updates on containment efforts for the novel coronavirus pneumonia. They learned that dozens of unusual pneumonia cases were being treated in two leading hospitals in Huanggang municipality (population six million), bordering Wuhan. However, diagnostic capabilities were lacking in Huanggang.[41] A retrospective study dated January 17 as a tipping point of the epidemic, when the number of confirmed cases outside Wuhan began to surpass that for Wuhan.[42] At the Hubei Provincial Health Work Conference the following day, Party Secretary Zhang Jin of the Hubei Provincial Health Commission stated that the containment of novel coronavirus pneumonia was the top priority of the provincial health system.[43]

Despite Zhang's internal statement, a sense of normalcy prevailed in Wuhan outside of hospital ICUs and respiratory wards. The Institute of Safety Evaluation of the Hubei Provincial CDC held its Lunar New Year gatherings as planned on January 15.[44] An infectious disease expert at a leading Wuhan hospital recalled a relaxed atmosphere at a Lunar New Year gathering on January 17. This expert traveled from Wuhan to Guangdong on January 18 without noticing any significant differences at the airport.[45] Professor Linfa Wang from Singapore was part of a scientific gathering of researchers on bat-borne viruses at the Wuhan Institute of Virology from January 14 to 18, 2020. He remembered that scientists dined at restaurants and took no additional precautions. However, for his return flight to Singapore, he had his temperature checked three times before boarding because Singapore had implemented temperature screening for passengers coming from Wuhan in early January 2020.[46]

Wuhan authorities showcased high-profile events and programs to demonstrate that everything was under control in the city. The Culture and Tourism Bureau announced that residents could apply for 200,000 free passes to visit landmark sites such as the Yellow Crane Tower.[47] A particularly noteworthy event was the 20th annual Ten Thousand Family community feast held at the Baibuting Community, which boasted over 110,000 residents (plus more than 60,000 non-residents during normal times) and was located about 6 miles from the Huanan Seafood Market. Although some community staff suggested postponing or canceling the feast as early as January 15, it proceeded as planned on January 18, coinciding with offerings to the kitchen god ahead of the Lunar New Year.[48] The event attracted more than 40,000 families and over 100,000 participants across one main venue and nine branch venues.[49]

Upon receiving the second edition of the NHC documents on January 18 and learning that a high-profile expert team was en route to Wuhan, the city's health leadership went into self-defensive blame avoidance mode and made a last-ditch effort to defend Wuhan's anti-epidemic record. In the wee hours of January 19, the WMHC released interviews with Vice Mayor Chen Xiexin, Wuhan CDC director Li Gang, and Dr. Huang Chaolin. Despite the increasing number of cases and their awareness of medical staff infections, Chen and Li maintained that there was little cause for concern. Chen Xiexin boasted that Wuhan "has built a multi-level joint-action mechanism, formed a strong task force, quickly responded to and dealt with the epidemic, and made every effort to treat patients and prevent the spread of the epidemic."[50] Li Gang reiterated the reassuring message that many had taken as a guarantee of safety:

> Considering all factors, our initial impression of this outbreak is that the infectivity of the novel coronavirus is not strong. While the possibility of limited human-to-human transmission cannot be ruled out, the risk of sustained human-to-human transmission is low. With the implementation of various prevention and control measures, this outbreak is preventable and controllable.[51]

The NHC Refocuses on Stewarding National Health

While the NHC and Wuhan/Hubei authorities faced a deadlock, the NHC leadership received vital new data, including insights from the second NHC expert team, compelling evidence from Guangdong, and the identification of new cases internationally. Before discussing these significant developments, it is crucial to acknowledge that the NHC's regained focus on its stewardship role was partly due to the expanding scope of front-line activities undertaken by the NHC working team in Wuhan.

During the time the second expert team was in Wuhan, various division directors and staff members from the NHC joined the NHC front-line working team there. Jiao Zhenquan and his colleagues from the NHC Bureau of Disease Prevention and Control visited municipal and district CDCs, hospitals, train stations, communities, and other locations. They also "attended working meetings of the local authorities and regular meetings of the prevention and control team."[52]

Li Dachuan, director of the Medical Management Division, and Ma Xudong, deputy director of the Medical Quality and Assessment Division, both from the NHC Medical Administration Bureau, arrived in Wuhan on January 12. They spent considerable time visiting key hospitals, with Ma Xudong focusing on fever clinics in various facilities. While providing expert staffing, Ma Xudong also interacted with medical staff and patients. Following these visits, he helped Wuhan implement a mechanism to put together the total number of outpatients visiting fever clinics in over 60 hospitals each day. In mid-January, the number of such outpatient visits increased from 1,600 per day to approximately 5,000 per day in about a week's time.[53] For context, this figure would surpass 13,000 on January 22.[54] In retrospect, the number of outpatients visiting fever clinics was a critical indicator of epidemic spread.

Li Dachuan played a valuable role in helping to secure resources for treating the growing number of severely ill patients at Jinyintan Hospital. Through his visits and consultations with medical staff, he "guided" Jinyintan Hospital in reconfiguring ward layouts and transforming three floors of wards into ICU wards. Meanwhile, he steered the Hubei Provincial Health Commission to have the Tongji and Union Hospitals and People's Hospital to assume responsibility for these three ICU wards (S5–7) on January 15.[55]

The involvement of Li Dachuan, Ma Xudong, and others in these crucial developments provided them and their superiors with a more accurate understanding of the situation in hospitals and fever clinics. Consequently, they supplied the NHC leadership with essential information on the escalating outbreak in Wuhan, even though the official number of confirmed cases remained at 41.

The Assessment of the Second NHC Expert Team

Members of the second NHC expert team returned from Wuhan and met with NHC officials on January 16 to assess the epidemic situation. Although the team could not verify cases of medical staff infections in Wuhan, they gathered substantial information during their visits to fever clinics and emergency rooms in hospitals. The team unanimously agreed that the Hubei and Wuhan authorities were "underestimating the epidemic."[56]

After his January 10 interview with Xinhua, Dr. Wang Guangfa of Peking University First Hospital risked exposure by visiting crowded fever clinics and emergency rooms and checking on patients.[57] He observed many patients with fevers and other symptoms were visiting fever clinics with minimal protection, raising concerns that these clinics could become centers for new infections. After reviewing patients' computed tomographic scans, he recognized similarities with novel coronavirus infections. Dr. Wang felt that the situation was reminiscent of the 2003 SARS crisis. On January 16, he assessed the epidemic as "fairly serious" and the situation as "very NOT optimistic."[58]

Dr. Wang later expressed frustration over the China CDC's failure to share information.[59] However, he noted that approximately 13 of the 41 officially confirmed novel coronavirus cases had no exposure to the Huanan Seafood Market, an issue that Chinese CDC epidemiologists had mishandled thus far.[60] Consequently, there was either human-to-human transmission beyond the Huanan market or other sources of infection. Unfortunately, even thogh he had put on N95 facemasks and taken other precautions during his hospital visits in Wuhan, Dr. Wang himself contracted the coronavirus during his Wuhan trip and began showing clinical symptoms on the evening of January 16.[61]

At the meeting, some team members were more cautious about pushing the underestimation assessment to its limits and making recommendations for action. Not Dr. Wang Guangfa. Utilizing a rough estimate, Wang made a compelling assessment of the outbreak's scale, overcoming some hesitancy from fellow team members. He noted that Thailand identified its first case among approximately 11,000 passengers from Wuhan. Assuming one in 20,000 people in Wuhan was infected with the novel coronavirus and the city's population was only eight million (rather than the official figure of over 10 million), there would still be about 400 cases in Wuhan, roughly 10 times the officially announced number of 41 cases.[62] Using the ratio of 1 out of 11,000 multiplied by Wuhan's official population, the estimate would rise to just under 1,000. This figure was close to the estimate made by a research team at Imperial College London, which the China CDC was aware of.[63]

Alarm Bells from Guangdong: A Familial Cluster of Infections

At this juncture, the findings about a familial cluster of infections and the intellectual leadership from Dr. Yuen Kwok-yung and Dr. Zhong Nanshan became particularly significant.

The extended family at the center of attention resided in Shenzhen. The family consisted of a couple (husband H and wife W), their two children (son and daughter), the wife's parents (WF and WM), and the husband's mother (HM). Between December 29, 2019, and January 4, 2020, all family members, except for HM, visited Wuhan to see relatives. Upon returning from Wuhan, the family members began to exhibit fever and other symptoms, and they were subsequently diagnosed with novel coronavirus infections.

HM, the 63-year-old mother of H, was the first to seek medical attention, from Dr. Li Tianhao, a general practitioner at the Xueyuan Community Health Center of Shenzhen Traditional Chinese Medicine Hospital.[64] Owing to the heightened infectious disease preparedness in Guangdong and Dr. Li's vigilance, the situation involving the extended family garnered attention from the hospital and then the district and municipal CDCs.[65] After contact tracing and testing, family members who had also developed symptoms sought treatment at the University of Hong Kong-Shenzhen Hospital (HKU-SZH) on January 10, 2020.[66]

Professor Yuen Kwok-yung of the University of Hong Kong, a leading expert on infectious diseases including coronaviruses, also supervises the Microbiology and Infection Control Section of HKU-SZH. Using a test kit developed in Yuen's lab, his team was able to confirm on January 12 that the patients were infected with the novel coronavirus.[67] Contrasting with the reassuring updates from the WMHC, the Yuen team was initially in disbelief: "When the first test was positive, [we] didn't dare to believe it at the time, and did the testing again. But by January 12, we thought the [positive result] was real," Yuen recalled.[68]

In accordance with Shenzhen's prevention and control protocols, suspected cases of novel coronavirus infections were transferred to Shenzhen No. 3 People's Hospital, the designated facility. Teams from the Shenzhen No. 3 People's Hospital, the Shenzhen Municipal CDC, and the Guangdong Provincial CDC swiftly mobilized to conduct their own diagnostic tests and investigations.

The research staff at Shenzhen No. 3 People's Hospital began testing for the novel coronavirus without waiting for authorization or the availability of China CDC–authorized diagnostic test kits. They utilized the published genomic sequences of the novel coronavirus to create primers and probes for their own diagnostic test kit. In the early hours of January 14, a sample taken from Patient WF tested positive for the novel coronavirus.[69]

Interestingly, later on the same day of January 14, the Shenzhen Municipal CDC used a newly received China CDC–allocated test kit to verify the diagnostic results. This development raises questions about Wuhan's claims regarding test kit availability. On the same day, just before midnight, the Guangdong Provincial CDC laboratory confirmed the results using genomic sequencing. The sample from Patient WF was then sent to the China CDC for reconfirmation and final determination by an NHC expert panel.[70]

Subsequent tests, investigations, and consultations were conducted on all members of the extended family. The investigations in Shenzhen by specialists from the provincial, municipal, and district CDCs, as well as HKU-SZH, focused on the significance of Patient HM, who had not traveled to Wuhan but had tested positive for the novel coronavirus. Despite official WMHC updates repeatedly stating that no human-to-human transmission had been discovered, the HM case was proof positive of human-to-human transmission. The discovery was both a eureka moment and a cause for alarm. This revelation coincided with the distribution of the first edition NHC documents on January 15. That evening, the Shenzhen municipal leadership activated its "joint prevention and control mechanism" for major infectious diseases.[71]

Enter Dr. Zhong Nanshan and Dr. Yuen Kwok-yung

The Guangdong provincial leadership was keenly engaged and sought advice and leadership from Dr. Zhong Nanshan. As the director of the Guangzhou Institute of Respiratory Diseases, Dr. Zhong played a crucial role in helping Guangdong manage the SARS crisis in 2003, not only in treatment but also in initial outbreak response, in disease identification, and in reaching out to the public. He was greatly admired for his courage and political astuteness as he resisted misguided directions from Beijing and refused to downplay the severity of the epidemic when SARS intensified in Beijing. Following the SARS crisis, he was honored with the presidency of the Chinese Medical Association (2005–2009), a position previously held by either current or former health ministers since 1989. Seventeen years after SARS, the 83-year-old Dr. Zhong continued to be active on the front lines of clinical practice. A strong athlete in his youth, he looked 20 years younger with his hair dyed black.

On January 16, 2020, Dr. Zhong Nanshan discussed details of patients with novel coronavirus infections with Dr. Liu Lei, president of the Shenzhen No. 3 People's Hospital.[72] He then joined members of the Guangdong provincial leadership, most likely Vice Governor Zhang Guangjun, for briefings at the Guangdong Provincial CDC. While Hubei leaders were preoccupied with their annual "two sessions," the Guangdong provincial leadership relied on their SARS response experience and established a provincial leading group and an expert group for novel coronavirus epidemic control.[73] Dr. Zhong headed the expert advisory team.

The next morning (January 17), Dr. Zhong, accompanied by Guangdong vice governor Zhang Guangjun and Duan Yufei, the head of the Guangdong Provincial Health Commission, traveled to Shenzhen and visited the Shenzhen No. 3 People's Hospital to see patients and review the situation. He praised Shenzhen's efforts in patient care and infection prevention.[74] Concurrently, Guangdong Provincial CDC researchers obtained the whole coronavirus genome and compared it with the published genome from Wuhan.[75] The observation of clinical symptoms and the genomic analysis results provided evidence for Dr. Zhong and the Guangdong CDC that the patients in Shenzhen had contracted the same virus as those in Wuhan and that human-to-human transmission was occurring.[76]

Professor Yuen Kwok-yung and his team reached the same conclusion but with more comprehensive evidence and analysis.[77] On January 17, Yuen visited Wuhan to assess the situation firsthand.[78] Late that evening, he sent an "URGENT" email to the Guangdong Provincial CDC, providing supporting evidence for person-to-person transmission and recommendations for public health measures. With the report from Yuen's team and their own investigations and test results, the Guangdong Provincial CDC leaders and experts convened a late-night meeting and recommended that Guangdong elevate its epidemic control measures to address "human-to-human transmission and community spread." The Guangdong CDC recommendation was submitted to the provincial health commission leadership on January 18.[79]

That same evening, Professor Yuen Kwok-yung also sent his urgent message, which included supporting evidence on person-to-person transmission, to China CDC director general Gao Fu.[80] As the Guangdong CDC had previously sent the patient sample and genomic sequencing results to the China CDC for verification, Yuen's message served as a potent reinforcement of the communication through official channels and a catalyst for action.[81]

The NHC Shifts into Action Mode

China's health leadership faced increasing challenges as the situation escalated since the secretive January 14 teleconference and the January 15 epidemic control documents. In addition to the analysis and new findings mentioned earlier, there were significant developments abroad. Japan confirmed its first case on January 16, a patient who had visited Wuhan but not the Huanan Seafood Market. Thailand confirmed its second case, also a traveler from Wuhan. Meanwhile, the US CDC announced enhanced screening of flights from Wuhan at three airports.[82] These developments heightened concerns among China's health policymakers about potential international travel restrictions and WHO intervention.

Sources close to the NHC front-line team in Wuhan reported that NHC officials in Wuhan and Beijing recognized the epidemic situation as increasingly severe, in terms of both severity and number of cases. The initial optimism about the novel coronavirus pneumonia—that it was relatively mild compared to SARS—had given way to alarm as the number of patients with symptoms, if not confirmations, continued to grow. The situation at Jinyintan Hospital was particularly distressing and already in turmoil.[83]

January 17–18, 2020, marked a significant turning point for the NHC. The confluence of events, including the critical information on human-to-human transmission from Guangdong backed by two of the most respected scientist-doctors, shook the national health leadership out of its increasingly uneasy comfort zone. One source close to the NHC working team even suggested that the team leadership "knew everything" by this time, namely that the novel coronavirus was contagious and spreading and needed to be controlled.[84] It was the SARS crisis revisited.

Without a public announcement, the NHC shifted to a multi-pronged attack mode on the novel coronavirus epidemic between January 17 and 18. Firstly, the NHC issued an updated second edition of the epidemic control documents, not for public access, just 3 days after the January 15 edition. The updated Diagnosis and Treatment Protocol, citing information on cases under observation and confirmed cases, plainly states that "the number of cases without a history of exposure to the Huanan market is increasing, and there have appeared clustered cases that lack such exposure history; moreover, two countries have identified three confirmed cases that came from Wuhan but have no definite exposure history." The document goes on to say that the protocol is revised to "better control the epidemic outbreak, reduce and lower its chance of [the epidemic] spreading domestically and overseas, and further strengthen early discovery."[85] In essence, this document indicated that the health leadership's concern was no longer about whether human-to-human transmission was occurring but the extent of the viral spread. It was effectively an admission that the epidemic situation was not under control but spreading.

Secondly, while the NHC had previously focused on bringing respiratory medicine and infectious disease experts to Wuhan, it became clear that Wuhan hospitals needed assistance in treating patients in critical care, especially expertise in pulmonary and critical care medicine (PCCM). Between January 18 and 19, the NHC invited three of China's most prominent PCCM specialists to go to Wuhan to provide help and clinical leadership: Dr. Du Bin, vice president of the Peking Union Medical College Hospital; Dr. Tong Zhaohui, vice president of Beijing Chaoyang Hospital; and Dr. Qiu Haibo, vice president of the Southeast University Zhongda Hospital in Nanjing.

Thirdly, even though human-to-human transmission had become an a foregone conclusion, the national health leadership decided to organize yet another team of distinguished experts to travel to Wuhan and assist in assessing the epidemic situation, including the infectivity of the novel coronavirus.[86] After all, it had been less than a week since the NHC had acknowledged the possibility of limited human-to-human transmission. These experts could not only offer their expertise but also provide scientific justification for actions, helping to break through political inertia and chart a path forward.[87] One can imagine the flurry of calls and discussions involving NHC officials, Director General Gao Fu, and possibly Vice Premier Sun Chunlan and her staff on the evening of January 17 and the early morning of January 18, reminiscent of the events on December 30, 2019. The ad hoc Senior Advisory Panel, officially known as the Highly-Ranked Experts Mission or Group (高级别专家组) in Chinese, comprised six members, who are listed in Table 10.1.

Most of these six experts played significant roles in China's battle against SARS in 2003, except for Gao, who was abroad at the time. Four of them—Gao, Li, Yuen, and Zhong—are academicians of the Chinese Academies of Sciences and Engineering. This group's composition, with members from different regions, helped mitigate the possibility of groupthink. Gao Fu and Zeng Guang of the China CDC were on standby, while Dr. Du Bin had already arrived in Wuhan on January 18 as a member of the critical care specialist team. Dr. Yuen Kwok-yung, a compelling choice for the team due to his strong ties to Guangdong, urgent message, and world-class stature, reached Wuhan on January 17.[88]

The participation of Dr. Li Lanjuan and Dr. Zhong Nanshan warrants further elaboration. Dr. Li Lanjuan (b. 1947) has been a vice chair of the National Expert Advisory Committee on Public Health Emergencies for a long time. She served as director general of the Zhejiang Provincial Health Bureau for a decade and worked with Xi Jinping, then the Zhejiang provincial party secretary, to address SARS. Dr. Li closely monitored the situation after the so-called VPUE outbreak in Wuhan in late 2019. On January 17, she learned that healthcare worker infections with the novel coronavirus appeared to have occurred in Wuhan. Believing the epidemic situation in Wuhan was likely grave, Dr. Li proposed to the NHC that she would like to go to Wuhan to

Table 10.1 The Senior Advisory Panel to Wuhan, January 19, 2020

Dr. Du Bin, vice president and chief of the ICU, Peking Union Medical College Hospital
Gao Fu (George), director general, China CDC
Dr. Li Lanjuan, director of the State Key Laboratory of Infectious Disease Diagnosis and Treatment, the First Affiliated Hospital of Zhejiang University
Zeng Guang, chief epidemiologist, China CDC
Dr. Yuen Kwok-yung, chair of Infectious Diseases, Department of Microbiology, University of Hong Kong and director, State Key Laboratory of Emerging Infectious Diseases
Dr. Zhong Nanshan, director of the National Clinical Research Center for Respiratory Disease, The First Affiliated Hospital of Guangzhou Medical University

help assess the epidemic situation there.[89] Her involvement, especially given her connection to General Secretary Xi Jinping, was another factor that propelled the NHC leadership to assemble this distinguished team of experts. Her self-nomination spared the NHC leadership from asking a 73-year-old woman to go to the epidemic front as Chinese society is heavily gendered. On the morning of January 18, Dr. Li was instructed to go to Wuhan, and she boarded the train with two associates without assigned seats due to ticket unavailability.[90]

The national health leadership's anxiety and political judgment led them to request the 83-year-old Dr. Zhong Nanshan to lead the team in Wuhan. Dr. Zhong's gravitas and sterling national reputation, along with his independence and willingness to speak the truth during the SARS crisis in a politically acceptable manner, made him the ideal person to lead the team. For Minister Ma Xiaowei, Vice Premier Sun Chunlan, and others, Dr. Zhong would not only help confirm the epidemic situation but also help break the bad news to the national leadership and the public, 3 weeks after the initial outbreak garnered attention.

Jiao Yahui, deputy director general of the NHC Medical Administration Bureau, served as the NHC liaison for organizing and contacting experts. When the call for help came, Dr. Zhong had just returned from visiting Shenzhen No. 3 People's Hospital the previous day and was in a meeting about the cluster of cases in Shenzhen with other experts.[91] Dr. Zhong Nanshan's secretary, Su Yueming, recalled receiving the call from an NHC official at 11 AM on January 18. The call requested assistance with the Wuhan outbreak, which they had anticipated. Academician Zhong was asked to "go to Wuhan personally, regardless of [obstacles]."[92] Su remembered the NHC official mentioning that the situation in Wuhan was "a bit tense there."[93] It is evident that Dr. Zhong was treated not as a typical octogenarian but as a respected expert on active duty.

Dr. Zhong informed the NHC official through Su Yueming that he had another meeting scheduled at the Guangdong Provincial Health Commission that afternoon. He suggested flying to Wuhan early the next morning.[94] However, an hour later, Jiao Yahui, on behalf of the NHC leadership, urgently insisted that academician Zhong travel to Wuhan that same day.[95] Keenly aware of Dr. Zhong's reputation and expertise, Chinese health leaders, including Vice Premier Sun Chunlan and Minister Ma Xiaowei, emphasized their need for Dr. Zhong's assistance during this critical juncture.

Jiao personally spoke to Dr. Zhong, explaining that the NHC was assembling a team of distinguished experts to go to Wuhan and assess the epidemic situation. Minister Ma Xiaowei wanted Dr. Zhong to join the team.[96] Jiao emphasized that all experts were asked to report to Wuhan that day and urged Dr. Zhong, "Please reach Wuhan by tonight, no matter what." Aware that obtaining last-minute train tickets during the Lunar New Year holiday season would be challenging, she added, "We will help coordinate to arrange [transportation]."[97] According to his authorized biography, Dr. Zhong Nanshan told Su Yueming, "The country needs us to go, we must go today!"[98]

This call to action came almost exactly 17 years after Dr. Zhong's involvement in the fight against SARS in Guangdong in 2003. Dr. Zhong and Su boarded a fully occupied Wuhan-bound train without tickets. With the assistance of the NHC and Guangzhou South Station leadership, train staff accommodated Dr. Zhong and Su in the dining car for the journey. They arrived in Wuhan and checked into a hotel close to midnight.

Conclusion

While adhering to the thesis of limited human-to-human transmission and working within political constraints seemingly dictated by China's national leadership, the NHC advocated for increased prevention and control efforts in Wuhan and nationwide case surveillance in mid-January 2020. Conversely, Hubei/Wuhan authorities relied on the healthcare sector to treat those infected with the novel coronavirus. In another manifestation of China's fragmented authoritarianism at work, the Wuhan/Hubei authorities also aimed to dispel the notion of an epidemic outbreak and maintain the appearance that all was well in Wuhan in spite of a growing number of medical staff infections.

As the spreading outbreak necessitated population-wide public measures, neither the NHC nor the Wuhan/Hubei authorities were prepared to warn the public about the severe risks or initiate robust responses to the outbreak publicly. Consequently, they both contributed to downplaying the risk from the novel coronavirus and failing to respond effectively during that period. The Chinese public evidently discerned obfuscation and mismanagement. In an uncommon development on Weibo, a Twitter-esque microblogging platform known for its harsh content moderation, critical sentiments noticeably outweighed supportive ones on January 18, 2020, following the announcement of new confirmed cases.[99]

The substantive enhancements to prevention measures during this period occurred confidentially. In response to the surge of new cases and mounting international pressure, the NHC introduced the first edition of the prevention and control documents on January 15 and the second edition on January 18, 2020. With the first edition, the NHC expanded the case definition and aimed to prepare provincial health administrations for surveillance and testing of suspected novel coronavirus infections. With the second edition, the NHC plainly stated that cases that lacked a history of exposure to the Huanan market were growing and essentially admitted that the epidemic was spreading. Yet neither set of documents was issued publicly.

As more new cases emerged outside of Wuhan and convincing evidence of human-to-human transmission surfaced, the NHC began taking a more proactive approach as the institutional guardian of national health. It organized a senior expert panel led by Dr. Zhong Nanshan to conduct a field mission to Wuhan, aiming to break the political deadlock. We will explore this pivotal visit in the next chapter.

11
The Decision to Seal Off Wuhan

The decision to lock down Wuhan, a city with a population exceeding 10 million, marked one of the most extraordinary events during the COVID-19 pandemic. This chapter delves into the pivotal developments that led to the implementation of the cordon sanitaire in Wuhan, starting with the Senior Advisory Panel's visit on January 19 and culminating in the imposition of the cordon sanitaire in Wuhan on January 23, 2020.

We begin by examining the crucial moments during the Senior Advisory Panel's visit to Wuhan on January 19, particularly the confrontation spearheaded by Dr. Zhong Nanshan that resulted in the confirmation of significant medical staff infections in the city. The chapter also explores the experts' key deliberations and interactions with National Health Commission (NHC) officials.

Next, we discuss the State Council Executive Meeting (SCEM) on January 20, which ultimately classified novel coronavirus pneumonia as a new infectious disease. The response of Wuhan and Hubei authorities to the rapidly escalating epidemic proved insufficient as the Chinese leadership attempted to stave off the World Health Organization's (WHO's) decision to declare the outbreak a public health emergency of international concern (PHEIC). In light of these circumstances, Xi Jinping intervened on January 22, prompting the Wuhan leadership to enforce the cordon sanitaire, commonly referred to as the "Wuhan lockdown." The rest of the chapter tells how Chinese leader Xi Jinping, the WHO, and other authorities made the challenging decision to impose strict containment measures on the city.

The Senior Advisory Panel's Visit

In contrast to the second NHC expert team's ambiguous mission during a lull in the outbreak, the NHC leadership provided the Senior Advisory Panel with a clear objective: to "assess the infectivity of the disease and the degree of its spread."[1]

Upon arriving in Wuhan, Dr. Zhong learned more about the Shenzhen cases from Yuen Kwok-yung and received phone calls from his former students, who were now front-line clinicians in Wuhan.[2] They informed him of medical staff infections at a major hospital, indicating that the situation was more severe than anticipated.[3]

In reality, as more patients displayed symptoms of novel coronavirus infections in Wuhan's major hospitals, an increasing number of medical professionals realized they were dealing with a highly contagious disease. Members of the Wuhan University Zhongnan Hospital community were disappointed that the second expert team would not visit their hospital, thereby missing their insights and warnings about the epidemic. Dr. Wang Xinghuan, president of Zhongnan Hospital, learned on the evening of January 18 of the visit by the senior experts the next day. He and Dr. Li Lanjuan knew each other well, and they arranged to meet for breakfast on January 19, a Sunday. Dr. Wang recalled,

> As soon as I saw Academician Li Lanjuan, I began explaining that the situation was far more serious than imagined, with the number of novel coronavirus patients much larger than the figures announced in the [Wuhan Municipal Health Commission, WMHC] Updates. It was likely a repeat of SARS [severe acute respiratory syndrome]. As [we talked], Academician Zhong Nanshan also entered the dining hall for breakfast, and I reiterated [my earlier points] about the backlog of suspected novel coronavirus patients and infections among medical staff. I also mentioned that based on our medical visits, the situation in other Hubei cities and counties beyond Wuhan was equally dire. However, no cases had been reported due to the lack of nucleic acid testing in those locations. After hearing me, both Zhong Nanshan and Li Lanjuan appeared deeply concerned.[4]

Consequently, even before their official itinerary began, the experts had already gathered evidence of human-to-human transmission from multiple sources. As part of their meticulously planned schedule, they first received briefings from Hubei Provincial Health Commission (HPHC) and WMHC leaders on the epidemic situation and the containment measures implemented. Next, they visited Jinyintan Hospital to learn about patient treatment, although they didn't see the patients due to time constraints. They proceeded to the Wuhan Municipal CDC to understand diagnostic testing before being driven around the closed Huanan Seafood Market to observe the surrounding areas.[5]

The visiting experts, led by Dr. Zhong Nanshan, were accompanied or met by Hubei and Wuhan health officials, including Vice Governor Yang

Yunyan, Party Secretary Zhang Jin of the HPHC, Vice Mayor Chen Xiexin, Party Secretary and Director Zhang Hongxing of the WMHC, and a working team led by NHC vice minister Yu Xuejun. However, as Vice Governor Yang Yunyan was not a Communist Party member, he had limited influence within the Hubei and Wuhan leadership. Neither the governor nor the mayor, not to mention the provincial and the municipal party secretary, met with the team. Zeng Guang later publicly expressed his disappointment that their team of experts "did not see the main people in charge.... Thus, our proposals... didn't get heard by those who had real power" in Wuhan or Hubei.[6]

Dr. Yuen Kwok-yung observed that the Wuhan and Hubei officials and experts who met and briefed the visiting experts seemed "well prepared." "The organizations we visited in Wuhan were probably all 'model units.' Whatever we asked, they appeared to have replied with prepared answers."[7] Dr. Zhong agreed: "The local authorities, they didn't like to tell the truth at that time."[8]

However, Dr. Yuen noted that Vice Mayor Chen Xiexin, responsible for Wuhan's health portfolio and host of the lunch with Dr. Zhong and the experts, "looked laden with a heavy heart." "They should know from the arrival of the third expert team that something truly serious was up," Yuen remarked.[9] The HPHC leadership also understood the severity of the situation. While the NHC Senior Advisory Panel was visiting Wuhan, the HPHC sent an expert team to Huanggang to assess the local conditions, following the NHC's example.[10] The Hubei experts took 23 samples from patients at the Huanggang Central Hospital. 12 of them tested positive for the novel coronavirus that evening.[11]

Dr. Zhong's Questions

Yuen Kwok-yung and Zeng Guang commended Dr. Zhong for his assertive and probing questions.[12] With evidence of human-to-human transmission of the novel coronavirus from Guangdong and knowledge of medical staff infections in Wuhan, Dr. Zhong recalled asking his Wuhan hosts three key questions:

> Zhong: First, please clearly tell us, how many people are infected? Second, tell us, how many have died of [this disease]? Third, please also tell us, are there medical staff infected or not?
>
> Answer (as retold by Zhong): We now have 198 people who are infected [by the novel coronavirus]. There are 13 medical staff infections in the Neurosurgery

Department of [Union Hospital]; they were infected by patients.[13] [The number of infected medical staff was 15 when officially announced.]

Despite their efforts to maintain an appearance of normalcy, the Hubei and Wuhan health officials offered no resistance when confronted by Dr. Zhong.[14] In the presence of the esteemed Dr. Zhong, the local health leaders likely found it relieving to finally speak the truth, although they remained defensive and cited extenuating circumstances, such as the Hubei Centers for Disease Control and Prevention (CDC) not receiving the test kits developed by the China CDC until January 16, which delayed confirmation of medical staff infections.[15] Dr. Zhao Hongxiang, chief of Neurosurgery at Wuhan Union Hospital, later claimed credit for having the medical staff in his section tested as soon as possible, thus contributing to the national decision-making on the outbreak: "If we had not reported the results a few days earlier [than expected], the lockdown of Wuhan might have been delayed, and the epidemic might have been even more serious."[16]

For Dr. Zhong and his colleagues, learning about the substantial number of medical staff already infected with the novel coronavirus was alarming. Despite the China CDC leadership's initial suspicion of person-to-person transmission in early January, the expert assessment process had evolved into a search for and verification of medical staff infections by expert teams. For many others, including Hu Xijin, editor-in-chief of the *Global Times*, the question remained: "If Zhong Nanshan did not tell, is it possible that the Wuhan Health Commission would continue to conceal the 15 medical staff infections?"[17]

The Expert Deliberations

At 2 PM on January 19, members of the Senior Advisory Panel gathered at the Wuhan Conference Center to discuss their findings, joined by officials from the NHC, Hubei, and Wuhan. By this point, there was no doubt about human-to-human transmission. The real concern was about the presence of transmission but the severity of the novel coronavirus's spread. The knowledge of a substantial number of medical staff infections, the number of severe cases, and the expected increase in the number of confirmed cases following diagnostic tests provided indisputable evidence of the virus's high contagiousness, even though most experts could not yet imagine the Wuhan outbreak would escalate into a global pandemic.

After sharing information and engaging in discussions, the group "essentially concluded" that the source of the viral infections for current patients was linked to the wildlife sold at the Huanan Seafood Market.[18] China CDC director general Gao Fu had demonstrated unwavering leadership in collecting samples from the market and tracing the virus's origin. However, the experts knew through Gao that only environmental samples—and none of the animal samples—taken from the market had tested positive for the novel coronavirus by that time.

Dr. Li Lanjuan was asked to speak first during the team deliberations. With her decade-long experience as the director general of the Zhejiang Provincial Health Bureau, she knew how to address the key issues and policy implications at this critical juncture. First, she stated that human-to-human transmission was present, and the infection of medical personnel was a significant indicator. The disease, caused by the novel coronavirus, should be managed as a Class A infectious disease, with infected individuals identified and quarantined. Second, because Wuhan was the epidemic's source and due to the peak travel associated with the Lunar New Year, efforts should be made to control the epidemic in Wuhan under the principle of "no entry, no exit." Third, she suggested that many more people might have been infected. Jinyintan Hospital would not be sufficient, and more hospitals should be made available to accommodate infected patients "as much as possible," allowing medical professionals to engage in infection control more effectively. Fourth, in treatment, the experiences with H7N9 infections might be valuable for reducing the fatality rate.[19]

When Dr. Li Lanjuan called for "no entry, no exit," it does not seem that she advocated for a strict lockdown of the entire city but rather expected people to willingly comply with a government order. However, someone on the team did raise the possibility of a strict lockdown of Wuhan. According to Yuen Kwok-yung's recollection, that someone was "a professional, top-notch scientist in epidemiology."[20] The person who best fit this profile was Zeng Guang, the China CDC chief epidemiologist. Zeng later confirmed that he initially suggested the recommendation, but he also emphasized that it was the team's consensus recommendation for the national leadership to act on.[21]

The NHC Works with the Experts to Prepare for the SCEM

The NHC leadership eagerly awaited the expert team's assessment. They had established the expert advisory system to provide expertise and to confer legitimacy on as well as to lighten the political burden of key decisions on the NHC leadership. However, there was a sense of frustration among key NHC leadership members and the NHC working team in Wuhan as the expert advisory system seemed to slow down urgently needed decisions during this critical period when every hour counted.[22]

Before the expert team concluded their deliberations, their key findings on human-to-human transmission and the need to adopt Class A infection control measures, in accordance with the Law on Infectious Diseases Prevention and Treatment (as done with SARS in 2003), were clear. Zhang Zongjiu (张宗久), the director general of the NHC's Medical Administration Bureau, briefed the NHC leadership on these key conclusions by phone. The NHC leadership, presumably Minister Ma Xiaowei, immediately reported to Vice Premier Sun Chunlan.[23]

It is also worth noting that while the Senior Advisory Panel members were visiting Wuhan, a Guangdong team, including Guangdong vice governor Zhang Guangjun, health commission director general Duan Yufei, and Guangdong Provincial CDC deputy director Song Tie, flew to Beijing and reported to the NHC leadership on the cases in Guangdong. Besides the familial cluster of cases in Shenzhen, they also had information on another family cluster in Zhuhai identified on January 18. Drawing on Guangdong's experience with SARS, the Guangdong team also recommended more vigorous responses.[24]

Beijing was now at the center of dealing with the health emergency. Although the Chinese government had promoted the standardization of health emergency responses at different government levels in previous years, crucial decisions still had to be made at every step. Even by official accounts, 3 weeks had elapsed since the national leadership first learned of the initial outbreak in Wuhan at the end of December 2019. For these 3 weeks, the public had been reassured repeatedly that there was not much to worry about regarding the unusual pneumonia cases in Wuhan, even after scientists confirmed the novel coronavirus as the pathogen. Remarkably, while the Senior Advisory Panel members were meeting in Wuhan, the *Global Times*, a newspaper of the *People's Daily* Group, editorialized that "There won't be a repeat in China of the kind of late reporting and concealment that were characteristic of SARS in China."[25]

The emergence of a consensus expert opinion on the outbreak's severity provided a compelling reason for the national leadership to act. It also required the party-state leadership to manage the 180-degree turn in the official position after downplaying the situation's severity and cracking down on doctors who spoke up.

As the next step, the national leadership wanted to hear from the experts face to face. The Senior Advisory Panel members boarded the 5:55 PM Hainan Airlines flight bound for Beijing and met with NHC officials late that evening. By this time, the number of confirmed cases in Wuhan had tripled in just the last 2 days. The NHC also confirmed that the first case of novel coronavirus pneumonia from Shenzhen was positive and that there were another eight cases in Guangdong.[26] These cases highlighted the urgency of controlling the viral spread. The Senior Advisory Panel members joined senior NHC administrators to continue their discussion and assessment, as well as to prepare for presenting their findings and recommendations to the State Council leadership.[27]

Around midnight, Minister Ma Xiaowei met with Zhong Nanshan and Li Lanjuan to discuss their findings face to face.[28] He invited both Dr. Zhong Nanshan and Dr. Li Lanjuan to attend a special premier's SCEM as guests the following morning. Dr. Zhong was officially the team leader and thus a natural choice. Dr. Li Lanjuan, who had experience dealing with the SARS crisis in Zhejiang under Xi Jinping's leadership, brought unique administrative and political expertise to the meeting.[29] According to Jiao Yahui from the NHC Medical Administration Bureau, the NHC team worked overnight to prepare presentations for the SCEM.[30]

The experts now faced a significant challenge: determining what measures to recommend to the national leadership to control the novel coronavirus outbreak, which was rapidly spreading due to Wuhan's status as a transportation hub. The morning meetings with Vice Premier Sun Chunlan and the presentations at the SCEM would be among the most consequential of their lives.

The SCEM and Disease Recognition

The SCEM is a weekly institutionalized meeting convened by the premier and attended by the State Council vice premiers, state councilors, secretary generals, and officials from the relevant government departments. It is rare, though not unprecedented, for special guests to be invited to the SCEM.[31] Premier Li Keqiang, who had experience handling the AIDS and SARS crises in Henan Province, agreed to include the novel coronavirus pneumonia epidemic on the SCEM agenda on Monday, January 20, and to invite two of the most distinguished experts to the meeting.

Members of the Senior Advisory Panel took a special bus to the Zhongnanhai leadership compound. Before the SCEM, Vice Premier Sun Chunlan met with all members of the Advisory Panel at 8:30 AM. Having started her career at a clock factory in Liaoning Province in the late 1960s, Vice Premier Sun demonstrated her political acumen and street smarts by rising to serve as the party secretary of Fujian Province and Tianjin municipality and as the only woman on the powerful Politburo for 2017–2022. Appointed vice premier in spring 2018, her portfolio of responsibilities included education and health. While she may not have known that she was facing the toughest fight of her political career, Yuen Kwok-yung recalled that she and the NHC officials present "were all very frank" as they confronted the escalating public health crisis head on.[32]

Vice Premier Sun asked each of the six experts for their assessments of the epidemic situation. According to Yuen, the experts unanimously agreed that there were cases of human-to-human transmission, that the situation was serious, and that prevention and control measures must be taken immediately.[33] Yuen emphasized that the window for prevention and control was already very narrow and that the situation would become severe if drastic measures were not taken in the next few days.[34] Zeng Guang referred to the lessons of the 1967 meningitis outbreak, which killed more than 160,000 people during a Spring Festival travel season amid the Cultural Revolution.[35] He asserted that "the tragedy of 1967 must not be repeated," emphasizing the importance of taking decisive measures.[36]

At 10 AM, China Central Television news reported that Zhejiang had identified five suspected cases of coronavirus infection. The five individuals had returned from Wuhan and, alarmingly, were in four different cities, providing another powerful indication of the virus's potential to spread.[37] Notably, the Zhejiang Provincial Health Commission announced these cases without waiting for formal verification by the China CDC and final determination by an NHC expert panel. The Zhejiang Provincial Health Commission likely consulted Dr. Li Lanjuan, its former director, on the release and was thus able to warn the public several days earlier than if it had followed all the procedures the NHC required.[38] The timing of the release heightened the sense of urgency felt in Zhongnanhai.

The SCEM took place later in the morning.[39] By then, General Secretary Xi Jinping, who had been on a brief state visit to Myanmar on January 17–18 and was in Yunnan Province, had been briefed on the severity of the epidemic situation. Recognizing that the novel coronavirus pneumonia outbreak that he and the Politburo Standing Committee had initially discussed in early January threatened to spiral out of control, Xi emphasized in his instructions the urgency of epidemic control during the Lunar New Year peak travel period and called for "making full effort at the work of prevention and control." He now demanded that party committees, governments at all levels, and relevant departments "prioritize people's safety and physical health, formulate well-thought-out programs, organize all forces for prevention and control, and take practical and effective measures to resolutely curb the momentum of epidemic spread."[40]

Xi Jinping also stated that the government should "release information on the epidemic in a timely manner and deepen international cooperation." Yet, much like his predecessor during the 2003 SARS crisis, Xi concluded with an emphasis on maintaining control: "strengthen the guidance of public opinion, strengthen the work of propagating and elucidating the relevant policies and measures [to the public], resolutely maintain the overall stability of society, ensure that the masses have a peaceful Chinese New Year festival."[41] Xi's "important instructions" on the epidemic in Wuhan were broadcast to the entire country on prime evening news on January 20, 2020.

Chairing the SCEM, Premier Li Keqiang conveyed General Secretary Xi Jinping's "important instructions" to "prioritize people's safety and physical health . . . [and] resolutely curb the momentum of epidemic spread." He and the SCEM members then heard updates on the epidemic situation from NHC minister Ma Xiaowei and Hubei governor Wang Xiaodong. Consistent with the Hubei and Wuhan leaders' response to and handling of the outbreak, Governor Wang Xiaodong displayed little sense of urgency in his briefing.[42]

For Governor Wang, who had extensive experience working closely with provincial leaders in three provinces for nearly three decades before becoming the governor of Hubei Province with a population of approximately 57 million people, the number of novel coronavirus cases, officially at 198 confirmed as of 10 PM on January 19, was small. He seemed to have genuine difficulty comprehending the enormity of the epidemic situation. For him, Wuhan mayor Zhou Xianwang, and even some trained epidemiologists, grappling with the consequences of exponential viral spread was a challenge. Psychologists have found that people tend to exhibit what is known as "exponential-growth bias," which leads to overconfidence in handling infectious disease situations and failure to take aggressive preventive measures.[43] Nonetheless, Governor Wang must have sensed the seriousness of the epidemic situation; otherwise, he would not have been asked to speak at such a meeting in Zhongnanhai. His update was also likely influenced by considerations of making the Hubei leadership appear less culpable.

Premier Li Keqiang then invited academicians Zhong Nanshan and Li Lanjuan to speak. In view of the stance of Governor Wang and by extension the Wuhan/Hubei leadership, having the expertise of the two academicians, two veterans of the SARS crisis and other infectious disease outbreaks, acquired enormous importance at this juncture. Premier Li acknowledged the importance of their input, stating, "Today we have invited two experts [to our meeting] so that [we can] make our assessment from the scientific perspective, and more effectively prepare for and respond to this epidemic."[44]

According to the SCEM summary, academician Zhong Nanshan made concrete recommendations on containing the epidemic's spread, while academician Li Lanjuan provided guidance on enhancing epidemic prevention, control, and treatment.[45] Dr. Zhong emphasized three crucial points to counteract the "exponential growth bias": evidence of human-to-human transmission, medical staff infections indicating strong infectivity, and the lack of widespread recognition of the outbreak's severity.[46] Drawing on his SARS experience, Dr. Zhong stressed the importance of informing the public, advocating for transparency, and for collective efforts to combat the epidemic.[47] It was a poignant moment for this SARS veteran to remind the Chinese leadership of a basic but fundamental lesson from the SARS crisis, namely, letting the public know the facts so that they can take preventive measures and join in the all-people's efforts to combat the epidemic.

Dr. Li Lanjuan reiterated key points she had made earlier, focusing on specific policy measures. She recommended legally recognizing the novel coronavirus infection as a Category B infectious disease requiring Category A infectious disease measures for prevention and control purposes. She also advised implementing a "no entry, no exit" policy for Wuhan.[48]

While experts initially favored reducing population mobility to curb the virus's spread, they did not immediately recommend imposing a cordon sanitaire on Wuhan or "sealing Wuhan off (*fengcheng*, 封城)," which was later mistranslated as "lockdown" in English. However, Zeng Guang later claimed that *fengcheng* was a consensus recommendation.[49] A video clip from a January 20 meeting of a China CDC risk assessment team showed them discussing control measures, including a potential cordon sanitaire for Wuhan.[50]

The Classification of Novel Coronavirus Pneumonia (COVID-19) as an Officially Recognized Infectious Disease

Based on expert recommendations and guidance from the NHC, the State Council leadership used the Law on the Prevention and Treatment of Infectious Diseases to officially recognize novel coronavirus pneumonia (新型冠状病毒感染的肺炎) as a new infectious disease. The NHC swiftly issued Public Notice No. 1, announcing that novel coronavirus pneumonia would be classified as a Class B infectious disease, requiring Class A prevention and control measures used for plague and cholera.[51] This legal recognition and classification meant that novel coronavirus pneumonia would be handled like SARS, pulmonary anthrax, and highly pathogenic avian influenza that infects humans. The NHC's administrative determination thus authorized and empowered authorities (including health administrations and other government departments) and medical institutions to quarantine novel coronavirus pneumonia patients and close contacts for medical treatment or observation, aiming to control the chains of infection transmission.[52] The determination also made novel coronavirus pneumonia a mandatorily notifiable infectious disease under the National Notifiable Diseases Surveillance System.

Premier Li Keqiang urged the city of Wuhan to strictly implement prevention and control measures following the principle of "early detection, early reporting, early isolation, early treatment, and centralized treatment." He specifically highlighted the importance of controlling hospital infections, protecting medical staff, and strengthening scientific research. In an acknowledgment of the credibility gap between previous official rhetoric and recent developments, Li also called for "timely and objective" public communication: "Proactively respond to public concerns and steadily enhance the credibility of prevention and control work."[53]

Breaking the Bad News to the Public

As late as January 19, 2020, the Wuhan leadership still reiterated that "the risk of sustained human-to-human transmission is low."[54] As Premier Li Keqiang's remarks indicated, the Chinese government faced a major credibility issue with the public on the situation in Wuhan. The credibility gap between official rhetoric and reality had become so large that it would be hard for the NHC or officials in Wuhan/Hubei to bridge or fill it without admitting errors of judgment, and admitting mistakes to the public is not among the strengths of Chinese officeholders.

In this critical moment involving another coronavirus, the NHC leadership turned again to Dr. Zhong Nanshan.[55] Many Chinese citizens remembered Dr. Zhong for his willingness to speak against the positions of the China CDC and the health ministry during the SARS crisis. Seventeen years later, having the esteemed 83-year-old Dr. Zhong publicly address the issue would convey the gravity of the situation, command authority and respect, and relieve officials of the difficult task of explaining the sudden shift in their stance. As noted earlier, in the introductory chapter, Dr. Zhong was interviewed live on China Central Television on January 20.[56]

Dr. Zhong did not mince words. Referring to the Guangdong cases, he stated that the novel coronavirus pneumonia "is certainly transmissible from human to human." He reiterated this message several times for emphasis, contradicting and correcting the official stance of the previous 3 weeks. To drive his point home, he also mentioned that some medical staff had become infected. The epidemic was "just starting, still in the stage of sloping up," but it was developing "relatively fast" in parts of the country. "This is the time for us to be vigilant," Dr. Zhong said. As he did during the SARS crisis in February 2003, Dr. Zhong exuded calm and authority.[57]

Dr. Zhong observed that patients infected by the novel coronavirus exhibited similar but somewhat milder symptoms than SARS patients. He advised individuals with symptoms to visit the fever clinic, urged the public not to travel to Wuhan, and recommended wearing facemasks. He noted that even surgical masks, as opposed to the increasingly scarce N95 masks, could block most of the virus-carrying airborne aerosols.[58]

Dr. Zhong's message did more than inform and warn; it mobilized the public to take action. In a 180-degree turn for the propagdanda system, Dr. Zhong's message was accompanied by information about confirmed cases in Beijing, Guangdong, Shanghai, and Zhejiang and suspected cases in Sichuan, Yunnan, Guangxi, and Shandong and the announcement of cases in neighboring countries (Japan, South Korea, and Thailand). The entire country was put on alert. Dr. Zhong's advice on facemasks was particularly important and well received, encountering little cultural resistance.[59]

The Enforcement Gap in Wuhan

During the SCEM, Li Keqiang urgently called for Wuhan and Hubei to "resolutely contain the spread of the epidemic and implement territorial responsibility."[60] Senior Advisory Panel members Li Lanjuan, Zeng Guang, and Zhong Nanshan also appealed to the public to refrain from entering or leaving Wuhan.[61]

In response to the situation, the State Council Joint Prevention and Control Mechanism (JPCM) emerged as the institutional locus for coordinating and implementing *fangkong* policies. This health emergency response structure, which emphasizes both horizontal (inter-departmental) and vertical coordination, had previously been utilized during the SARS outbreak in 2003 and the Sichuan earthquake in 2008.[62] The JPCM involves 32 central government ministries and administrations, addressing a wide range of concerns such as treatment, scientific research, logistics, and propaganda.

Vice Premier Sun Chunlan announced the activation of the "joint prevention and control mechanism (JPCM) and public health emergency event response plan" during a national teleconference on January 20, 2020. Sun Chunlan supervised the JPCM; Minister Ma Xiaowei was appointed as the lead coordinator. Dr. Du Bin, who attended the teleconference, recalled a Hubei leader's report to the JPCM teleconference: "Frankly, judging from his report, I didn't think the situation had gotten unmanageable."[63]

Following the national leadership's intervention, the Wuhan municipal leadership established the Wuhan Municipal Command for Epidemic Fangkong of Novel Coronavirus Pneumonia. Mayor Zhou Xianwang served as the commander, and he convened the command's first meeting on the afternoon of January 20. Party Secretary Ma Guoqiang did not assume the role of co-commander until January 22 when he convened the municipal Party Committee to discuss and study General Secretary Xi Jinping's latest instructions.[64] Officials and staff at all levels in Wuhan were made responsible, layer by layer, for collaborating with community-level staff and health workers to supervise "close contacts."[65] However, these commands or aspirations far exceeded what could be realistically achieved at the time, especially due to the challenges of identifying close contacts when both the public and authorities were in panic mode.

In an interview on January 22, Mayor Zhou Xianwang explained that Wuhan, a significant transportation hub, would typically have around 30 million people living in or traveling through the city during the Lunar New Year period. He mentioned that temperature screening equipment was being installed at all entry and exit points. To prevent infected individuals from entering or leaving and to avoid placing additional pressure on other areas' prevention and control efforts, travelers with body temperatures of 37.3°C or above would be subject to quarantine for observation or treatment. The goal was to establish an "epidemic moat" before January 24, Lunar New Year's Eve.[66] Mayor Zhou opposed the idea of imposing a cordon sanitaire on the city, stating that the *fangkong* measures being taken "were not about denying entry/exit to the [entire] Wuhan population of more than 10 million people."[67]

Mayor Zhou later asserted that Wuhan's rank and file entered a "wartime status" against the epidemic on January 20.[68] However, the public perception was quite different. On January 20, Wuhan announced that it would distribute 200,000 free passes to encourage the public to visit 30 tourist attractions during the Lunar New Year holidays.[69] Despite Dr. Zhong Nanshan's high-profile interview, Hubei and Wuhan leaders continued with their Lunar New Year activities. The Hubei provincial leadership, led by Party Secretary Jiang Chaoliang and Governor Wang Xiaodong, proceeded with the Hubei provincial New Year's gala party. Official Hubei media even praised some performers for continuing despite being sick.[70] Various other Lunar New Year gatherings and celebrations took place throughout the city. The Hubei provincial leadership finally activated a public health emergency response at Level II in the early hours of January 22. The Wuhan municipal government issued an order on the evening of January 22 mandating the wearing of facemasks in all public spaces and institutions.[71]

Professor Guan Yi of the University of Hong Kong was a leading scientist in identifying the sources of the SARS and Middle East respiratory syndrome coronaviruses and a collaborator with Zhong Nanshan during the SARS crisis. In an interview on January 20, 2020, Guan relied on official Chinese reports and thought the outbreak situation in Wuhan was similar to the early phase of SARS in Guangdong in early 2003.[72] He then visited Wuhan the following day to assess the situation and explore potential assistance. Guan spoke with researchers and policymakers, visited wet markets, and observed crowded areas with shoppers preparing for the Lunar New Year holidays, most of whom were not wearing facemasks.[73] Others noted that few people on crowded subways and buses wore facemasks. Some counties in Hubei responded to the outbreak more vigilantly than Wuhan.[74]

Guan observed "inaction" by local authorities as of January 22 and admitted feeling "truly helpless." He concluded that Wuhan was still "an unguarded city" against the novel coronavirus and saw a viral explosion in progress. Guan estimated that "the size of this epidemic could end up at 10 times the size of SARS at least," adding, "I've been through so much and never felt scared, but this time I'm scared."[75]

Anguish in and Overwhelming Demand on Wuhan Hospitals

With few noticeable efforts to curtail virus transmission at the community level in Wuhan, the explosion in the number of infections was already apparent in the increasing number of patients rushing to hospitals by the time the NHC administrative notice recognized the novel coronavirus pneumonia as an infectious disease. To enhance diagnosis and treatment capacity and reduce cross-infections, the WMHC on January 21 designated seven municipal hospitals (Hankou, Red Cross Society of Wuhan, Pu'ai-West, No. 7, No. 9, Wuchang, and No. 5) for triaging and treating novel coronavirus pneumonia patients. Known as the "7+7" arrangement, these seven hospitals were paired with and placed under the "entrusted" management of seven top hospitals

(Tongji, Union, Provincial People's, Zhongnan, Municipal First, Wuhan Central, and No. 3).[76] Additionally, 61 hospitals were listed as having dedicated "fever clinics." However, with the explosion in the number of symptomatic people, demand far outpaced available hospital capacity. Even though the number of confirmed cases of coronavirus infections was less than 450 as of early January 22, long lines of patients formed outside fever clinics, waiting to be seen by doctors.[77] Dr. Du Bin, a member of the Senior Advisory Panel who was in Beijing on January 20, rushed back to Wuhan on January 21. He lamented that many hospitals in Wuhan had become "paralyzed and were no longer capable of fulfilling their mission. They had become places for virus transmission."[78]

Jinyintan Hospital was already the toughest battleground for leading Chinese clinicians in respiratory and critical care medicine. In just about 3 weeks, as waves of patients with novel coronavirus infections arrived at the hospital, most wards at Jinyintan Hospital had already been repurposed for patients infected by the novel coronavirus. On January 21, Zhang Dingyu transformed the last uncommitted floor, one that he had proudly earmarked for clinical trials, to combat the novel coronavirus pneumonia.[79]

Dr. Zhang was dealing with the biggest challenge of his life. Even though the HPHC had ordered three leading hospitals in Wuhan to take over medical care at three intensive care unit floors (S5–7) at Jinyintan Hospital in mid-January, Jinyintan still became too short-staffed to handle the increasing number of patients and provide the intensive care many patients needed.[80] The Jinyintan doctors had been on the front lines for more than 3 weeks non-stop and were exhausted. The staffing situation was exacerbated by the shortage in nursing staff and orderlies after many orderlies quit in mid-January. Each ward with 30-plus critically ill patients was staffed with only five or six doctors and a dozen nurses. The quality of care suffered when there were simply not enough staff to take care of patients needing constant care, an issue that would spread to many hospitals worldwide in the following months.[81]

For Dr. Zhang Dingyu, the danger of the novel coronavirus was also personal. His wife Cheng Lin, who worked at the Wuhan No. 4 Hospital, tested positive for the novel coronavirus on January 19.[82] Dr. Huang Chaolin, his hardworking deputy at Jinyintan Hospital, began to show symptoms on January 17 and was confirmed by diagnostic test on January 22.

Dr. Zhang Dingyu found himself much like a beleaguered ship captain in the midst of a perfect storm. Few were aware that he had been diagnosed with Lou Gehrig's disease over a year earlier, and his physical movements were now affected by the illness. Despite these challenges, Dr. Zhang continued his work with determination. His primary concern was the possibility of contracting the coronavirus, which would force him into isolation at a time when the hospital he had dedicated 6 years to needed him the most. After discovering his wife's infection on January 19, he tested himself and, fortunately, received a negative result.[83]

Dr. Zhang shared glimpses of the overwhelming burden and feelings of helplessness that consumed him during this time. One night, around January 20 or 21, as he drove home alone, he was filled with fear and sadness. He had witnessed many deaths but still did not understand how critical cases developed or progressed. His concern for his wife's well-being intensified his feelings of terror and helplessness: "I felt terrified while driving. I had tears in my eyes. [I was] really scared because you don't know how your loved one would fare with her illness."[84]

The emergency and respiratory sections of the major hospitals in Wuhan were in distress.[85] Wuhan Central Hospital (WCH) experienced a particularly heavy impact due to staff infections, including three hospital vice presidents. On January 21, the WCH Emergency Section alone had 1,523 patients—three times the usual number—with 655 of them presenting fevers.[86] Exhausting days ensued for the doctors and nurses working extended shifts. An emergency room doctor at WCH's Houhu Branch reported that, during this time, patients in the respiratory department struggled with an unreliable oxygen supply and a lack of intubation in the emergency room. Consequently, many patients died from hypoxia or oxygen deprivation.[87]

The smaller Wuhan Red Cross Society Hospital faced a dire situation. Designated as one of seven hospitals for fever patients on January 21, the facility discharged 330 regular inpatients in a single day to accommodate the change. However, the hospital had only one noninvasive ventilator, 13 protective suits, and limited access to N95 facemasks.[88] Under the leadership of 35-year-old President Xiong Nian, the hospital made the transition to a designated facility with the help of personal protective equipment sent from the Union, Youfu, and No. 1 Hospitals.[89] At 5:30 PM on January 22, doctors at the Red Cross Society Hospital began to see patients suspected of having symptoms of novel coronavirus infections. Compared with a designed capacity for 800 outpatients, they saw 1,700 patients that evening, 2,400 the next, and another 1,700 on January 24.[90]

By January 23, the Red Cross Society Hospital had already taken 340 inpatients with novel coronavirus infections and reached full capacity the following day. With many staff members becoming patients themselves, the Red Cross Society Hospital had only five doctors and nine or 10 nursing staff per floor. There was simply not enough manpower to address the patients' needs.[91] Dr. Lü Xijun, who had worked in the emergency department for a decade, likened these days to being on a battlefield. On January 24, the day before Lunar New Year, Dr. Lü was on duty from 8 AM until 4 AM on New Year's Day, traditionally the time for families to be together. He could hardly hold back tears when he took a meal break. "My life was no longer my own," he recalled.[92]

The large number of outpatients crowding hospitals turned these facilities into potential hotspots for further infections. On the evening of January 22, Xiao Hui (萧辉), a reporter for *Caixin*, visited the Wuhan Red Cross Society Hospital's waiting room and found it filled with coughing patients. Patients were eager to share their anxieties and complaints with her. Many had ground glass opacities on their computed tomographic scans and even diagnoses of viral pneumonia but could not be confirmed for novel coronavirus infections due to a shortage of diagnostic test kits. Even hospital medical staff with symptoms struggled to get tested. Consequently, many patients with milder symptoms were unable to be admitted to the hospital. Some patients acknowledged that they were "mobile sources of the virus."[93]

The Intervention of Xi Jinping, the WHO, and the Seal-Off of Wuhan

Xi Jinping left Beijing for a state visit to Myanmar on January 17, returning to China on the evening of January 18. Instead of going straight back to Beijing, he made an extended layover in Yunnan, the province bordering Myanmar. From January 18 to 21, Xi engaged in various appearances, connecting with ethnic groups and the armed forces. Official media highlighted his visit's significance in providing guidance for local and central government initiatives aimed at poverty alleviation and promoting ecological civilization in ethnic areas.[94] Xi's public activities revealed an itinerary that mixed work and leisure. Critics, like Ren Zhiqiang, later condemned Xi for not following up on the epidemic situation after his January 7 "requirements" and for his extended stay in Yunnan as the epidemic spiraled out of control.[95]

After the Senior Advisory Panel visit, Xi instructed the January 20 SCEM to support containment measures. Once back in Beijing on January 21, 2020, Xi Jinping's focus shifted to the coronavirus crisis while a surge in novel coronavirus pneumonia cases linked to Wuhan was reported.[96] The case of Dr. Wang Guangfa, who was the public face of the second NHC expert team to Wuhan, came as a major shock to many.[97] The growing numbers of cases in Beijing, Zhejiang, and elsewhere were more than just numbers to Xi. As data and analysis from the Ministry of Transportation made clear, the spread of the novel coronavirus was likely to accelerate due to massive numbers of travelers.[98]

Internationally, the WHO International Health Regulations Emergency Committee was scheduled to meet to consider whether to advise the WHO leadership to declare the novel coronavirus outbreak a PHEIC. Such a declaration on the eve of the Chinese Lunar New Year would be a major humiliation for China's leaders.

Xi Jinping, who has consistently promoted the doctrine of comprehensive national security, recognized the epidemic in Wuhan as a grave threat to both national and personal security. On the afternoon of January 22 (Beijing time), he directed that "strict closure of exit channels" for Wuhan and the rest of Hubei Province be implemented without delay.[99] Vice Premier Sun Chunlan, a Politburo member, represented Xi and the Party Central in Wuhan on January 22. She urged the leaders of Hubei and Wuhan to implement the strictest measures to stop the epidemic from spreading beyond Hubei.[100]

Most people in Wuhan still had little idea of the threat they faced. Late on January 22, Dr. Li Lanjuan got a phone call from Zhang Ping, director general of the Zhejiang Provincial Health Commission. Zhejiang is famous for having people engaged in business around the world, including in Eyewear City located on the upper floors of the complex that housed the Huanan Seafood Market in Wuhan. Zhang alerted Li Lanjuan that many more people were expected to return to Zhejiang from Hubei, bringing the virus with them.[101]

Li Lanjuan immediately reported her concerns to the NHC leadership and recommended an immediate lockdown of Wuhan.[102] "Based on the epidemic situation, Wuhan must be sealed off immediately," Li warned, "otherwise the consequences are unthinkable."[103] While Xi Jinping had already signaled his approval of "no exit" from Wuhan/Hubei in the afternoon, the advocacy from Li Lanjuan and probably others added urgency to the lockdown implementation.[104]

The WHO International Health Regulations Emergency Committee met hours later by teleconference in the evening (Beijing time; afternoon in Geneva). The meeting was inconclusive and adjourned, but it put China on the defensive. Xi and the Chinese leadership understood that the International Health Regulations Emergency Committee wanted more information about containment measures being taken in China.[105]

Representing the national leadership, Vice Premier Sun Chunlan made determined efforts to secure the imposition of cordon sanitaire, commonly known as "lockdown," in Wuhan while local officials struggled to comprehend the necessity of sealing off a city of more than 10 million people when infections were only in the hundreds. There were palpable public sentiments that such a lockdown would mean sacrificing Wuhan. According to Mayor Zhou Xianwang, Party Secretary Ma Guoqiang was concerned that issuing the unprecedented lockdown decision "would make us go down in infamy in history."[106] In the end, Ma shared with his colleagues that "for the sake of controlling the epidemic, we'd take whatever responsibility necessary."[107]

Finally, at 2:30 AM on January 23, Wuhan's leadership, in the name of the Wuhan Municipal Epidemic Fangkong Command, issued its Order No. 1 to stop all modes of transportation into or out of Wuhan, sealing the city off from the rest of the country at 10 AM. Dr. Li Lanjuan was notified of the lockdown decision at about 3 AM.[108]

A few hours later, the WHO secretary general reconvened the Emergency Committee to examine the information from China about the outbreak and containment measures implemented. The committee concluded its meeting at 3:10 PM Geneva time (9:10 PM in Beijing, on January 23, 2020). It outlined seven stipulations directed at China but refrained from declaring a public health emergency for the time being.[109] As a result, China successfully averted the PHEIC declaration on that day and before the Chinese Lunar New Year. The WHO eventually declared the PHEIC a week later, on January 30, 2020.

Despite the 2 AM announcement, word of the impending lockdown spread quickly. Between the announcement and the 10 AM lockdown, as many as 500,000 people managed to leave Wuhan on trains, airplanes, motor vehicles, and boats and by other means. Some individuals continued to exit the city, mostly by car and boat, for several more days before Wuhan tightened the restrictions and other provinces closed their borders to travelers, especially those from Hubei.[110]

For most people in Wuhan, the lockdown "came without warning, so abruptly," said Dr. Tong Jun of the Wuhan Mental Health Center.[111] The abruptness was all the more shocking to residents because the Wuhan authorities had been attempting to maintain an image of normalcy and "protect the [festive] atmosphere of the Lunar New Year."[112] At the Wuhan Institute of Virology, renowned virologist Shi Zhengli and Yuan Zhiming, president of the Chinese Academy of Sciences' Wuhan Branch and director of the Wuhan National Biosafety Laboratory, cried when they learned of Wuhan's seal-off.[113]

At 10 AM on January 23, 2020, what would have been one of the busiest days of the year, the Wuhan Hankou Railway Station, located less than a kilometer from the Huanan Seafood Market, locked its doors behind a ring of armed police officers. Established in 1898 during the late Qing Dynasty's reform period, Hankou Station had weathered wars and revolutions. This marked the first time it had closed during peacetime. Hubei party secretary Jiang Chaoliang convened the provincial Fangkong Command that morning, and three other cities near Wuhan quickly followed suit, sealing their borders on the same day. More cities followed, eventually isolating the entire province of 57 million people from the rest of the country.

Simultaneously, Wuhan Tianhe Airport suspended all passenger flights and fell eerily silent. A strong sense of suspense and abandonment pervaded not only the airport but also the entire city. Many people at the time believed that Wuhan was being sacrificed to save the rest of the country and, indeed, the world.[114] An article from the Chinese foreign affairs ministry referred to the move as "strongman putting a chokehold on his own arm."[115]

Each subsequent hour at the Wuhan Tianhe Airport seemed to drag on. It wasn't until 2:29 PM the next day (January 24) that Shunfeng 6956 landed at the airport, a Shunfeng Air Cargo flight carrying 16 tons of medical supplies. Typically unemotional in their communications with pilots, the air traffic controller went out of his way to express gratitude for the support being brought to Wuhan.[116] Such expressions became standard in the following weeks as planes delivered medical teams and supplies from across the country and around the world.

As news of the Wuhan lockdown spread, the provinces of Guangdong, Hunan, and Zhejiang activated the Level I public health emergency response, the highest level possible, on January 23. Zhejiang, which had announced novel coronavirus cases on January 20 without going through the NHC, reported that it already had 27 confirmed cases as of mid-day January 23.[117]

After belatedly activating a Level II emergency response on January 22, Hubei declared its Level I emergency response around noon on January 24. Fourteen other provincial units, including Beijing, Shanghai, Tianjin, Anhui, Chongqing, and Sichuan, made the same declaration that day. The rest of China, except for Tibet, followed suit on January 25, the Lunar New Year.[118] Public gatherings and social visits were canceled for the Lunar New Year holidays. As a result, China entered a nationwide state of emergency in the name of public health.

Conclusion

From a political perspective, the organization of the Senior Advisory Panel visit by China's national health leadership was a politically astute move. By leveraging the expertise and prestige of experts like Zhong Nanshan, the health leadership was able to communicate the gravity of the epidemic to the national leadership, inform the public about the outbreak, and utilize the national leadership and political authority to introduce and enforce the unprecedented cordon sanitaire in Wuhan and Hubei Province. It is clear, in retrospect, that the decisions leading to the implementation of the cordon sanitaire around Wuhan were not exclusively grounded in scientific understanding but were rather politically charged. Moreover, the decision to impose the cordon sanitaire on Wuhan was influenced not only by the assessment of the epidemic situation in Wuhan but also by the desire of Xi Jinping and other Chinese leaders to avoid an immediate WHO PHEIC declaration regarding the novel coronavirus epidemic.

Dr. Du Bin, a member of the Senior Advisory Panel, later reflected on the response in Wuhan, saying, "The most important decision is not to determine the life and death of an individual, but to decide the life and death of a group of people. The role of administrative agencies is truly the most consequential, as it can determine the life and death of a group of people."[119]

12
"The Battle for Wuhan"

With the sealing off of Wuhan and the declaration of Level I emergencies throughout the country, China implemented a nationwide containment strategy and initiated a "national general mobilization to combat the epidemic."[1] Journalists and scholars reflecting on the Wuhan lockdown often give the impression that it was effectively and swiftly enforced. On the first anniversary of the Wuhan lockdown, Emily Feng, a reporter for the American media outlet National Public Radio, aptly summarized the popular perception of the 76-day Wuhan lockdown:

> A year ago, on January 23, 2020, China imposed an absolute lockdown in the Chinese city of Wuhan. For more than two months, nearly all of its 11 million residents could not leave their apartments. Anyone displaying symptoms was taken to hastily-built quarantine centers to prevent family infections.[2]

However, the reality on the ground was far more chaotic and challenging. For both the leadership and the people of Wuhan, January 23, 2020, marked the start of a prolonged and painful process. In late January and early February, Wuhan and much of Hubei Province experienced cycles of distress and powerlessness. The crisis was multifaceted. Hospitals faced critical situations as China's top respiratory and emergency medicine experts struggled to treat severely ill COVID-19 patients. The city was under siege due to a severe shortage of medical facilities to treat and quarantine the increasing number of confirmed COVID patients. More generally for the Chinese people, this period surrounding the announcement of the cordon sanitaire around Wuhan marked a historical moment of profound uncertainty.

A study of public sentiments on Weibo revealed that *both* negative and positive sentiments peaked in the days immediately following the imposition of cordon sanitaire in Wuhan.[3] While the shortcomings in the official response and the resulting distress were linked to public dissatisfaction, the Chinese government swiftly garnered public support by initiating an extensive campaign to aid Wuhan during the lockdown.

This chapter and the next cover the extensive and severe COVID crisis that engulfed Wuhan during the lockdown period and the national efforts to support and rescue Wuhan. In launching the national campaign, Xi Jinping and the national leadership switched the Chinese party-state into performance mode, establishing a mission-oriented organizational structure to lead the front line and mobilize the resources needed for the arduous national campaign to assist and rescue Wuhan. Clinical experts rushed to accumulate and share expertise for disease treatment; medical aid teams from across the country arrived to help with treatment; and treatment and quarantine capacity expanded rapidly through the designation of existing hospitals for COVID treatment, the construction and acquisition of new facilities, and the conversion of public structures into field hospitals.

This extensive campaign showcased the strengths of the Chinese party-state in mobilizing resources on a national scale and enjoyed enormous public support. It proved effective within China because the Chinese system was able to overcome the severe problems of information suppression and hoarding that had characterized the pre–Wuhan lockdown period. As clinicians learned to treat novel coronavirus infections and epidemiologists gained a better understanding of the virus's transmission dynamics, the Chinese leadership incorporated new information into their epidemic response strategy and significantly increased the number of quarantine facilities by embracing the conversion of large-scale public structures into quarantine facilities.

Xi, the Party-State, and the Wuhan Rescue

Earlier, the Hubei and Wuhan leadership had attempted to rely on Wuhan's own considerable medical resources and "not trouble" the national leadership with the outbreak. This is a typical approach for provincial leaders concerned that asking for help would expose their weaknesses and potentially be held against them. Between January 22 and 24, national health leaders and the Wuhan leadership realized that the scale of the epidemic had grown far larger than they had anticipated. The imposition of the cordon sanitaire jolted the Wuhan and Hubei leadership out of their comfort zone. While the official statistics on confirmed cases remained relatively low, decision makers heard urgent appeals for assistance from medical professionals at Jinyintan and elsewhere. They also had access to analyses and projections from both international and domestic sources, indicating that the situation was much more severe, and they were now paying attention. Simultaneously, there was a strong sentiment that, with the lockdown, the people of Wuhan were sacrificing for the nation's benefit and that they needed and deserved assistance.

On the day of the Wuhan lockdown, the Hubei leadership formally requested national medical assistance during a Joint Prevention and Control Mechanism (JPCM) meeting convened by Vice Premier Sun Chunlan. That afternoon, National Health Commission (NHC) staff, operating within the JPCM framework, collaborated with province-level health commissions from around the country to organize and dispatch medical teams to Wuhan. In times of disaster, a popular Chinese saying is that the entire country must coordinate like pieces on the same chess board.

For example, Shanghai was asked to organize a medical aid team comprised of specialists in critical care, respiratory medicine, and infection control, as well as nursing and support staff. This team of 135 members included specialists from 52 Shanghai hospitals. Led by Dr. Zheng Junhua (郑军华), vice president of the Shanghai First People's Hospital, this first Shanghai team was en route to Wuhan on the evening of January 24.[4] Before the flight took off for Wuhan, Zheng Junhua learned that his team was assigned to help Jinyintan Hospital and was given Zhang Dingyu's phone number.[5] Guangdong sent its first team of 133 to Hankou Hospital the same day.

Military Medical Aid and Xi's Direct Involvement

As he decided to impose the condon sanitare on Wuhan, Xi Jinping faced enormous political peril from the exploding coronavirus epidemic.[6] The Chinese military has played major roles in helping to deal with disasters. During the severe acute respiratory syndrome (SARS) crisis, military medical units deployed 1,200 people to staff the Xiaotangshan SARS Hospital in Beijing. Since there was much public complaint about the delays and deficiencies in the official response to the Wuhan outbreak, sending in the military medical units would help win public support for Xi Jinping as well as for the military as an institution. There was eager public anticipation that Xi, as the Chairman of the Central Military Commission, would deploy the military's emergency medical units to Wuhan.

On the evening of January 24, Xi approved the deployment of three medical teams of 150 staff each, organized by the Army, Navy, and Air Force Medical Universities and their affiliated hospitals.[7] These teams reached Wuhan by military transport planes later that night.[8] For the Chinese public, the high-profile dispatch of the military medical teams to Wuhan was an extremely powerful statement. It was both an indication of General Secretary Xi Jinping's personal commitment to helping the people of Wuhan and a revelation of the severity of the epidemic situation.

Dr. Zhang Dingyu of Jinyintan Hospital recalled that "it's impossible [for us] to hold on any longer" around January 24–25.[9] When he heard from Zheng Junhua, captain of the first Shanghai medical team, Zhang Dingyu exclaimed, "Someone's here to save us."[10] At the Wuhan Red Cross Society Hospital, Dr. Xiong Nian learned on January 25 that a Sichuan medical team of 138 was on the way to his hospital. By then 35 of the hospital staff were confirmed to have been infected, and there were just as many who had not yet gotten tested. The hospital, according to Dr. Xiong, was on the verge of collapse. The moment the Sichuan team entered the hospital on January 26, many Red Cross Society Hospital staff were in tears.[11]

Xi and the Party Central in Command

January 25, Lunar New Year's Day, is typically a time for family gathering. However, that morning, General Secretary Xi Jinping convened the Politburo Standing Committee (PBSC)—consisting of Xi and six other members—to address the "serious situation of accelerated spread" of the novel coronavirus.

"I couldn't sleep on New Year's Eve," Xi stated gravely at the beginning of the meeting.[12] As civilian and military medical aid teams were deployed to Wuhan, Xi and his PBSC colleagues recognized that the epidemic in Wuhan/Hubei posed an existential threat to "the bigger picture" and vowed to "win the epidemic prevention and control (*fangkong*) battle."[13]

Although the State Council JPCM had been activated, the party leadership deemed it insufficient for the challenges, particularly given the sluggish responses in Wuhan/Hubei. Consequently, on top of the JPCM, Xi and the party leadership established the higher-powered Central Leading Group on Responding to the Novel Coronavirus Pneumonia Epidemic (中央应对新型冠状病毒感染肺炎疫情工作领导小组), also known as the Central Leading Group for Epidemic Response. Emphasizing that the epidemic *fangkong* battle must be fought under the unified leadership of the Party Central, the Party Central Committee issued an order to the entire party on strengthening Communist Party leadership and called on the party rank and file to provide firm political assurance for winning the anti-epidemic battle.[14]

Many were surprised when Xi, who had taken control of numerous party commissions, did not make himself leader of the Central Leading Group for Epidemic Response. Instead, he appointed Premier Li Keqiang as the nominal leader of the Central Leading Group for Epidemic Response. Wang Huning, the party's ideology czar (ranked fifth on the PBSC), was named the deputy leader. The other members of the Central Leading Group included Vice Premier Sun Chunlan, the party secretary of Beijing (Cai Qi), the party propaganda chief (Huang Kunming), the ministers of foreign affairs and public security, plus the director of the Central Committee General Office and the secretary general of the state council.[15] Health Minister Ma Xiaowei was notably absent, in part because he did not concurrently hold a higher-ranked appointment (such as state councilor). The composition of the Central Leading Group highlighted that the Chinese leadership viewed the novel coronavirus crisis as a significant political threat requiring a whole-of-party-state response.

The Central Leading Group was represented in Wuhan/Hubei by the Central Steering Group (中央指导组). This steering or guiding group setup was first used in fall 2019 for Xi's campaign to promote re-education in the original aspirations and mission of the Communist Party.[16] As the aspirations/mission campaign concluded, Xi transposed the steering group setup to another campaign, this time focused on epidemic *fangkong*. Members of the Central Steering Group included Ma Xiaowei and other NHC leaders as well as representatives from several other ministries. It established at least seven task forces. A vice minister each from the National Development and Reform Commission and the Ministry of Industry and Information Technology headed the materials supplies team or task force. This team worked tirelessly to arrange for the production and supply of protective gear and medical equipment and allocate these products across the country during a time of acute shortages. The team also made emergency purchases of large numbers of ventilators and extracorporeal membrane oxygenation (ECMO) machines.[17]

Known for his love of the language of "struggle," Xi Jinping led the charge in using war-like language and referred to the battle of Wuhan in various ways.[18] In early February he declared that China was fighting "a total war, all efforts must be made to provide support for winning the battle of interdiction in epidemic *fangkong*."[19] Local authorities eagerly invoked and embraced the "wartime control" language in pursuing *fangkong* objectives.[20]

Even though Premier Li Keqiang headed the Central Leading Group, Xi was decidedly in charge of the overall anti-epidemic efforts. He told Vice Premier Sun Chunlan to "feel free to call directly to discuss any difficulties or needs that the steering group may encounter."[21] According to his own account, Xi consistently monitored the epidemic situation and provided frequent oral and written guidance.[22] In addition to working with the Central Leading Group and the Central Steering Group, Xi authorized and oversaw medical aid from the People's Liberation Army and directed policy using the Politburo and the various Party Central commissions he controlled.

The Central Leading Group's and the Central Steering Group's Rescue Efforts in Wuhan and Hubei

As head of the Central Leading Group, Premier Li Keqiang visited Wuhan on January 27, where he went to Jinyintan Hospital, the Hubei Provincial Centers for Disease Control and Prevention (CDC), and the construction site of the Thunder God Mountain makeshift field hospital. During his visit to Jinyintan Hospital, he heard urgent pleas for personal protective equipment and nursing support, needs the Hubei provincial leadership had failed to grasp let alone effectively address.

Now that the national leadership had decided to reorient the entire country and especially authorities in Hubei and Wuhan toward the mission of epidemic *fangkong*, Li Keqiang was in Wuhan to get the message through. During a work meeting, he urged Hubei and Wuhan leaders to fulfill their responsibilities and truly prioritize epidemic *fangkong*: "release authoritative information timely, publicly, and transparently, respond to public concerns, strive to bring down the morbidity and mortality rates, vigorously and effectively control the epidemic, and protect the lives and health of the people."[23]

On behalf of General Secretary Xi Jinping and the Central Leading Group, Li Keqiang introduced and empowered Vice Premier Sun Chunlan, the only woman on the Politburo, as the leader of the Central Steering Group.[24] He also practically wrote a blank check on behalf of the national leadership. "Going forward," Li Keqiang stated, "whatever your needs, whether manpower, materials or funds, the national government will make special efforts in these special circumstances, mobilize forces, increase support. The [Central] Steering Group on the frontline will continue to provide strong coordination."[25]

Bolstered with direct lines to General Secretary Xi Jinping and Premier Li Keqiang, the Central Steering Group, equipped with task forces for medical care, materials supply, and so on, became the organizational driving force behind China's battle for epidemic *fangkong*. While her status as leader of the Central Steering Group gave her greater political clout over the local officials, Vice Premier Sun Chunlan continued to leverage the bureaucratic and organizational resources of the JPCM. Armed with these two conjoined mechanisms, Sun Chunlan became China's anti-epidemic czar. Health

Minister Ma Xiaowei maintained a low profile after visiting Wuhan in mid-January and did not reappear in Wuhan until early February (partly for health reasons).[26]

Initially, there was a division of labor between the Central Steering Group and the Hubei and Wuhan authorities. Ding Xiangyang, Vice Premier Sun Chunlan's lieutenant, explained that the Central Steering Group was responsible for supervising Hubei's implementation of central leadership measures; guiding the province while providing support in supplies, personnel, and technologies for combating the epidemic; and inspecting and demanding remedial actions for any failures to act and to take care of problems.[27] In practice, the Central Steering Group leadership made major decisions such as the development of *fangcang* shelter hospitals while the local authorities were responsible for implementation with support from the Central Steering Group and the JPCM.

Given the immense challenges and difficult epidemic conditions everyone had to face, it was unsurprising that tempers sometimes flared, personality clashes occurred, and other tensions arose. Due to health reasons, some senior officials such as Minister Ma were out of the spotlight for extended periods. To overcome the disparate organizational and political interests, Vice Premier Sun Chunlan encouraged officials from varied backgrounds and organizations by saying, "Let's seek truth from facts, discuss difficulties as they are; we're not 'facing off,' we are in the same boat."[28]

By mid-February 2020, as the epidemic situation improved and significant leadership changes occurred in Wuhan/Hubei, the Central Steering Group took center stage. Members of the group held a series of press conferences starting on February 20 that also highlighted the leadership role of the Central Steering Group.[29] Most members of the Steering Group also made their first public appearance together on February 23.

The Mobilization of Medical Rescue Teams

The State Council JPCM began to mobilize medical rescue teams to Wuhan on the day the city was sealed off. This urgent rescue operation intensified under the guidance of the Central Steering Group. In total, the national mobilization of medical assistance deployed 344 medical teams, comprising over 44,000 healthcare workers, to Wuhan and the rest of Hubei Province, making it the largest medical assistance mission in China's history (Table 12.1).

In addition to the involvement of armed forces medical institutions, which contributed around 4,000 military medical personnel, this massive effort

Table 12.1 Medical Teams to Wuhan and the Rest of Hubei

Province/institution	Doctors	Nurses	Other medical	Subtotal	Chinese CDC system
Armed forces				4,000	
NHC hospitals in Beijing	233	650	59	942	
National TCM	255	507	11	773	
Jiangsu	755	1936	80	2,771	39
Guangdong	767	1646	82	2,495	53
Liaoning	590	1348	99	2,037	64
Zhejiang	542	1363	113	2,018	47
Shanghai	511	1208	99	1,818	16
Shandong	499	1242	72	1,813	34
Chongqing	488	1085	53	1,626	36
Heilongjiang	404	1109	20	1,533	15
Shanxi	401	1049	66	1,516	9
Hunan	442	988	29	1,459	25
Sichuan	423	932	84	1,439	34
Guizhou	499	836	59	1,394	25
Fujian	361	963	57	1,381	31
Anhui	329	971	34	1,334	23
Tianjin	386	775	130	1,291	67
Henan	359	805	98	1,262	18
Jiangxi	341	850	27	1,218	32
Jilin	283	887	18	1,188	18
Yunnan	285	812	31	1,128	43
Hebei	245	767	71	1,083	21
Guangxi	231	683	38	952	37
Shaanxi	238	643	36	917	30
Hainan	201	603	51	855	23
Inner Mongolia	178	611	9	798	18
Ningxia	175	572	35	782	13
Gansu	174	593	9	776	20
Xinjiang	88	289	9	386	6
Beijing	80	131	50	261	12
Qinghai	41	194	4	239	
Xinjiang Production Corps	20	46	41	107	1
Tibet				3	3
Hong Kong				2	
China CDC					149
Total				43,597	962

Sources: "全国援鄂医疗队人员名单", 健康中国 2020-09-10, https://zhuanlan.zhihu.com/p/118130105; "军队援鄂医疗队圆满完成任务回撤," 新华社 2020-04-17, http://health.people.com.cn/n1/2020/0417/c14739-31677209.html.

included every provincial unit, rallying the country to the national cause of providing rescue amid criticism of the party-state's handling of the outbreak.[30] Guangdong and Jiangsu Provinces led the way in providing the most significant support, sending the largest contingents of aid teams from among the provinces.

Although the initial focus of the medical aid missions centered on Wuhan, the Central Steering Group's leadership was also concerned about preventing a similar crisis in other Hubei cities. Beginning on February 10, 2020, 19 provinces were assigned to support 16 Hubei municipalities, excluding Wuhan.[31] Guangdong sent the largest number of doctors (767), with its 26 medical teams being deployed to the cities of Wuhan (18 teams), Jingzhou (7 teams), and Yichang (1 team).[32]

Based on the recommendations of medical experts struggling to treat the large number of critically ill patients and driven by the urgency to save lives and reduce the fatality rate, significant efforts were made to bring intensive care unit (ICU) specialists from around the country to assist in treatment centers such as the Wuhan Jinyintan and Pulmonary Hospitals.[33] As the number of hospital facilities available increased, additional medical teams were deployed to treat patients with less severe symptoms.

Alongside the prominent role played by medical teams from the PLA military hospital system and NHC-controlled hospitals, traditional Chinese medicine (TCM) also received high and indeed outsized visibility during the rescue efforts in Wuhan and the rest of Hubei, as well as in China's global diplomacy. Dr. Zhang Boli, an academician and president of the Tianjin University of Traditional Chinese Medicine, was a strong proponent for using TCM in treating SARS in 2003. On January 21, 2020, Dr. Zhang proposed that, in the absence of vaccines and approved therapeutic drugs, specially selected TCM herbal soups could be made widely available for patients in quarantine. He believed this would help buy time and "soothe the emotions" of patients during a period of panic:

> The biggest problem [for quarantined patients] was not treatment, but panic; if I were put in isolation without any medication, I would feel helpless. It makes a difference between not being given any medication and receiving two to several [TCM] packs a day, thus making the patients feel that at least they are taking medication.[34]

Dr. Zhang essentially argued for the wide distribution of TCM herbal packs or soup among confirmed or suspected patients with novel coronavirus infections. He assumed that even if the medication acted as a mere placebo, it could still be very valuable for the large number of people in China, especially in Wuhan and Hubei, who trusted TCM. Zhang's proposal was embraced by the Central Steering Group, with strong support from national leadership, particularly Xi Jinping, who was known to be a champion for TCM. Dr. Zhang accompanied the Central Steering Group to Wuhan on January 27 and was entrusted with leading the TCM treatment effort, often combining TCM with modern medicine. Under the National TCM Administration, five contingents of TCM medical teams, totally over 4,900 medical staff, were deployed.[35]

Learning by Doing and the Updating of the Diagnosis and Treatment Protocol

Dr. Du Bin rushed back to Wuhan on January 21, 2020, to join other clinical experts in observing and caring for patients at Jinyintan Hospital. They were perplexed and frustrated because patients with severe symptoms were unresponsive to treatment.[36] These patients typically had ground glass opacities on chest computed tomographic (CT) scans and dangerously low blood oxygen levels (hypoxemia), which are usually associated with breathing difficulties (dyspnea). However, clinicians discovered that these patients could suffer from hypoxemia without experiencing dyspnea. This "silent hypoxemia" made the condition particularly dangerous.[37] Some patients seemed healthy but had serious low oxygen levels that went unnoticed, leading to sudden deterioration and the development of acute respiratory distress syndrome (ARDS) and organ complications.[38]

Doctors in Wuhan recalled with horror how some patients appeared to be doing well but suddenly succumbed to the virus: the aunt in the neighborhood who liked to dance in the square, was rarely sick, and was still on video chat when she died; the professor who had no illnesses previously.[39] It was crucial for these patients to receive medical interventions before developing ARDS, but this often did not occur during the early days of the pandemic. Many patients transferred to Jinyintan Hospital already had severe symptoms. "They were already drowning," the doctors used to say. These patients were difficult to treat even in the best of circumstances. One of these patients was Jinyintan's own Dr. Huang Chaolin, who needed no transfer. He was checked in as a patient infected by the novel coronavirus on January 23. With his blood oxygen level already quite low at that point, his condition did not stabilize until February 4, 2020.[40]

For the expert physicians at Jinyintan, treating patients with severe novel coronavirus infections was like "operating in the dark." Dr. Du Bin recalled spending a whole morning by a patient's bedside trying to improve the patient's stubbornly low blood oxygen reading. Despite his best efforts, he was still unsuccessful. "I felt so defeated," Dr. Du said. "You had no idea what you were doing and what effect you were actually producing."[41] Dr. Fang Minghao, deputy chief of Emergency and Critical Care Medicine at Tongji Hospital, worked in the Jinyintan Hospital ICU at the same time and felt very much the same.[42]

Dr. Xia Jian, the deputy chief of the Wuhan University Zhongnan Hospital ICU, is a renowned ECMO specialist. In late December 2019, he joined the expert team at Jinyintan Hospital with the goal of using ECMO machines to help save critically ill patients with the so-called viral pneumonia of uncertain etiology (PUE). Unfortunately, all five patients (four males and one female) who were placed on ECMO ultimately passed away.[43]

Before the Wuhan lockdown, prohibitions against unauthorized public disclosure of outbreak information severely hindered the sharing of prevention and treatment knowledge within and between medical institutions. For instance, Dr. Peng Zhiyong's ICU team at Wuhan University Zhongnan Hospital used fiberoptic bronchoscopy for sputum aspiration of the lungs and placed patients in the prone position. These crucial supportive treatments helped reduce the fatality ratio at the Zhongnan Hospital ICU but were not widely known until later.[44] In another case, Liu Weiquan, a nursing expert from Tongji Hospital assigned to Jinyintan Hospital, suggested using a hermetic suction tube to effectively mitigate the risk of infection to medical staff. Although Liu's recommendation was quickly implemented at Jinyintan ICU, it was not extensively circulated to other medical institutions and remained relatively unknown at Wuhan Tongji Hospital.[45]

Following the official recognition of novel coronavirus pneumonia as an infectious disease and the Wuhan lockdown, leading respiratory and critical care medicine experts embarked on a crash program of learning by doing. Besides evident respiratory failures, the experts identified within 10 days that many patients also suffered from kidney issues, though recognizing heart damage from COVID-19 took considerably longer.[46] Through experimentation, they devised strategies for enhancing non-invasive oxygen therapy effectiveness, such as placing patients in the prone position (i.e., lying on their abdomen).[47] They also adopted a strategy of "early" intubation for critically ill patients, with some hospitals like Union Hospital (West Branch) forming dedicated intubation teams in mid-February to perform the labor-intensive and risky procedure.[48] The term "early" is used in quotation marks because it was misinterpreted when removed from the context of Wuhan.[49] Most patients in Wuhan who required intubation had already experienced significant treatment delays in January–February 2020. From the physicians' perspective, intubation needed to be "early" or prompt, but the treatment was in fact not early for these patients.

It is now acknowledged that the Chinese name for COVID-19, which translates to "pneumonia caused by infection with the novel coronavirus," led clinicians to focus on lung functions rather than considering COVID-19 as a disease affecting multiple organs. Early on, clinical experts recognized the need for autopsies to help understand the novel coronavirus's impact on the human body. However, due to cultural and institutional factors, the first autopsy was not performed until February 15. When the first (unannounced) death from the unusual pneumonia occurred on January 6, 2020, Cao Bin, Huang Chaolin, and Wu Wenjuan attempted but failed to persuade the deceased's family members to consent to an autopsy.[50] By the time of the first COVID-19 autopsy in Wuhan on February 15, 2020, around 1,500 people had already died from the disease in the city.[51] Nonetheless, subsequent autopsies significantly contributed to the global pursuit of knowledge about COVID-19.[52]

As clinical experts learned through experience, they made roving visits to designated hospitals to offer guidance and provide triage.[53] They also advised Sun Chunlan and Central Steering Group members on key policy and decision formulation.[54] Meanwhile, experts helped train the medical teams from across the country. Dr. Jiang Rongmeng alone trained over 3,600 medical staff in treatment and infection control within a 6-week period.[55] While many medical staff in Wuhan contracted SARS-CoV-2 early on, partly because they risked infection performing intubation and other hazardous procedures, the medical aid teams that joined in the rescue of Wuhan/Hubei had dedicated infection control specialists and took strict precautions to prevent staff infections.

The Updates to the Diagnosis and Treatment Protocol and the Significance of the Fifth Edition Protocol

Hard-earned clinical experiences, along with epidemiological (incubation period, contact history) and virological updates on the novel coronavirus, were integrated into successive editions of the Diagnosis and Treatment Protocol. These became publicly available starting with the delayed release of the second edition on January 22, 2020. On the same day, the NHC distributed the provisional Diagnosis and Treatment Protocol for Severe and Critical Novel Coronavirus Infected Pneumonia Cases, which was also updated repeatedly. The protocol for severe and critical cases emphasized oxygen therapy, ranging from oxygen masks to mechanical ventilation (including intubation), coupled with circulatory support.[56] These treatment protocols were crucial for disseminating the clinical experiences not only in Wuhan, Hubei, but also to the rest of China and beyond China's borders.

Excluding the January 2, 2020, protocol for the so-called viral PUE, the NHC distributed eight editions of the Diagnosis and Treatment Protocol between January 15 and April 14, 2020 (Table 12.2).[57] Among these, the fifth edition, released on February 4, was especially influential on *fangkong* strategy. Under NHC auspices, Zhong Nanshan, Li Lanjuan, and Wang Chen led the lengthy discussion sessions with experts to review and finalize the text of this revised protocol.[58] In addition to the existing categories of "ordinary, severe, and critical," the fifth edition expanded the classification of disease severity levels to include a "light" category and acknowledged the possibility of asymptomatic transmission.

By the beginning of February, clinical researchers not only had gathered ample and alarming evidence of high mortality among the critically ill in Wuhan but also had gained useful experiences for supportive treatment and preliminary indications from ongoing clinical trials.[59] The China CDC had also moved beyond its earlier missteps in keeping track of and analyzing the early cases and regrouped. Among the co-authors of the late January China CDC study on early transmission dynamics were Hong Kong researchers, who paid particular attention to asymptomatic transmission and the possibility of under-ascertainment and underestimation.[60] With a focus on a broader range of potential transmission routes, the study, published in the *New England Journal of Medicine*, concluded that "urgent next steps include identifying the most effective control measures to reduce transmission in the community."[61]

Table 12.2 Editions and Dates of the Diagnosis and Treatment Protocol

1. Viral PUE Diagnosis and Treatment Protocol, January 2, 2020, not publicly disclosed
2. Novel Coronavirus Pneumonia Diagnosis and Treatment Protocol
   First edition, January 15, 2020, not publicly released
   Second edition, January 18, not publicly released until January 22
   Third edition, January 23, publicly released immediately beginning with this edition
   Fourth edition, January 27
   Fifth edition, February 4
   Sixth edition, February 18
   Seventh edition, March 3
   Eighth edition, April 14

The fifth edition of the protocol reflected advances in epidemiological assessment. It stated that sources of infection were primarily patients infected with the novel coronavirus and that the main transmission routes were respiratory droplets and contact. However, it recognized the need to understand aerosol and gastrointestinal transmission routes. Contrary to the earlier impression that young people were unaffected, the protocol noted that children with COVID-19 tended to have mild symptoms. Importantly, having learned that asymptomatic individuals had tested positive for the novel coronavirus, the experts, who disagreed on the degree of asymptomatic infectivity, stated in the fifth edition that "asymptomatic infected persons may also become infectious."

Despite the restrained language, the updated understanding of virus transmission called into question the practice, and indeed the de facto strategy, of allowing individuals with mild symptoms, not to mention the asymptomatic, to remain at home and in the community. If the goal of containing the epidemic was based on the dual approach of reducing infection through isolation and reducing fatality through effective treatment, the realization that transmission and thus infection could be asymptomatic and more widespread signaled a need for more stringent *fangkong* measures. As we will describe below and in the next chapter, this understanding led directly to more aggressive efforts to expand quarantine capabilities and impose *fangkong* measures at the community level.

The Dire Need for Treatment and Acute Shortage of Hospital Beds

Following the January 20 announcement, long lines of patients outside fever clinics became the most visible signs of the disaster that had struck Wuhan. The next day, the Wuhan Fangkong Command announced that the government would cover all medical costs for patients with confirmed diagnosis of novel coronavirus infection.[62] The Wuhan Municipal Health Commission also announced the "7+7" hospital-pairing arrangement to increase the total number of hospital beds for treating patients with coronavirus infections to more than 3,000. Yet, even before the lockdown, it was evident that these hospital beds were woefully inadequate for the surging demand. Furthermore, the constructing and commissioning of new field hospitals took time.

Due to the severe imbalance in capacity to treat patients with novel coronavirus infections, triage of patients for treatments had to be done. Staff from provincial and municipal commands and health commissions worked directly with hospitals and doctors to arrange patient admissions, thus determining their fate. Volunteers from the *People's Daily*, among others, helped screen patients who most urgently needed treatment.[63] However, the task was so emotionally draining that some volunteers struggled to continue. An unnamed staff member from the Hubei Provincial Health Commission who managed the phone bank at the Command Headquarters for Epidemic Response referred to the week of February 7–13 as the "dark week" and described it as the most challenging time at the command. It was particularly devastating for staff to finally arrange for a critically ill patient to be taken to a hospital, only to be informed by the family that the patient had passed away.[64]

With hospital admission often making the difference between life and death for patients, administrators and doctors faced difficult choices when deciding who to admit for treatment. Dr. Peng Peng, president of the Wuhan Pulmonary Hospital, recalled working with doctors to allocate the limited number of available hospital beds each day and having to choose from a long list of patients waiting for admission. "It was really very hard, because a hospital bed meant the chance for survival."[65] The Hubei Provincial Hospital of Integrated Chinese and Western Medicine, where Dr. Zhang Jixian works, was among this third group of designated hospitals. "[I've] never seen an infectious disease like this, never seen so many patients rush to the hospital like this," Dr. Zhang recalled. In one of the most memorable remarks during the Wuhan lockdown, Dr. Zhang said, "I shed all the tears of my life this time!"[66]

The large number of healthcare worker infections further strained the healthcare system in Wuhan and the rest of Hubei. According to the NHC, as of February 11, Wuhan had 1,103 infected healthcare workers, while the rest of Hubei had another 400.[67] This resulted in a reduction in the healthcare workforce and the commitment of significant medical resources to care for infected healthcare workers, who received priority (but no guarantee) for in-hospital treatment.

However, from late January to mid-February, it was exceedingly challenging for the family members of healthcare workers to secure admission for in-hospital treatment. The Wuhan Central Hospital (WCH) community experienced numerous dark days for both staff and their families. Dr. NM served on the front lines in the Ultrasound Section of WCH. Four members of her extended family—her grandparents, father-in-law, and uncle—contracted the virus and required hospitalization. When the 120 Medical Emergency Center could not assist them, Dr. NM sought help from WCH. She was informed that over 100 family members of WCH staff were already on the waiting list, preceding her and her family. Unable to access hospital care, her grandmother, father-in-law, and grandfather succumbed to the illness in succession during the first half of February 2020.[68]

Table 12.3 presents a daily update on the number of hospital beds in designated hospitals from January 31 to February 25, 2020. Except for the last column, which represents the difference between newly added hospital beds and vacant beds, the remaining columns contain the raw data released by the Wuhan Municipal Health Commission. I have labeled the last column "Hospital capacity indicator," which is a negative value when patients occupy

Table 12.3 Hospital Resources Available for Treating COVID-19 Patients

Date	Number of designated hospitals	Total number of beds available	Occupied	Vacant	Hospital capacity indicator
2020-01-31	23	6,641	6,414	389	
2020-02-01	23	6,754	6,808	175	62
2020-02-02	26	7,259	7,332	131	-374
2020-02-03	28	8,199	8,279	139	-801
2020-02-04	28	8,254	8,182	305	250
2020-02-05	28	8,574	8,759	120	-200
2020-02-06	28	8,895	9,105	142	-179
2020-02-07	28	9,057	9,198	123	-39
2020-02-08	29	9,312	9,269	236	-19
2020-02-09	31	10,300	10,087	378	-610
2020-02-10	35	12,437	12,077	720	-1,417
2020-02-11	35	12,922	12,822	473	-12
2020-02-12	38	14,269	14,004	645	-702
2020-02-13	38	15,018	14,625	776	27
2020-02-14	38	15,985	15,446	880	-87
2020-02-15	42	17,262	17,082	678	-599
2020-02-16	46	18,816	18,037	1,212	-342
2020-02-17	45	19,161	18,086	1,452	1,107
2020-02-18	45	19,927	18,393	1,845	1,079
2020-02-19	46	19,989	18,955	1,257	1,195
2020-02-20	48	20,989	19,313	1,828	828
2020-02-21	48	21,722	19,003	2,853	2,120
2020-02-22	48	22,681	19,099	3,672	2,713
2020-02-23	48	23,435	19,335	4,100	3,346
2020-02-24	48	23,532	19,275	4,311	4,214
2020-02-25	48	24,378	19,425	5,024	4,178

Source: "全市定点医院病床使用情况," Wuhan Municipal Health Commission (https://wjw.wuhan.gov.cn), various dates.

more beds than are newly added (some patients may temporarily be placed in makeshift beds). This indicator reveals that it was not until February 17 that COVID-19 patients in Wuhan could consistently secure admission to a designated hospital. In the following section, I briefly outline the various efforts undertaken to increase hospital capacity.

Expanding Treatment and Quarantine Capacity

On the day before the Wuhan lockdown, the city's leadership, with approval from Vice Premier Sun Chunlan and the national leadership, decided to follow Beijing's SARS experience by building an emergency field hospital, the Fire God Mountain Hospital. They also converted general hospitals into designated hospitals. This marked the beginning of an extensive program to construct and deploy new hospital facilities for isolating and treating coronavirus-infected patients. As the scale of the epidemic grew, so did efforts to build new hospital facilities, including *fangcang* shelter hospitals, and to repurpose hotels and school dormitories for quarantine purposes. In this section, I briefly summarize these efforts, with a particular focus on how they helped alleviate the shortage of hospital beds.

Commissioning of the Fire God Mountain and Thunder God Mountain Hospitals and Other Medical Facilities

Wuhan's leadership announced the decision to build the *Huoshenshan*, or Fire God Mountain, Hospital, with 1,000 beds, on the day of the lockdown. Two days Mountain, later, they decided to construct a second, larger *Leishenshan*, or Thunder God Hospital, with a capacity for 1,600 beds. The invocation of the fire and thunder gods represented a reference to the mythic founding figure of the Chu people, who inhabited present-day Hubei.

China Construction Third Bureau deployed over 12,000 workers to construct the Fire God Mountain Hospital in just 9 days and 10 nights and an additional 22,000 workers to build the Thunder God Mountain Hospital in 10 days and 10 nights.[69] Due to the Lunar New Year and lockdown-induced transportation difficulties, tremendous efforts were necessary to overcome obstacles and bottlenecks in securing production and deliveries for these projects.[70] It is no exaggeration to say that China's construction workers, mostly contract workers, heroically rose to the occasion.

To minimize nosocomial infections, special emphasis was placed on constructing negative pressure units for patients and maintaining spatial separation between patients and medical staff.[71] Learning from the difficulties many hospitals faced in maintaining steady oxygen supplies amid demand surges, extra oxygen storage tanks were installed at these new facilities.[72]

The construction of the Fire God Mountain and Thunder God Mountain Hospitals was televised and streamed live to the public, showcasing China's capabilities for executing such complex projects as well as symbolizing China's national resolve to combat the epidemic.[73] As the hospitals—at least parts of them—began operating on February 4 and 8, 2020, they provided hope for desperate patients, their families, and the general public.

The Fire God Mountain Hospital was staffed by a combined military medical team of 1,400 people. The entire Army Medical University medical team at Jinyintan Hospital, along with members of the Navy and Air Force medical teams at Hankou and Wuchang Hospitals, were transferred to the Fire God Mountain Hospital.[74] Dr. Zhang Sibing of the PLA General Hospital served as president of Fire God Mountain Hospital. Wang Xinghuan, president of the Wuhan University Zhongnan Hospital, took on the stewardship of Thunder God Mountain Hospital. My interviewees in Wuhan saw Dr. Wang's appointment as a recognition of Zhongnan Hospital's superior response and performance in January 2020. Between February 3 and April 15, 2020, Fire God Mountain Hospital admitted 3,059 COVID-19 patients and successfully discharged 2,961 of them. Thunder God Mountain Hospital admitted 2,011 COVID-19 patients and successfully treated 1,918.[75]

Two nearly completed hospital complexes, the Taikang Tongji Hospital and the Guanggu Branch of the Hubei Maternal and Child Health Care Hospital, were rapidly transformed into infectious disease hospitals to operate like the Thunder God Mountain and Fire God Mountain Hospitals.[76] The Taikang Tongji Hospital, with 1,060 beds, was staffed by a combined military medical corps of 1,402 personnel drawn from multiple military hospitals. It treated 2,060 COVID-19 patients between February 14 and April 5, 2020, ranking just behind Fire God Mountain Hospital and Jinyintan Hospital.[77] The same model was adopted for the Hubei Maternal and Child Health Care Hospital (Guanggu Branch). It was staffed by 1,200 military medical staff and took in 639 COVID-19 patients between February 19 and 25.[78]

The *Fangcang* Shelter Hospitals

While the Fire God Mountain and Thunder God Mountain Hospitals were announced with great fanfare and boosted morale in Wuhan and nationally, they only added 2,600 beds and did not make a significant difference in meeting the urgent need for hospital beds until they were completed in February. Complicating matters, amid public talk about the timing of a turning point for the epidemic, the Chinese leadership received a reality check in early February from a group of distinguished experts led by academician Wang Chen, president of Peking Union Medical College (PUMC) and the Chinese Academy of Medical Sciences (CAMS). A respiratory and critical care specialist, Wang Chen led the expert team during the SARS crisis in Beijing in 2003. Once mentor to Dr. Cao Bin, he was well informed about patients suffering from novel coronavirus infections in Wuhan from early on.

Wang Chen arrived in Wuhan on February 1, 2020. Based on his observations and findings, he candidly reported to the leadership and did not sugarcoat his message to the public. In line with the updated epidemiological understanding of virus transmission, he noted that the epidemic situation in Wuhan remained serious because many patients could not receive timely care in hospitals, and they were also sources of further infections in households and communities. Contrary to the official messaging that strove to be reassuring aimed to reassure, Dr. Wang admitted that he, and by extension the authorities, did not have a good grasp on the number of infected people, and that the sources of infection were still not cut off. Consequently, there was not enough evidence to predict when the epidemic might plateau and reach a turning point.[79] Testing problems further compounded the challenges as many probable cases still could not get tested. According to a vice chair of the Hubei Medical Imaging Professional Committee, polymerase chain reaction nucleic acid testing tended to produce false negatives in the range of 30%–40%; in fact, Dr. Li Wenliang tested negative on his first two tests.[80]

Faced with the dire need to quarantine, treat all infected individuals, and cut off chains of transmission in households and communities, multiple experts led by Dr. Wang Chen recommended converting large-scale structures, such as sports stadiums and convention centers, into field hospitals.[81] The recommendation played to Wuhan's strengths as a regional hub city, with many public structures recently refurbished for hosting the World Military Games. These hospitals would be called "*fangcang* shelter hospitals"; in Chinese, *fangcang* (方舱) takes after *fangzhou* (方舟) or "ark" as in "Noah's ark." Since Dr. Wang Chen is the president of PUMC/CAMS, two of China's most prestigious medical institutions, the proposal came with strong credibility.

The Central Steering Group's leadership embraced the *fangcang* idea as it offered a feasible, if not ideal, route to the goal of "admitting all who needed to be admitted" for treatment and cutting off community transmission. On February 3, the day before the Fire God Mountain Hospital began accepting patients on a limited basis, Vice Premier Sun Chunlan ordered the conversion of major public structures into *fangcang* shelter hospitals.[82] That evening, the Central Steering Group meeting at the Wuhan Convention Center lasted into the early hours.[83] Teams from Wuhan and the NHC quickly identified an initial list of more than a dozen structures for conversion and made plans for staffing the field hospitals.

Under the guidance of medical experts led by Dr. Wang Chen and NHC staff, Mayor Zhou Xianwang spearheaded the massive effort to convert existing structures into *fangcang* hospitals.[84] He received substantial support from various quarters for design, supply, and interior reconstruction, including numerous volunteers who assisted in setting up beds.[85] On February 5, the 1,600-bed Jianghan Fangcang Hospital (located in the Wuhan International Convention Center) and the 800-bed Wuchang Fangcang Hospital (housed in the Hongshan Sports Stadium) began operations. Within 30 hours, 2,380 medical personnel from over 20 emergency medical teams took responsibility for the initial 4,000 *fangcang* beds.[86]

Public Skepticism about *Fangcang* Hospitals

Chinese officials and social media often showcased communal activities and interactions, such as group dancing, as a hallmark of life in the *fangcang* hospitals. They also highlighted patients, whose symptoms had receded, volunteering to help staff serve others.[87] While these images captured an important aspect of life in *fangcang* hospitals after conditions and patients had improved, it is important to remember that these were makeshift facilities deployed during a time of crisis and scarcity of medical resources. Dr. Wang Chen emphasized that *fangcang* hospitals were implemented because they were "desirable, realistic, and doable" when the best options were not available.[88]

The spartan camp-like conditions at the shelters presented challenges for patients, medical staff, and management. In the first days after the initial *fangcang* hospitals began operations, Wuhan experienced cold and snowy weather, leading to issues with access to basic facilities such as water, heating, and sanitation in some shelters.[89] One clinical study found a high prevalence of diarrhea among patients admitted to the Dongxihu Fangcang Hospital, suggesting that common environmental factors at the shelter hospital contributed to the issue.[90] Dr. Wan Jun, a vice president of the Wuhan University People's Hospital, was the president of the 800-bed Wuchang Fangcang Hospital between February 5 and March 10. He admitted that "every day is really tough" at the *fangcang* hospital.[91]

As patients shared videos from *fangcang* hospitals on platforms like Douyin/TikTok, public skepticism grew both domestically and internationally. Critics likened *fangcang* hospitals to a "new type of refugee camp" and called for halting further construction and use.[92] Despite the criticism, Wang Chen remained steadfast and reiterated the importance of building the *fangcang* hospitals with Wuhan party officials in this time of health emergency and scarcity.[93]

In theory, careful screening of patients should take place before admitting them to *fangcang* hospitals. Moreover, patients in *fangcang* hospitals whose symptoms worsened would be evaluated and transferred to designated hospitals for treatment if needed. However, due to the shortage of beds at designated hospitals, it was initially challenging for patients in need to secure transfers. For those who did manage to move to designated hospitals, the transfer process was often marked by uncertainty and anxiety.[94]

Nonetheless, the process of admission, quality of life, and care in *fangcang* hospitals improved over time.[95] By February 15, the nine operating *fangcang* hospitals had admitted 5,606 patients. By February 22, 16 *fangcang* shelter hospitals were operational, providing 13,000 beds. In total, between February 5 and March 10, *fangcang* hospitals cared for 12,000 patients, approximately one in four of the COVID-19 patients treated in Wuhan.[96] As the epidemic situation eased, the Qiaokou Wuti Fangcang Hospital became the first to suspend operations on March 1. All 16 *fangcang* hospitals had transferred their remaining patients to designated hospitals and ceased operations by March 10, 2020.

Conclusion

As the cordon sanitaire was imposed in Wuhan/Hubei and emergency rule implemented nationwide for public health purposes, the Chinese party-state, under Xi Jinping's leadership, utilized its organizational and disciplinary power to mobilize medical and other forms of aid and support for Wuhan/Hubei. Both clinical and public health professionals, as well as decision makers overseeing the overall epidemic response efforts, learned through hands-on experience. Initially, authorities attempted to replicate the SARS-era experience by constructing the Fire God Mountain and Thunder God Moutain Hospitals but soon realized that such a response was woefully inadequate for the novel coronavirus epidemic in Wuhan. Instead, they managed to dramatically increase the availability of hospital beds and quarantine spaces by converting existing structures, particularly public facilities like convention centers and stadiums. The *fangcang* shelter hospitals, in particular, played an essential role in Wuhan's efforts to ensure that no confirmed COVID-19 patient went untreated.[97] Each patient housed in a *fangcang* hospital also reduced the potential sources of infection within the community. We now shift our focus to the struggles faced on the community front.

13
The Real Wuhan Lockdown

The efforts to rapidly increase the capacity for treating COVID-19 patients in hospitals would not have been effective without the concurrent implementation of robust community epidemic control measures aimed at curbing virus transmission. Chinese official media has underscored the fundamental importance of the Communist Party–led community governance structure, particularly the grid management mechanism, in successfully executing Wuhan's lockdown and containing the COVID-19 epidemic in China in 2020.[1] Numerous community leaders have been hailed for their role in safeguarding the health and security of their respective communities.[2] The initial wave of academic papers on grassroots responses in China has likewise emphasized the significance of preexisting party-lead community and grid governance structures in combating the epidemic.[3]

In reality, the situation in communities with novel coronavirus cases closely mirrored the struggles encountered in hospitals. Amid the acute shortage of hospital resources in Wuhan, the highly regarded grid management mechanism at the grassroots level provided limited assistance initially. Many communities were plagued by chaos and disarray as community staff grappled with offering help, let alone providing proper care, for their infected residents. As a result, a community's resilience and fate during the burgeoning epidemic became intrinsically linked to the capabilities of the local health sector and the judgment of political and health leaders, who operated at a distance from the grassroots level.

This chapter delves into the politics of community-level epidemic control actions. The eventual success in containing the virus hinged critically on community-level efforts, but this success was achieved after arduous struggles. I begin by discussing the community-level distress and disarray during the first 2 weeks of the lockdown period, with a particular emphasis on the situation at the Baibuting mega-community and the epidemic control weaknesses at the community level during this time. Following this, I describe the cries for help from Wuhan and connect them with the national efforts to revamp leadership in Wuhan and Hubei. I then outline the significant measures undertaken by the new leaders of Wuhan and Hubei to shift the fight against the epidemic to the community level as shortages in hospital and quarantine capacity eased. This transition ultimately led to a true lockdown focused on home confinement, which not only contributed to the end of the Wuhan lockdown but also became central to China's prolonged pursuit of a zero-COVID strategy.

Grassroots Governance and the Epidemic Control Challenge in Wuhan

As mentioned in Chapter 2, the city of Beijing pioneered the application of grid management to govern urban societies that had undergone significant transformation and diversification.[4] Since the 2010s, the grid governance model, under party leadership, has spread across the country as part of the stability maintenance regime. This model divides urban neighborhoods into smaller spatial grids. Under the Street Office leadership and staff, community grid managers or staffers (社区网格管理员) act as handymen or handywomen for the party-state hierarchy, tasked with various responsibilities ranging from collecting statistics to providing public services, or more generally connecting with and getting to know residents within a block or part of a block.

The grid governance model has been promoted as a mechanism for collaborative party-state-society governance, aiming to mobilize residents, provide services, reduce crime, and address conflicts and challenges.[5] Although official language emphasizes "governance" and "service," the grid governance model, combined with existing street bureaucracy in urban areas and villagers' committees in rural areas, has undoubtedly strengthened top-down monitoring and supervision of residents, with special emphasis on the migrant population.[6] The grid, represented by the grid manager, acts as a supplementary mechanism within an organizational setup that includes the party branch committee, a residents' committee, and, in newer residential areas, a property management and property owners' committee. Positioned at the lower end of the vast party-state hierarchy, community grid workers are typically contract staff who report to leaders and staff in the Street Office or township and face very limited opportunities for upward mobility.

Prior to the novel coronavirus outbreak, Wuhan had gained national recognition for promoting "red" grassroots governance by combining party-building at the grassroots level with initiative in urban social governance.[7] As of 2019, Wuhan had staffed urban communities with approximately 12,000 grid workers (compared to a total of 170,000 for Hubei Province).[8] It also selected 10,000 police, 1,000 lawyers, and representatives from government or business "units"—mostly Communist Party members—to work closely with street- or community-level institutions.[9] Thus, when the Central Committee General Office called for strengthening and improving party-building at the grassroots level in 2019, including at the grid level, Wuhan was already steps ahead.[10] In December 2019, the Central Political and Legal Affairs Commission (CPLAC), the Communist Party's institutional minder for stability maintenance, convened the first national work conference on urban social governance modernization in Wuhan. Wuhan was the only provincial capital city given the honor of presenting its experience in social governance innovation.[11]

Grassroots Governance and the Coronavirus Outbreak in Wuhan

Before the lockdown, the Wuhan municipal leadership relied on the "red" grassroots governance structure to reinforce official messages of reassurance. Street Office leaders and staff participated in efforts to dispel "rumors" about the viral outbreak, downplaying the severity of the situation. They also discouraged preventive measures, such as wearing facemasks, in the weeks leading up to the lockdown.[12]

Resourceful urban communities inadvertently further helped the novel coronavirus spread by organizing social gatherings. Baibuting community, Wuhan's model for red social governance, was most notable for organizing large-scale communal banquets ahead of the Lunar New Year. This also explains why Baibuting and city leaders found it difficult to cancel the community's nationally famous mass banquet. It was on a pedestal and had to perform its expected role, serving as an example for Wuhan and beyond.

The difference between Baibuting and other communities was a matter of degree, not of kind. Shuiguohu, or Fruit Lake Street (水果湖街道), in Wuchang District is located near the heavily guarded compound for the Hubei Provincial Communist Party Committee and Provincial Government. It is home to many officials, staff, and retirees from provincial party and government offices. Comprising 23 communities (社区) and 28 residents' committees (居委会), Fruit Lake Street is known as Hubei's First Street and has been named a national model of party-led community innovation and Harmonious Community Building.[13] In the weeks leading up to the Lunar New Year, multiple parties and social gatherings were held for residents, particularly retired cadres, with little attention given to protection against the novel coronavirus. Consequently, the number of COVID-19 cases in the Fruit Lake Street communities was quite high.[14] Community staff bore the brunt of the spreading infections. In Shuiguohu's Fangyingtai community, only 7 of the 15 community staff members remained on duty in early February to cope with the skyrocketing demand.[15]

Distress, Disarray, and Call to Action

Following imposition of the lockdown, the mood and tempo in the communities changed drastically. The leaders, staff, and volunteers in the street offices and neighborhood and residents' communities were just as stunned as most of the people in Wuhan. They were also immediately asked to play indispensable roles in epidemic prevention and control.

On the day of the Wuhan lockdown, the Wuhan Municipal Health Commission outlined its expectations for grassroots leaders and staff to contribute to epidemic control and ensure that all infected individuals and their close contacts would be helped and supervised. The goal was to "not miss a single person." "Close contacts should be promptly and accurately referred to the residential district for management."[16] In a striking illustration of the mismatch between the party's top-down governance style and the explosive epidemic situation, Party Secretary Ma Guoqiang emphasized these points and directed district leaders to ensure that the ill received treatment promptly.[17] Community grid management teams, comprising community staff, medical staff, and grid workers, were ordered to conduct daily medical observations on close contacts. Those close contacts with a fever of 37.3°C (99.14°F) or above, cough, and other symptoms had to be immediately reported so that they could be promptly transferred by ambulance to designated hospitals for treatment.[18]

Chen Jun, a mother of two, was one of the 12,000 community grid workers in Wuhan. She was ordered to report for duty on January 23 immediately. Bringing a few single-use facemasks from home, she was given a thermometer for checking her own temperature. Her initial task was to phone residents in her community grid of 966 people for fever symptoms. It was only a few days later that she and her colleagues began to receive protective gear for their duties. Fortunately, her community grid did not have a resident with fever and other symptoms associated with COVID-19 until the end of January.[19]

In the Baibuting mega-community, the atmosphere turned somber abruptly after Dr. Zhong Nanshan's January 20 interview. Suddenly, the grand community feast at Baibuting became a massive cloud hanging over the entire community. For at least the 2-week incubation period, Baibuting residents lived in anxiety, worrying that they might have caught the novel coronavirus during the mass gathering. Mao Yonghong, a well-known entrepreneur and long-serving party secretary of the Baibuting community, went quiet.[20] Wang Bo, head of the Baibuting Community Management Committee, sank into a psychological "bottomless whirlpool."[21]

Mr. Liu (pseudonym), who chaired one of the nine residents' committees at Baibuting, was asked on January 21 to help trace confirmed or suspected cases. He discovered that the cases or people he needed to track had recently left Baibuting and even Wuhan for treatment.[22] The next day, January 22, Liu was asked to help persuade a resident with fever—Patient BD—to go to a designated hospital for further investigation. BD went to the hospital that afternoon. When BD returned the next morning, he reported that the hospital was crowded with patients; he was found to have bilateral infections in his lungs but was told to return home to self-isolate because the hospital had no bed available to admit him.

By then, Wuhan was in lockdown and the Baibuting Community Health Service Center had a line of outpatients waiting. Liu received information on another five suspected cases. He learned that all five individuals were like BD: their computed tomographic (CT) scans showed bilateral lung infections, but the hospitals had no room to admit them. Consequently, they had returned home to self-isolate and were thus back in the community.

On January 24, Liu called to inquire about BD and learned that his symptoms appeared to have eased. That evening, to his astonishment, he received the distressing news from BD's family that BD had passed away at home. "From that night to noon the next day, feelings of fear, helplessness, and guilt rushed repeatedly through me," Liu recalled.[23]

Because BD had not had his coronavirus infection confirmed by polymerase chain reaction (PCR) testing, his death was not counted as a COVID-related death. In the early weeks of the epidemic, a large number of COVID-19 deaths were registered as deaths from "ordinary pneumonia" because the deceased could not get tested for the novel coronavirus.[24]

Amid this atmosphere of grief and fear, Liu and his colleagues helped BD's widow contact the relevant departments and the crematorium. For BD's widow, who had lost her and BD's only daughter to suicide in the Yangtze River a few years earlier, and the many families caught up in the epidemic, their agonies were compounded by the severe emergency restrictions on funerary arrangements during the lockdown.[25] Family members were not permitted to go to the crematorium to say farewell to loved ones, nor were they allowed to pick up the cremated remains until a yet-to-be-determined time, which turned out to be the end of March 2020.[26]

To some extent, diarists like writer Fang Fang, whose daily journals attracted enormous attention, gave voice to those who were suffering or in mourning during the pandemic, offering some symbolic rites of passage for families who had lost loved ones and experienced disruptions to mourning rituals.[27] Unfortunately, Fang Fang also attracted vicious attacks from nationalists who viewed her candid reports—often made to disappear in Chinese cyberspace—as providing ammunition for China's critics and enemies.

In the days that followed, Liu and other community leaders and staff in Baibuting and elsewhere were inundated with calls for help with medical care. When residents managed to contact community staff, the typical response they received was that their case had been filed and reported to a higher level of authority, but there were no diagnostic test kits or hospital beds available; they were instructed to wait at home.[28]

The stresses at the community level were joined at the municipal level. The Mayor's Hotline and the 120 medical emergency service were overwhelmed with calls for help in the first weeks of the lockdown but had precious little assistance to offer. Residents also turned to social media for healthcare information and help. Large numbers of people in need used the "#COVID-19 Patient Seeking Help" hashtag on Weibo but faced the same bottlenecks and frustrations.[29] A volunteer at the 120 emergency center recalled that the most distressing situations involved elderly couples in their 70s or 80s with no children at home to help them and limited ability to obtain information online. "We were in pain and anxious [about them] but had no way to solve [their problem]."[30]

Consider the case of the Y family at Baibuting. Both of Y's parents showed symptoms on January 21, 2020, and were told to isolate at home. Y's 63-year-old mother, YM, urgently needed professional medical care because she had a high fever and difficulty breathing. The best the community staff could do was to arrange a CT scan for YM at Hankou Hospital, which revealed infections in both lungs. Community staff then informed YM and her family that she was first in line among patients with severe symptoms for diagnostic testing and admittance to in-hospital treatment. However, it wasn't until around February 4, 2020, that YM was finally admitted to the hospital.[31]

YM's experience was far from unique. Due to the massive increase in the number of people infected, patients and their families seeking help through various channels to gain access to in-hospital care faced frustration and disappointment.[32] Forced to stay at home without medicine or proper medical care, patients had to rely on themselves. While many recovered thanks to their own immune systems, it was extraordinarily challenging for those whose conditions worsened suddenly to survive.[33] Those in serious or critical conditions required more intensive treatment and were more likely to be fatally ill by the time they reached hospitals. Survivors were also more likely to suffer from long-lasting damage.

Confronted with a long list of demands from the Wuhan Command, community staff and grid workers struggled with the scarcity of hospital beds and transportation, on the one hand, and residents in dire need, on the other, all while risking infection themselves.[34] Liao Jianjun, a leader of a neighborhood committee in Qiaokou District, tragically died in early February 2020 after contracting the virus while assisting a suspected patient to hospital.[35] Yet, community staff faced complaints and anger from exasperated residents who were sick but couldn't access proper medical care or were simply frustrated by being forced to shelter in place.[36] Some community staff and grid workers quit.

Despite the increasing number of residents who tested positive and others who had yet to be tested but were suspected cases, the Baibuting community leadership remained silent and did not disclose the community infection information for about 2 weeks. Fearful of being ostracized, infected individuals and their families also kept quiet. "Some bitterness you've got to bear on your own," said one interviewee.[37]

The eerie silence surrounding the Baibuting community was finally broken on February 4, when a staff member informed a media source about the existence of numerous confirmed cases in the area.[38] An uproar ensued about problems in the community's response to the epidemic and fears that the virus continued to spread because many residents still entered and left the community for shopping and other activities.[39] The uproar culminated in highly public appeals for help on February 9, 2020.[40]

According to the Wuhan Command, the Baibuting community had 87 confirmed cases and 112 suspected cases on February 8 (out of a population of about 110,000).[41] In hindsight, considering the total number of residents in this large community, the number of confirmed and suspected cases was not as alarming as initially feared, although some infections had not yet been identified. By then, with more hospitals opening, including *fangcang* shelter hospitals, hospital beds had started to become available for infected individuals. On February 6, Liu and his colleagues in their part of Baibuting managed to send four COVID-19 patients to hospitals for treatment; six more followed on February 7 and then eight on February 8.[42]

The Push on Community-Level Epidemic Control in Early February 2020

As described in the previous chapter, the official response during the first 2 weeks of the lockdown in Wuhan focused on enhancing treatment capabilities by bringing in medical teams from around China and increasing the number of hospitals for treating and quarantining infected patients. Authorities also hoped that the number of new cases would drop significantly toward the end of the estimated 2-week incubation period following the lockdown. However, when the number of confirmed cases continued to rise rapidly in early February (see Figure 13.1), it became clear that the lockdown measures had failed to break the chains of transmission within households and communities.[43]

On February 3, Vice Premier Sun Chunlan and members of the Central Steering Group began regularly visiting the Wuhan Fangkong Command. With a better understanding of the need to prevent new infections and reduce fatalities, as well as the weaknesses at the community level, Sun led the Central Steering Group to urge Wuhan's municipal authorities to achieve the goal of "admitting all who should be admitted."[44] Although the Wuhan Fangkong Command made quick promises to admit patients by February

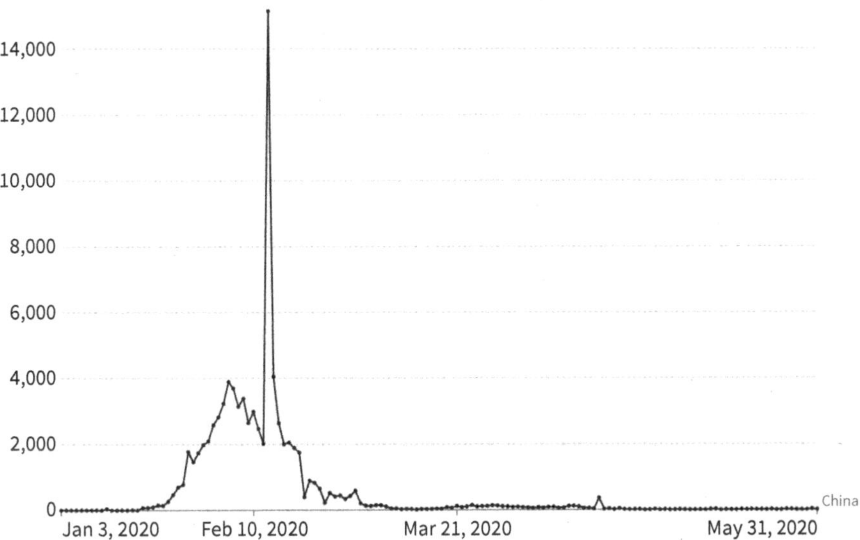

Figure 13.1 Daily New Confirmed COVID-19 Cases

Generated with COVID-19 Data Explorer at Our World in Data site (https://ourworldindata.org/explorers/coronavirus-data-explorer). Used with permission under the Creative Commons BY license.

5 and complete PCR testing of all suspected cases by February 7, it was unable to deliver on these promises.[45] In response, Sun and the National Health Commission (NHC) leadership strongly intervened in the community front, and on February 6, the NHC organized a team of community infection *fangkong* experts to come to Wuhan to provide advice.

The community infection *fangkong* experts were drawn from community health service centers in Beijing and Jiangsu Province, as well as the Institute for Communicable Disease Control and Prevention (ICDC) of the China Centers for Disease Control and Prevention (China CDC). Dr. Wu Hao, director of the Fangzhuang Community Health Service Center in Beijing and a professor at Capital Medical University, served as team leader.[46] As noted earlier, the Fangzhuang community in Beijing had activated its grid governance mechanisms in mid-January 2020, even before many communities in Wuhan began taking serious action. In Fangzhuang, teams of three, with representatives from the neighborhood office, the community, and the community health center, were formed by community grids to assist the district CDC in conducting contact tracing, managing suspected cases, and preventing the introduction of infections.[47]

By this time, the epidemic in China outside Hubei was under control. With relatively few cases, local authorities in most areas outside Hubei were able to mobilize both the rank and file and grassroots communities to focus on prevention, primarily by closing off communities and limiting interactions with the outside. Using data from disease surveillance points covering around 300 million people, a team of researchers later found that the strict anti-contagion policies in the rest of China not only helped stop the spread of COVID-19 but also significantly reduced non-COVID-19 mortality during the lockdown period and in the following months.[48]

In contrast, Wuhan was still focused on providing care for patients with confirmed or likely coronavirus infections.[49] The team of community health experts brought to Wuhan was shocked by what they saw. "The grassroots *fangkong* system was in a state of chaos," said a member of the team.[50]

On February 7, Dr. Wu Hao and his two teammates went to Jiang'an District, which had 800,000 residents and had suffered especially badly from the epidemic. Wu noted that the district had 18 venues for isolation. Yet he saw that "the supermarkets were full of people" shopping. He observed,

> the communities were not practicing closed-off management at that time. Household waste that might be infected was scattered all over the place. Those with mild symptoms went out for grocery shopping and activities; those who had more serious symptoms went out to seek medical treatment and admittance into hospitals. There were many people in close contact with the infected.[51]

Dr. Wu and his colleagues also noted that some cadres in management positions focused on collecting data and preparing reports for superiors, rather than supervising work on the front lines in the communities. The repeated demands for data and reports added to the burdens on grassroots staff and volunteers, affecting their morale.[52] Front-line employees who braved the virus and the cold weather resented the office managers. Dr. Wu and his colleagues questioned how the sources of infection could be controlled when the sick were like mobile sources of infection. "If the disorderly scenario in front of our eyes continues and the pathways of community transmission are not cut off," Dr. Wu concluded, the number of new infections "will eventually engulf all the hospital beds in the city."[53]

That evening, in a WeChat discussion group, Wu Hao and his colleagues on the community health expert team shared their observations and concerns. Based on these observations and local experiences, as well as his experience combating severe acute respiratory syndrome (SARS) in Beijing in 2003, Dr. Wu articulated a community-based disease control strategy centered on strictly closing off residential communities and asking residents to shelter in place at home. Meanwhile, as part of a people's war against the epidemic, there would be door-to-door screening for infected individuals within each community. Staff from party-state bureaucracies would also be asked to go into the communities to help ensure compliance with the community-centered lockdown, unleash the potential of grid management, and achieve the goals of epidemic *fangkong*.[54] In short, this strategy played to the political and institutional impulses and capabilities of the Chinese party-state system.

A limited number of Wuhan communities had already put such measures into practice beginning in late January.[55] Some elements of this community strategy, such as dispatching party and government staffers to help targeted communities, were part of Wuhan's "red" social governance experience. Starting around February 5, some members of the provincial party-government apparatus were dispatched to selected communities to help solve problems.[56]

Beginning on February 7, Wu Hao and his colleagues formed teams of three, which included one community health expert, a China CDC specialist, and one local representative, to visit the 13 districts in Wuhan. On February 8, armed with additional information, Wu Hao reported the community team's assessment and recommendations to the Central Steering Group leadership. Dr. Wu's community-centered strategy for infection control was eagerly embraced. In the afternoon, the Jiang'an District leadership agreed to implement the strategy starting the next day.[57]

Over the following 7 weeks, the community health teams led by Wu Hao visited and reviewed more than 500 residential communities, 161 community health centers, and 377 "neighborhoods," identifying 1,275 issues in anti-epidemic work that required attention.[58] Members of the China CDC–ICDC who participated in these reviews and investigations reported that their suggestions on a broad range of issues, including community disease prevention and control, disinfection, patient transfer, and reviews of specific locations such as quarantine quarters, retirement homes, and detention and detox centers, were quickly incorporated into guidance for the district or directly resolved by community staff or through the coordination of the district *fangkong* commands.[59] These researchers were impressed that their suggestions were promptly embraced as directives and swiftly translated into action.

Xi Jinping, Public Anger, and the Revamping of the Wuhan/Hubei Leadership

Dr. Li Wenliang, aged 34, was admitted to Wuhan Central Hospital with clinical symptoms on January 12, 2020. After several tests, he was finally confirmed to have contracted the novel coronavirus on February 1. By then, his condition had already worsened. When the public learned about the severe reprimand he received from the police and Wuhan Central Hospital in early January, his illness became a symbol of the government's mishandling of the outbreak and abuse of power. Dr. Li Wenliang's quote "A normal society should not have only one voice" resonated and reverberated across the country.

On the evening of February 6, 2020, tens of millions of Chinese people anxiously waited online as doctors attempted to resuscitate Dr. Li after he had gone into cardiac arrest earlier in the evening. Authorities officially pronounced Dr. Li dead in the early hours of February 7.[60] The Chinese public, having been confined to their residences for 2 weeks and uncertain when their ordeal would end, shared a collective grief at Dr. Li's unjust treatment. In Wuhan, residents opened their windows and joined in a chorus of shouts, united in anger at how the authorities had handled the coronavirus crisis.[61] Despite stringent post moderation and frequent account suspensions, critical sentiments reached another plateau on Weibo.[62]

Unknown to the public, Dr. Li's death was followed on February 8 by that of Dr. Xiao Jun, a 49-year-old surgeon at the Wuhan Red Cross Society Hospital who had worked tirelessly on the front lines and became infected with the novel coronavirus in mid-January. Concerned about the sociopolitical repercussions of announcing Dr. Xiao's death so soon after Dr. Li Wenliang's, authorities pressured Dr. Xiao's family to agree to postpone the announcement of his death.[63]

Meanwhile, the deaths of four members of the Chang Kai family garnered enormous national attention and added to the prevailing atmosphere of acute crisis. Mr. Chang Kai was a film producer and the director of External Relations at a subsidiary of the state-owned Hubei Provincial Film Studio. He was repeatedly recognized as a model employee. Chang's parents, both retired professors of Tongji Hospital, likely contracted the coronavirus during holiday social gatherings at the hospital. On Lunar New Year's Day (January 25), Chang's father began showing symptoms of novel coronavirus infection. Chang Kai attempted to admit his father to various hospitals, but none could accommodate him. Eventually, his mother also fell ill and was admitted to Wuchang Hospital on February 4 but passed away 4 days later. Chang and his wife began to show symptoms as well. He finally secured a bed at the district hospital on February 9, but, exhausted and grief-stricken from caring for his parents, he was in a somnolent state by that time. He died on February 14, age 55. His elder sister also passed away the same day.[64]

The misfortune that struck the Chang family encapsulated the excruciating agony many families in Wuhan/Hubei experienced during this period. Millions of people read Chang Kai's heart-wrenching "farewell message" on social media. The sense of shock was "incomparably intense," wrote Wuhan resident Yang Shengwei.[65]

China is commonly known as a country of relationships, and it was no surprise that patients and their families tried to pull strings to gain admittance into designated hospitals. "A hospital bed was truly hard to come by, more precious than gold or diamonds," said a staffer in the office of the Hubei Provincial Party Committee. He tried to get help for his parent through a director general but failed. He lamented that "the common types of ties or connections all ceased to work."[66] After all, if a well-connected upper-middle-class family like Chang Kai's was so defenseless, who stood a chance against the novel coronavirus?

Leadership Revamp to Boost Control and Implementation

Recognizing the public outrage over Dr. Li's mistreatment and the official handling of the epidemic, national authorities sought to placate the public by announcing that the National Supervisory Commission would immediately head to Wuhan to conduct "a full investigation." Simultaneously, Xi Jinping made several key appointments in Hubei between February 8 and 13 to capitalize on public sentiment and enhance the implementation of anti-epidemic measures centered on social control. This dramatic makeover of the leadership unfolded in a series of carefully orchestrated moves.

The first move in the Wuhan/Hubei leadership reshuffle occurred on February 8, the day after Dr. Li's death. There were three appointments, two of which were major additions to the Central Steering Group. Chen Yixin, the secretary general of the CPLAC and thus a key leader overseeing the stability maintenance regime, became deputy head of the Central Steering Group.[67] Chen had become a trusted assistant to Xi Jinping during Xi's tenure as Zhejiang provincial party secretary. Xi later brought Chen to Beijing to help manage the office for reform and then assigned him to positions in Wuhan (party secretary, December 2016–March 2018) and Hubei Province (deputy secretary, February 2017–March 2018) to give him more substantial experience in governing a major metropolitan area. Chen was then recalled to Beijing to become the secretary general of the powerful CPLAC, making him extremely well positioned to be sent back to Wuhan/Hubei to help gain control of the epidemic situation. Sun Lijun (孙立军), a vice minister of Public Security with a public health degree from Australia, was also appointed to the Central Steering Group, although Sun would fall from grace and be given a death sentence with reprieve partly for his behavior in Wuhan that remain a mystery to the public.

Also on February 8, Wang Hesheng, an NHC vice minister and Central Steering Group member, was appointed concurrently as a Standing Committee member of the Hubei Provincial Party Committee. While Chen Yixin's and Sun Lijun's appointments reflected the national leadership's concern for social stability and desire for social control, Wang's appointment aimed to integrate the Central Steering Group and the Hubei provincial administration in managing the health emergency response. Two days later, Wang was made both party secretary and director general of the Hubei Provincial Health Commission, replacing Zhang Jin and Liu Yingzi.

The sidelining of Zhang and Liu foreshadowed the much anticipated sacking of Jiang Chaoliang and Ma Guoqiang and the installation of their replacements. Because this involved the two top party leaders in Hubei, this second part of orchestrated personnel moves was likely to have been set in motion at the same time as the first set of appointments but took more time to work through.

On February 13, the Party Organization Department carried out Xi Jinping's and the central leadership's decision to replace Jiang Chaoliang and Ma Guoqiang as the party secretaries of Hubei and Wuhan. The national leadership made the replacements without publicly blaming the sacked officials. Nonetheless, the public viewed the sackings as evidence of the national leadership's responsiveness to their anger over Dr. Li's mistreatment and the earlier mishandling of the outbreak. Dr. Li was later named a martyr, and his Weibo account has remained active, serving as a digital "wailing wall" for numerous visitors. These moves were part of a complex and nuanced blame or blame avoidance game between central and local authorities and between the party-state leadership and the public.[68]

Taking the places of Jiang and Ma were Ying Yong, the Shanghai mayor, and Wang Zhonglin, the party secretary of Jinan, capital of Shandong Province. Both came from areas that Xi Jinping had repeatedly tapped for loyal talent. Ying and Wang, following Chen Yixin, had backgrounds in policing before assuming generalist government and party leadership roles and were known for their detail-oriented, no-nonsense leadership styles.[69] As commander-in-chief, General Secretary Xi Jinping dispatched two generals from two of China's most important cities to take over the leadership of Hubei and Wuhan and carry the Wuhan campaign to its conclusion.

Xi Emphasizes Community-Level Engagement in the People's War on Coronavirus

With the formation of the Central Leading Group, Xi Jinping recognized the Wuhan campaign as more than just a public health issue. At a Politburo meeting on February 3, he discussed key aspects of the epidemic prevention and control work, placing significant emphasis on maintaining social stability, effective propaganda, public education, and guiding public opinion.[70] In the published version of his speech, Xi called for soothing public anxiety, promoting positivity, rallying public support, and "taking the initiative and effectively influencing international public opinion."[71]

On February 9, a heartrending plea for help from a Baibuting resident gained widespread attention and captured the nation's interest. The resident disclosed that despite the presence of numerous suspected cases and fever patients confined to their homes, each community grid in Baibuting was allotted only one nucleic acid test per day. The resident exposed the reluctance of local leaders to report the truth out of fear for their positions and implored central authorities to intervene and save the Baibuting Community.

"We, the residents of Baibuting, are in a state of desperation and hope the central government learns of our situation at Baibuting! Please save the Baibuting residents."[72]

The following day, Xi Jinping made his first public appearance since the Wuhan lockdown, visiting the Anhuali community in Chaoyang District, Ditan Hospital, and the Chaoyang District CDC in Beijing. He emphasized the importance of community-level infection control and social governance during his visit to Anhuali. Xi highlighted that communities were the first line of defense against the epidemic, supporting door-to-door screening and monitoring key groups. He urged directing resources and particularly "*fangkong* forces" to the community level to help with infection control.[73]

In a video call with Sun Chunlan and Jiang Chaoliang in Hubei, Xi reiterated the need to "comprehensively strengthen management and control of the societal front." He urged officials to "strengthen social governance, properly deal with all kinds of issues that arise in epidemic *fangkong*. [Carry out] the various tasks thoroughly and meticulously, do well the work of supplying life necessities, medical treatment, psychological intervention, and so on, and maintain the overall stability of society."[74]

Two days later, Xi declared at a Politburo Standing Committee meeting that the epidemic prevention and control campaign had entered a critical stage and that there should be no let-up in efforts to "win the people's war, overall war, and battle of containment."[75]

In response to Xi's call, the Wuhan Fangkong Command issued Notice No. 12 on February 11, directing all residential communities to control infection sources by further reducing human mobility and implementing "enclosed management."[76] Each family was allowed one person to go outside for purchases every 3 days.

The day after newly appointed Ying Yong and Wang Zhonglin took over, the Wuhan Fangkong Command tightened "enclosed management" even further. Residents were prohibited from leaving their homes except for medical treatment, *fangkong* duties, and limited essential services.[77] Major cities in the rest of Hubei, particularly Huanggang and Xiaogan, followed suit and declared "wartime" controls.[78]

"The General Offensive"

After Xi Jinping announced that the epidemic prevention and control efforts had reached a critical stage, Sun Chunlan, during a visit to the Hubei Fangkong Command, demanded a "comprehensive general offensive with firmer confidence, more tenacious will, and more decisive measures."[79] The objectives of the remaining mission were now clear. In his speech to the Hubei Provincial and Wuhan Municipal Fangkong Commands, Ying Yong called for "meticulously screening all residents" to identify confirmed and suspected patients and their close contacts. He exhorted, "Do not miss a single household, do not leave out a single person, isolate all who should be isolated, admit all who should be admitted, treat all who should be treated."[80]

With new leaders in Wuhan and Hubei, the party-state apparatus refocused on strengthening leadership, tightening organizational control, and mobilizing party-state members to ensure strict enforcement of home confinement while providing necessary provisions. Ying Yong restructured the Hubei Provincial Fangkong Command on February 16, adding teams for propaganda and social stability alongside disease control and treatment and logistics.[81] Chen Yixin, deputy head of the Central Steering Group, implemented a mechanism requiring districts in Wuhan to report progress to the Wuhan and Hubei Fangkong Commands every hour. District representatives were encouraged to truthfully report problems and difficulties for prompt resolution.[82]

Over the next month, the Central Steering Group leadership, joined by Chen Yixin and the new leadership of Ying Yong and Wang Zhonglin in Hubei and Wuhan, used promotion and demotion to ensure the success of the effort to treat and quarantine as many people as necessary to "turn off the spigot" of community infections. Party members and their organizations in the communities were expected to play exemplary roles. Capable performers were given more responsibilities and promoted, while underperformers were replaced or demoted. Interviewees likened the situation to a battlefield, with lives on the line and success measured in lives saved and infections avoided. Between February 9 and March 16, 2020, 55 officials were promoted, while 245 division-level cadres and 10 bureau-level cadres were disciplined by the Communist Party Organization Department.[83] Gao Yu, a member of the Central Steering Group and head of the Supervision Team, publicly reprimanded Wuhan vice mayor Chen Xiexin and Wuchang District mayor Yu Song (佘松) on February 10.[84]

Intensified Measures and the Great Inspection in Wuhan

While Hubei party secretary Ying Yong addressed the entire province with a mix of praise and urgency, Wuhan party secretary Wang Zhonglin acted like a general on the front line, showing no patience for lax attitudes and actions.[85] In various meetings, Wang complained that implementation of the community lock-in still fell short and emphasized the need for strict home confinement, urging residents to protect their communities by staying home. "Wuhan is the place for waging the decisive battle," he declared. "It's time to concentrate forces to fight a war of annihilation, not to let it drag out in a protracted war."[86]

With leaders possessing extensive police backgrounds installed, the police force, utilizing lockdown-exempt vehicles, took over transporting patients to hospitals in the latter half of February to prevent further infections.[87]

As the focus shifted to enforcing strict home confinement, Wuhan entered the most intense phase of the lockdown, seeking 100% compliance on key prevention and control indicators (residential "enclosed management," isolation of close contacts, testing of fever patients and of suspected patients, and admittance of confirmed patients). Over February 17–19, 2020, Wang launched a 3-day "Great Inspection" characterized by "dragnet-style door-to-door inspection and screening [集中拉网式大排查]." District leaders were directed to guarantee no confirmed or suspected cases were left at home. "If another case is found, the district party secretary, district mayor will be held responsible for it."[88]

Besides grassroots leaders and staff in street offices, community centers, and police precincts, over 55,000 party cadres and members from party-government apparatuses in Wuhan joined in the "street barricade battles" against the epidemic in the communities.[89] They participated in the Great Inspection and Screening, enforced home confinement, and helped provide groceries and essentials to locked-in residents.[90] Older residential communities without walls/gates were fenced in, and strict rules on the disposal of household waste were implemented.[91]

The Great Inspection led to the resolution of some complicated situations, such as the case of 71-year-old Madame Wang. Madame Wang received confirmation of her novel coronavirus infection on February 10 but was kept waiting for admittance to a hospital. Following her daughter's public appeal for help on Weibo, community staff, the street office, and district government intervened; but her case remained unresolved due to a tangle of makeshift rules. Although Madame Wang exhibited mild symptoms, warranting admission to a *fangcang* shelter hospital, these facilities did not admit patients over 65 years old. Pressured by the Great Inspection deadline, the District Command ultimately arranged for Madame Wang's admission to the newly opened Hubei Provincial Maternal and Child Health Hospital (Guanggu Branch), providing her with treatment and removing a potential source of infection from the community.[92]

On the evening of February 19, all 13 districts in Wuhan submitted updated reports on the Great Inspection efforts. Most districts provided details on the number of households and residents screened, while some also included information on the extra staff deployed and various types of cases identified. In Hongshan District, which had garnered the attention of the Central Steering Group for its deficiencies, 1,213,161 people in 535,457 households were screened, identifying 30 confirmed cases, 122 clinical cases requiring further testing, 133 patients with fever, and 152 close contacts. The district reported that arrangements had been made for each identified case. Of the 30 confirmed cases, 8 were admitted to designated hospitals, 11 were admitted to *fangcang* hospitals, and 11 had recovered and were under observation at home. All close contacts were taken to quarantine facilities.[93]

The push to tighten "enclosed management" of residential areas, combined with the Great Inspection, led to the strict enforcement of home confinement for residents in all areas of Wuhan. However, officials such as Party Secretary Wang Zhonglin, who had risen from the grass roots and were familiar with tactics of subterfuge and feigned compliance, were not in the mood for bureaucratic games. Immediately following the Great Inspection, community and grid workers were asked to conduct follow-up reviews and maintain their efforts in epidemic control.[94] The Wuhan Health Code also made its debut on February 22, allowing authorities to digitally track and manage residents' mobility.[95] The digital health code would become a ubiquitous element in Chinese life as the country pursued a zero-COVID strategy.

By the end of February and early March 2020, the multi-pronged expansion of treatment facilities, combined with "enclosed management" and the screening of residents, led to a significant decrease in confirmed cases compared to the beginning of February. Those confirmed to have COVID-19 were taken to different types of hospitals for treatment depending on the severity of symptoms. As shown in Table 12.3, Wuhan finally reached a point where there were more hospital beds than patients with COVID-19. With strict infection control measures maintained in residential communities, transportation, and hospitals, the prospect of epidemic containment began to appear within reach.

The Role of Grassroots Workers and Essential Services

The strict community-level lockdowns and increased availability of hospital beds dramatically elevated the workload for grassroots staff and volunteers in Wuhan. These individuals had to step up to facilitate or provide services that were previously performed by efficient commercial providers.[96] They became incredibly busy arranging and assisting with grocery deliveries, often through group buying.[97] Due to the prolonged home confinement, many seniors started running out of medications for chronic conditions and urgently needed help. With limited supplies, staff and volunteers went from pharmacy to pharmacy to obtain the necessary medications.[98] A photo of a community grid worker adorned with bags of medications for residents went viral on February 24, showcasing their efforts and reassuring the public that help was available.[99]

The Baibuting mega-community consists of a mix of buildings, ranging from low-rent public housing to high-end commercial housing. The Wenhuiyuan compound has 15 low-rent buildings, many of whose residents received state assistance and faced significant pressure due to increased prices for groceries and other necessities during the lockdown. As the crisis began to ease, special attention was given to caring for these residents.[100]

Community workers noticed a shift in the city's mood around mid-February. Chen Jun (陈珺), a grid worker and secretary of the Communist Youth League branch in a community in Wuhan's Hanyang District, recalled,

> After the *fangcang* hospitals began to open, visits from and calls for help from community residents increased our workload sharply. But this was good, as confirmed and suspected patients got admitted and treated, and the sense of panic among residents eased.[101]

A major lesson from the lockdowns in Wuhan and other Chinese cities is that top-down restrictions on residents' activities must be combined with measures to ensure the continued availability of essential services. Despite the efforts of grassroots staff and volunteers, makeshift services from ill-equipped community personnel often fell short of expectations compared to well-run commercial providers. In Wuhan, the inconveniences and even dire shortages induced by the lockdown coupled with the official insistence on accentuating the positive spin—the spreading of "positive energy"—in the official media and the heavy censorship of negative vibes on social media bred dissatisfaction among residents who had been subjected to weeks of home confinement.[102] Many residents aired their grievances and stories of struggles on social media and in online dairies.[103] While netizens aired their suffering, they directed much of the blame toward "the lies, negligence, and censorship" by the authorities.[104]

One moment of public frustration and discontent revealed the multiple games played during the lockdown by the central leadership, local authorities at different levels of the political-administrative hierarchy, community leaders, and residents. When Vice Premier Sun Chunlan visited a high-rise community on March 5, 2020, residents shouted "It's fake! It's fake!" to complain about the food and grocery deliveries in their community.[105] The Central Steering Group's leadership quickly utilized the incident to demand improvements in local services.

Easing and Healing

After enduring the immense challenges of the previous month and a half, grassroots staff began to feel a decrease in pressure by the end of February 2020. One community volunteer observed that February 25 was the first time in weeks that staff in his community experienced a normal work shift and were able to finish work at the end of the day.[106] By then, the weather in Wuhan had also improved, transitioning from snowy conditions in early February to a balmy 25°C (77°F) on February 25.

On March 6, 2020, the municipal leadership of Wuhan started arranging for community workers to take days off. Grid worker Chen Jun got her first day off on March 7, 43 days after the cordon sanitaire was imposed.[107]

Wuhan residents are well known for their love of fish. Throughout much of February, as the city battled to survive the epidemic, having fish to eat was not a top priority for the leadership or the residents. However, as the epidemic situation began to ease, the Wuhan municipal leadership organized fish deliveries to every family in mid-March as a goodwill gesture to residents. The responsibility of delivering the fish to families once again fell on the shoulders of community staff and particularly grid workers, who remarked that they had never handled so many fish in their lifetimes.[108]

A Look Back at the Wuhan Epidemic in Numbers

Wuhan reported no new suspected COVID-19 cases for the first time on March 17, 2020. As these results were consolidated, the lockdown was finally lifted on April 8, 2020, 76 days after the imposition of cordon sanitaire. According to the Wuhan Fangkong Command, correcting for inaccuracies in the early statistics, Wuhan had 50,333 confirmed COVID-19 cases and 3,869 deaths due to COVID-19 as of April 16, 2020.[109]

Although Wuhan hospitals were free of COVID patients by April 26, the rest of China continued to treat Wuhan and Hubei with caution. Residents from Hubei faced discrimination when seeking jobs outside the province.

Even within Wuhan, those who had contracted the virus continued to live under the shadow of their previous infections and were stigmatized. Wuhan psychologist Du Mingjun noted that many who had suffered from the disease felt "a sense of shame about having contracted the disease."[110]

Between May 14 and June 1, Wuhan conducted a high-profile citywide PCR testing campaign for residents aged 6 years and above, screening just under 9.9 million people for SARS-CoV-2 infections. The program identified and quarantined 300 asymptomatic cases and 1,174 close contacts.[111] By June 15, 2020, the last three asymptomatic cases were certified to have had two consecutive negative PCR tests for SARS-CoV-2 and were released from quarantine.[112] This allowed Wuhan to declare that it had achieved zero-COVID status.[113] Despite some questions about the utility and cost of such mass testing, the results provided valuable information and helped Wuhan residents cope with the emotional scars of the epidemic.

Since the number of confirmed COVID cases was only a fraction of the total number of infected individuals, a seroprevalence survey based on blood samples was carried out as part of a project under the direction of Dr. Wang Chen. This program used multi-stage, population-stratified random sampling and took blood samples from 3,599 families with 9,702 individuals. The study found that 6.92% of the sample population of Wuhan had developed antibodies against SARS-CoV-2 (rising to 6.96% if the official number of COVID deaths is included).[114]

Using the total population for citywide PCR testing of about 10.6 million, it can be estimated that among the surviving population in Wuhan, the total number of people who had antibodies against SARS-CoV-2 was approximately 737,425 as of April 2020. Since antibodies among some infected individuals had waned to undetectable levels and the number of COVID-19-releated deaths might still be undercounted, the ballpark number of the total number of people who were infected in Wuhan, including those who died from COVID-19, would be around 750,000.

Conclusion

The massive national campaign to rescue Wuhan and Hubei initially focused on mobilizing medical resources from across China to provide treatment for the infected. While it is well known that authorities relied on the party-dominated grassroots governance structure, including grid workers, to implement epidemic control policies in communities, this structure did not become activated and effective immediately. Amid the shock and challenges of the lockdown, fissures, fragilities, and deficiencies emerged during the early days and weeks of Wuhan's lockdown. With overwhelmed hospitals and a paralyzed city, many residential communities struggled for understandable reasons in the early days of the lockdown period. The extraordinary circumstances placed demands on the grassroots governance structure that went beyond its capabilities.

It was not until early February that the leadership for the Wuhan rescue began to refocus their efforts on cutting the chains of virus transmission in communities while they dramatically ramped up the capacity for treatment and quarantine by opening new hospitals and repurposed *fangcang* shelter hospitals. Fortuitously, the relatively relaxed enforcement of community controls in the first 3 weeks allowed households, communities, and service providers to adjust to the abrupt impositions. As hospital capacities vastly improved, enforcing confinement in the community appeared less draconian in relative terms. Given the objective of stopping viral transmission in households and communities, community-level actions could not have succeeded without the capacity to quarantine and treat the infected and vice versa.

In simple terms, suppressing SARS-CoV-2 depended on controlling the known and suspected human carriers of the virus through community-level efforts. With renewed leadership and organization, the party-state tightened "enclosed management" of residential areas, enforcing home confinement by utilizing and reinforcing the grassroots governance structure. As the party-state demonstrated an unrivaled capacity to control society at the grassroots level, it also justified the party-dominated community governance structure as essential in the fight against the epidemic.[115]

However, it is important to acknowledge that while the Chinese leadership mobilized the party-state and residents' committees, the goal of epidemic control in communities was to demobilize society into mostly household units, forcing compliance with home confinement. Chinese society complied with the party-state's demands with a level of acquiescence and discipline that would be difficult to achieve in other parts of the world. This effort was facilitated by fear of the virus, digital apps that helped users stay connected, the hard work of dedicated grassroots staff, and efficient logistics from companies like Alibaba and JD.

The intensification of community-level efforts to cut off infection sources became a campaign for the party-state to exercise its unrivaled capacity to dominate society at the grassroots level. As the number of new infections was curtailed, Xi Jinping convened an unprecedented teleconference on February 23, 2020, and directly addressed approximately 170,000 cadres from across the country to emphasize the crucial need for integrating epidemic control measures with socioeconomic development. Nonetheless, many of the mechanisms and tactics used in Wuhan were adopted in other cities, including Xi'an and Shanghai, during China's persistent pursuit of the zero-COVID strategy, setting China apart in the global response to the pandemic.

14

Was the COVID-19 Pandemic Inevitable?

Fragmented Authoritarianism, Leadership, and the Question of Preventability

The COVID-19 pandemic is an immensely complex and pressing "wicked problem" that has eluded technocratic solutions.[1] Moreover, it has defied simple explanations regarding the relationship between regime type and governance quality. Scholars studying governance have found that existing theories and frameworks fall short in addressing the unique challenges posed by the COVID-19 pandemic.[2] Although the type of political regime appears to be connected to governmental policy responses and pandemic performance, the outcomes depend on the indicators used to evaluate performance.[3] Even within a single country, governance practices that are effective during one phase of the pandemic may prove inadequate in another.[4] The most competent leaders and systems in pandemic response are those that rapidly adapt to leverage new knowledge about virus mutations and transmission, embrace advances in technologies such as vaccines and therapeutics, and maintain the trust of their populations.

China occupied a unique position during the COVID-19 pandemic. As Hubei Provincial Party Secretary Jiang Chaoliang stated, "Wuhan is both the epicenter of the outbreak and the point from which the epidemic spread."[5] Consequently, China's management of the initial outbreak was of utmost importance, not only for Wuhan and the rest of China but also for other nations confronting the spreading virus in subsequent stages.

In the cases of both the severe acute respiratory syndrome (SARS) outbreak in 2003 and the SARS-coronavirus 2 (SARS-CoV-2) outbreak in 2020, the initial outbreaks escalated into crises that required extraordinary efforts to address. Once the crises were acknowledged for what they were, the Chinese party-state showcased its immense capacity to mobilize resources in handling crises and disasters. In 2020, following the imposition of a cordon sanitaire in Wuhan on January 23, China distinguished itself with its aggressive and comprehensive containment strategy, both in Wuhan and across the country.[6]

In cross-country comparisons, China stands at one end of the spectrum, pursuing its zero-COVID strategy through late 2022.

As the intense politicization surrounding discussions and research on the COVID-19 pandemic has subsided in China and globally, we can now reflect more objectively and calmly on the earlier phases of China's response, benefiting from the clarity that hindsight provides. This not only enables us to gain a better understanding of what transpired but also allows us to assess which actions could have been more effective and what deficiencies should have been avoided and to draw lessons that China's outbreak response can offer for managing and preventing future pandemic outbreaks.

This concluding chapter underscores two critical aspects in managing the outbreak before the imposition of the cordon sanitaire in Wuhan. First, contrary to popular perceptions of China under the centralized control of the party-state led by Xi Jinping, the underlying fault lines and tensions of fragmented authoritarianism, typically concealed or minimized in more stable times, significantly weakened the health emergency response during the initial weeks of the COVID-19 outbreak. These dynamics resulted in deliberate concealment, distortions, and blockages in epidemic information flows; defensive avoidance by organizational leaders; shirking of responsibility; and efforts to assign or shift blame to other authorities. The intricate relationship between the National Health Commission (NHC) and Hubei/Wuhan authorities became evident during the Senior Advisory Panel's visit to Wuhan, revealing the challenges of addressing the COVID-19 outbreak within the context of fragmented authoritarianism.

Second, modern bureaucratic hierarchies tend to promote specialists into leadership roles whose qualities may be ill-suited for situations requiring decisive leadership. Regrettably, during the early weeks of the Wuhan outbreak, effective public health leadership was desperately needed to tackle political, organizational, and psychological vulnerabilities but was largely absent. There was a failure to rise above routine with purpose. Key decisions by Chinese health authorities, such as not associating the outbreak with "infectious atypical pneumonia" (SARS), not allowing disclosure of information about the novel coronavirus until it had gone through bureaucratically organized verification, and strict adherence to a case definition that focused narrowly on exposure to the Huanan Seafood Market, led to consequences that could have been avoided with more open communication and consideration of alternative perspectives. Nonetheless, it should be noted that significant variations in governance quality exist in China.

Operating within a political-administrative structure that suppressed information and particularly discussions of potential risks, dismissed anomalies, and discouraged proactive measures, the viral spread in Wuhan and beyond Wuhan seemed almost predestined. As missteps and erroneous judgments accumulated, an air of inevitable banality pervaded. Nevertheless, the substantial knowledge and experience held by China's medical professionals and health policymakers at the end of 2019 suggested a promising future of effective containment. Similarly, China's triumph in containing SARS-CoV-2 in the spring of 2020, subsequent to the Wuhan lockdown, stands as a testament to the country's remarkable capabilities.

In the final section of the chapter, I invite the reader to join me in exploring a thought experiment regarding whether and to what extent the COVID-19 pandemic might have been preventable in a scenario where China had not practiced "censorship and limits on free flow of information." It is suggested that, in such a scenario, major missteps and deficiencies would likely have been avoided or significantly mitigated, and there would have been a real and non-trivial chance of containing the initial outbreak early on.

Central–Local Dynamics and Tensions in Fragmented Authoritarianism

Studies of Chinese politics and policy often employ the concept of fragmented authoritarianism to describe the structural fragmentation of authority that arises from the party-state's organization into bureaucratic systems and territorial divisions.[7] Efforts to strengthen central control typically result in superficial compliance, while local authorities simultaneously strive to advance their own interests using a variety of strategies. The post-SARS efforts to establish and strengthen the health emergency response regime exemplify official efforts to counteract the pathologies of fragmented authoritarianism.

Nonetheless, bureaucratic and territorial fragmentation significantly undermined the effectiveness of the health emergency response regime during December 2019 and January 2020. Although the NHC and Wuhan/Hubei authorities ostensibly cooperated to manage the so-called viral pneumonia of uncertain etiology (PUE) health emergency and control the epidemic information available to the public, a closer examination reveals that their interests were markedly divergent from the beginning of the outbreak. For instance, China Centers for Disease Control and Prevention (China CDC) director general Gao Fu first learned of the outbreak in Wuhan through social media instead of official channels. Overall, epidemic information flows suffered from severe distortions and blockages during the early weeks of the outbreak, grievously undercutting the effectiveness of the health emergency response.

Initially, the National Notifiable Disease Surveillance System (NNDSS) and the associated PUE surveillance program, often lauded for its effectiveness, was not employed for reporting the first PUE or SARS-like pneumonia cases when identified by front-line clinicians, infectious disease specialists, hospital administrators, and district, municipal, and provincial CDCs and health commissions in Wuhan/Hubei during December 2019. Technically, any of these individuals or organizations should have been able to report the unusual pneumonia cases to the China CDC via the disease reporting system, but none did so before December 31, 2019, a striking fact since Hubei prided itself on ranking among the very best on the disease reporting metric. Hubei, through Jinyintan Hospital, finally reported some cases to the China CDC using the disease reporting system on December 31, 2019, after NHC/China CDC teams had arrived in Wuhan and conducted visits. However, such reporting was suppressed again in the following weeks, despite efforts by the NHC front-line team to request such reporting.

This non-reporting or non-submission from Wuhan/Hubei to the national health authority was evidently a form of localist concealment that delayed the involvement of the national health authority initially. If there were PUE cases that were reported to the local CDCs in Wuhan much earlier than officially indicated, say in mid-December 2019, it is worth discussing to what extent the reporting of such cases, had they been filed into the national disease reporting system, might have affected the course of the outbreak response. However, raising such questions has been strongly discouraged in China. Remarkably, even though it is widely known that Gao Fu first learned of the Wuhan outbreak from social media on December 30, 2019, publications from the China CDC have falsely claimed that it was reporting from the Hubei provincial health authority on December 30, 2019, that "triggered the dispatch of a rapid response team from Beijing."[8] Such rewriting of history is part of an effort to conceal the multiple organizational failures in national disease reporting and health emergency response.

In the following weeks, the interactions between the national health authority (NHC/China CDC), Hubei Province, and Wuhan municipality continued to reflect the characteristics and tensions of fragmented authoritarianism, severely affecting the outbreak response. Most prominently, the Hubei/Wuhan leadership preferred not to have an infectious disease outbreak disrupt the peaceful atmosphere of the "two sessions" season. For Hubei party secretary Jiang Chaoliang, the outbreak barely registered on his public schedule from the end of December 2019 to January 20, 2020.[9]

When organizational leaders are preoccupied with maintaining the status quo, they tend to adopt a defensive avoidance mode and avoid identifying new problems.[10] In Wuhan, health and provincial/municipal officials went even further. They ignored requests by NHC officials to use the NNDSS to report viral PUE cases and broke their promise to the second NHC expert team to disclose the number of suspected patients with novel coronavirus infections. In another instance, the China CDC activated a Level II emergency response on January 6, but neither the Hubei provincial CDC nor the Wuhan municipal CDC followed suit.[11] The Hubei provincial leadership could theoretically have invoked the Emergency Response Law (2007) to take proactive measures against the outbreak. Instead, according to Professor Shen Kui of Peking University, the recommendation from the China CDC for Wuhan or Hubei to activate a Level II health emergency response "was tied up in a bundle and put on a high shelf."[12]

Powerful systemic, institutional, and organizational forces created a tight net in Hubei/Wuhan to discourage voicing concerns and maintain silence about cases that contradicted the prevailing discourse of no sustained human-to-human transmission in Wuhan. The more committed provincial and municipal officials became to preserving the status quo, the more difficult it was for them to break free from it on their own, even when they were made aware of the growing epidemic dangers. The provincial health authority prevented using the national disease reporting system for reporting viral PUE/novel coronavirus cases through January 23.[13] In mid-January 2020, the health authorities and administrations in Wuhan/Hubei were actively engaged in efforts to keep new evidence of cases from being submitted and to conceal medical staff infections. Medical professionals and administrators who followed established procedures to repeatedly submit new cases were criticized.

The complex relationship and tensions between the NHC and the Hubei/Wuhan authorities were on public display on January 19, 2020. Ahead of the Senior Advisory Panel's arrival, Wuhan's health leadership adopted a self-defensive blame avoidance mode. In the early hours of January 19, the Wuhan Municipal Health Commission (WMHC) released interviews with Wuhan vice mayor Chen Xiexin, Wuhan CDC director Li Gang, and Dr. Huang Chaolin, vice president of Jinyintan Hospital. Despite the growing number of cases and their knowledge of medical staff infections, Chen and Li still spoke as if there was little cause for concern. Vice Mayor Chen Xiexin strongly defended Wuhan's anti-epidemic performance, stating that Wuhan "has built a multi-level joint-action mechanism, and formed a strong task force." He claimed that Wuhan had "quickly responded to and dealt with the epidemic and made every effort to treat patients and prevent the spread of the epidemic."[14] Wuhan CDC director Li Gang maintained that "with the implementation of various prevention and control measures, this outbreak is preventable and controllable."[15]

Meanwhile, Dr. Huang Chaolin commended national research organizations, particularly the China CDC, for their prompt development and subsequent optimization of virus nucleic acid test kits. Echoing an earlier explanation provided by the WMHC, he mentioned that the Hubei provincial CDC received these test kits on January 16 and started testing for viral PUE cases.[16] Despite acknowledging and appreciating the assistance from the central government, notably the China CDC, these comments seemed to overlook the failure to report suspected cases through the disease reporting system and to utilize locally available resources for testing suspected cases. Furthermore, these statements implicitly suggested that the delayed reporting of newly confirmed cases was primarily the responsibility of the central government, a situation driven by the availability of diagnostic test kits from the NHC/China CDC.

As tensions mounted during the Senior Advisory Panel's visit to Wuhan, the NHC prepared its own statement. It stated that, upon learning of the outbreak, the NHC promptly sent a national work team and expert groups to Wuhan "to jointly study and implement epidemic prevention and control measures in accordance with *the principle of territorial management*" (italics added). The NHC enumerated various actions it had taken and said that a leading group chaired by Minister Ma Xiaowei "provided timely guidance and support to Hubei Province and Wuhan Municipality for treatment of patients, epidemic prevention and control, and emergency response."[17]

Released on the evening of January 19, 2020, ahead of the State Council Executive Meeting on the Wuhan epidemic situation, the NHC used the statement to defend its own performance in responding to the outbreak and essentially rebut the indirect criticism found between the lines in the interviews from Wuhan. By invoking the principle of territorial management, the NHC statement reminded its readership that the NHC leadership operated based on the idea that Hubei/Wuhan authorities bore primary responsibility for implementing epidemic prevention and control measures in Wuhan. The NHC cited expert assessment to say that the epidemic situation "is still preventable and controllable," but it was most likely with a sense of foreboding that the NHC leadership put together and released its statement. In hindsight, the NHC's actions during the first 3 weeks of January 2020 were a mixed bag of useful responses and counterproductive moves that failed to prevent the initial outbreak from spreading beyond Wuhan and spiraling out of control.

The question of blame persisted during the Wuhan lockdown. In an interview on January 27, 2020, Wuhan mayor Zhou Xianwang admitted to widespread "dissatisfaction with our disclosure of [epidemic] information. On the one hand, our disclosure was untimely, on the other hand, there was inadequacy in utilizing effective information to improve our work."[18] However, Mayor Zhou went on to argue that, as a local government, Wuhan must follow the Law on Infectious Disease Prevention and Treatment and leadership by higher levels of political authority. "After I obtained the information, I can only disclose it after I am authorized."[19] Mayor Zhou thus implied that Wuhan's actions were limited by the constraints imposed by higher levels of authority. He further noted that the State Council Executive Meeting of January 20, 2020, not only gave the novel coronavirus pneumonia legal standing as a new infectious disease but also stipulated the principle of territorial responsibility, thus allowing Wuhan to become more proactive in dealing with the epidemic.[20]

Variations in Governance Quality within China

Organizational theorists have long noted the difficulty for organizations to break out of a climate of silence from within.[21] It took powerful alerts from outside of Wuhan/Hubei, particularly from Thailand and Shenzhen/Guangdong, to get the NHC/China CDC leadership out of tunnel vision. The varying performances of Wuhan and Shenzhen have led to speculation about whether the COVID-19 outbreak would have been contained had it started in Shenzhen, Shanghai, or Zhejiang instead. Assessing governance quality in China requires attention to such variations.

While it is difficult to answer such hypothetical questions conclusively, we do know that early cases from Hubei that reached Guangdong (Shenzhen) and Zhejiang (Wenzhou) did not lead to widespread epidemic spread.[22] The public health system in Shenzhen properly managed early cases and avoided the information blockages and concealment that plagued Wuhan. Shenzhen also demonstrated significant initiative by quickly developing its own diagnostic testing for the novel coronavirus, showing less delay in verifying human-to-human transmission than Wuhan. Moreover, Guangdong Province significantly increased testing capacity, conducting over 320,000 reverse-transcription polymerase chain reaction (RT-PCR) tests in approximately 30 days between January and February 2020 to identify and isolate infected cases.[23]

While Wuhan and Shenzhen varied in pandemic preparedness and control capabilities, they operated within the same overarching political framework.

It is essential to note that authorities in Shenzhen/Guangdong were also secretive about early COVID-19 cases, operating with the same discretion that facilitated the spread of SARS beyond Guangdong in 2003. On January 16, 2020, the Guangdong provincial leadership began setting up structures for addressing the novel coronavirus epidemic and organized designated hospitals to conduct an epidemic response exercise.[24] Publicly, however, the leadership emphasized the importance of seasonal infectious disease control work and awaited NHC authorization to announce the first confirmed novel coronavirus infection identified in Guangdong.

Cognition, Information, and the Challenges of Leadership

Studies of crisis preparedness and response have long noted that organizational leaders must contend with political, organizational, and psychological vulnerabilities.[25] Often, they engage in decision processes such as groupthink, which narrows the search for information, limits the number of alternatives considered, and fails to update their conclusions and policies.[26] Due to the difficulty of understanding and communicating the risks of invisible pathogens, decision-making during an infectious disease outbreak is especially prone to cognitive biases.[27] Consequently, the need for effective leadership becomes paramount. In the context of fragmented authoritarianism, the complexities and tensions in the relationship between the national health leadership and local authorities raise the following question: who was responsible for overseeing the situation and providing proactive leadership in such a critical health emergency situation?

While the NNDSS and associated disease reporting systems failed to function as intended, the NHC, led by Minister Ma Xiaowei, and the China CDC, led by Gao Fu, responded to the Wuhan outbreak in late 2019 as soon as they learned of it from unofficial sources. They dispatched experts and emergency response teams to Wuhan, resulting in the shutdown of the Huanan Seafood Market and the implementation of the action program. As the number of newly confirmed cases appeared to have stabilized, the sense of crisis that had initially gripped the national health leadership dissipated. By the time the novel coronavirus was officially confirmed, leading scientists, led by academician Xu Jianguo of the China CDC, believed the outbreak was under control.

Meanwhile, Wuhan hospitals experienced a surge in new novel coronavirus infections in the first half of January 2020, but the identification and submission of such cases through the health administrations were virtually halted, keeping vital alerts from reaching the China CDC/NHC. The Hubei and Wuhan authorities and the NHC adopted a multitude of political and administrative restrictions that hampered epidemic information collection and flow. Within the confines of the party-state, the Chinese health emergency regime turned into a bureaucratic-pathological deadwood in handling epidemic information. As a result, Wuhan and subsequently the rest of Hubei became a massive virus incubator.

Chinese health policymakers and experts, led by the China CDC leadership, adopted the zoonosis-in-the-Huanan-market thesis as the framework for understanding and responding to the novel coronavirus and the disease it causes. Scientists like China CDC director general Gao Fu emphasize the importance of evidence and were open to reconsidering their theories or hypotheses based on new evidence. However, the zoonosis-in-the-Huanan-market thesis and framework proved especially resilient to challenge for much of January 2020 when the authorities enforced strict control on the submission of new suspected cases and the sharing and disclosure of epidemic information in the entire health sector.

First, the thesis was used to support the restrictive inclusion–exclusion criteria, which included a Huanan market exposure requirement. Through mid-January 2020, enforcement of the exposure requirement thwarted the inclusion of new cases that lacked exposure to the Huanan market. The prevailing understanding about the novel coronavirus, coupled with the absence of new cases from Wuhan, served to reinforce the commitment to the zoonosis-in-the-Huanan-market thesis. Along with the anti-epidemic measures adopted, the thesis contributed to an illusion of manageability in Wuhan.

Second, the zoonosis-in-the-Huanan-market thesis suggested that the transmissibility of the novel coronavirus would evolve in stages and be limited before it could transmit efficiently. Consequently, suspected human-to-human transmission cases, particularly the initial family clusters known at the end of December 2019 and in early January 2020, were not considered indications of significant transmission. They were not even regarded as examples of limited human-to-human transmission until representatives of the Chinese health leadership heard persistent questioning by visiting epidemiologists from Taiwan and Hong Kong. Even after Wuhan was sealed off, senior health officials continued to rely on key assumptions of the zoonosis thesis when assessing the epidemic situation. In his first press event after the imposition of cordon sanitaire in Wuhan, Minister Ma Xiaowei stated that the virus may have initially jumped from wildlife to humans and had now gradually begun adapting to humans, entering the stage of human-to-human transmission.[28]

When these considerations were combined with efforts by Wuhan and Hubei officials to delay the submission of suspected cases and maintain silence about medical staff infections during the "two sessions period," Wuhan became, as Guan Yi described it, an "unguarded city." To the great surprise of scientists and policymakers, SARS-CoV-2 was more contagious than the SARS coronavirus. Shortly after the cordon sanitaire was imposed in Wuhan, Minister Ma Xiaowei acknowledged that the novel coronavirus behaved "very differently" from the SARS coronavirus and was transmissible even during the incubation period.[29] As is now well known, asymptomatic transmission made SARS-CoV-2 infections harder to detect and control. Gao Fu later repeatedly referred to SARS-CoV-2 as a "cunning virus" and thus a scientific challenge.[30]

The zoonosis framework assumptions and the information clampdowns and bottlenecks reinforced each other in a political culture that tends to "report only the good news, not the bad." Motivated reasoning in the Chinese political system is not merely a cognitive issue but a matter of everyday political practice. Wang Xinghuan, president of the Wuhan University Zhongnan Hospital, noted in an atmosphere that

> demand[ed] experts put emphasis on political considerations, some experts understood "talking politics" to mean trying to minimize the epidemic situation, saying that it was preventable and controllable, that there was no human-to-human transmission, and then that limited human-to-human transmission could not be ruled out. As a result, the [higher political] leaders came to believe [such rhetoric] and instead doubted the reports [of new infections] that came from hospitals on the front-line.[31]

The Leadership Vacuum

By invoking the principle of "territorial management" to defend its performance, the NHC's January 19, 2020, statement exposed the fault lines within China's party-dominated political-administrative system and the tendencies toward buck passing and blame shifting. It also paradoxically revealed the limitations of adhering to that principle when dealing with an outbreak caused by a highly contagious virus that respected no provincial boundaries. The situation underscored the need for proactive leadership. No other than Xi Jinping lamented, "I write my instructions to guard the last line of defense; if I don't give instructions, will [these officials] not do any work at all?!"[32]

As China's national health authority, the NHC leadership, with advice and support from the China CDC and expert panels, was expected to provide effective national leadership. China CDC director general Gao Fu played crucial roles in uncovering and eliciting the initial NHC-led national response to the Wuhan outbreak at the end of December 2019 and in spurring the NHC to orchestrate the Senior Advisory Panel visit on January 19, 2020. This visit confirmed medical staff infections and helped persuade the national leadership to publicly respond to the epidemic. Minister Ma Xiaowei was involved in responding to the SARS crisis as the youngest vice minister of health in 2003 and his response at the end of December 2019 and on January 1, 2020, showed that he knew well time was of the essence in responding to the novel coronavirus outbreak. Later, Ma played a major role in leveraging on the Senior Advisory Panel visit to reorient the national and subnational authorities toward fighting the epidemic. While these two junctures saw stronger national intervention, various other decisions by the China CDC and the NHC leadership in the intervening period were counterproductive.

First, as observed, infectious atypical pneumonia (SARS) is categorized as a Schedule B infectious disease, requiring Class A prevention and control measures according to the Law on Infectious Disease Prevention and Treatment. When clinicians initially submitted the so-called PUE cases in December 2019, they reported that patients exhibited SARS-like symptoms. Genomic sequencing results also indicated a novel coronavirus, approximately 80% like the SARS coronavirus. For all practical purposes, health authorities implemented SARS-style prevention and control measures, except for public involvement and mobilization. Therefore, it seems reasonable to classify the viral PUE cases in Wuhan as "infectious atypical pneumonia." Some clinicians in Wuhan told me emphatically that this should have been done.

One memorable line from *The Plague* by Camus is that "all our troubles spring from our failure to use plain, clean-cut language."[33] The decision not to associate the viral PUE cases with "infectious atypical pneumonia" may have been the most consequential decision during the initial outbreak response. If the novel coronavirus infections in Wuhan had been recognized early as "infectious atypical pneumonia," in other words, a new iteration of SARS, more rigorous responses would have been required, including mandatory reporting of cases through the NNDSS, in accordance with the Infectious Diseases Law, and disclosure of disease information to the public. This might have changed the course of the pandemic. However, the Wuhan/Hubei authorities and the NHC, supported by the China CDC, decided against this association and instead used police powers to suppress doctors who shared information about patients with SARS or SARS-like coronavirus infections.

China also strongly opposed international efforts to associate the novel coronavirus pneumonia with SARS. In February 2020, the International Committee on Taxonomy of Viruses officially named the virus "severe acute respiratory syndrome coronavirus 2" (SARS-CoV-2) because it is "genetically related to the coronavirus responsible for the SARS outbreak of 2003."[34] China objected to this name, with Gao Fu and other China CDC experts advocating for a completely different name to differentiate it from SARS-CoV.[35] China's influence was more evident in the disease name, which the World Health Organization (WHO) named "coronavirus disease 2019" (COVID-19) instead of "severe acute respiratory syndrome 2019" (SARS-19). In announcing the disease name, the WHO, alluding to resistance from Asia (implicitly China), stated that "using the name SARS can have unintended consequences in terms of creating unnecessary fear for some populations, especially in Asia which was worst affected by the SARS outbreak in 2003."[36] According to this convention, however, the 2003 SARS outbreak would be "coronavirus disease 2003" (COVID-03).

Second, China's official Strategy for the Prevention and Control of Emerging Infectious Diseases (2007) stipulates that the NHC and provincial authorities should adopt the strictest Class A prevention and control measures to address emerging infectious diseases in compliance with the Infectious Diseases Law. Reflecting the painful lessons of the SARS experience, the strategy further states that the NHC should "promptly recommend the State Council to include emerging infectious diseases into the schedule of statutory infectious diseases in accordance with the needs of prevention and control."[37]

These provisions raise questions about the appropriate timing for presenting the novel coronavirus pneumonia to the State Council, particularly because the WHO began to use "2019-nCoV" as the interim disease name on January 11, 2020, in offering its guidance, including case definition.[38] Should the NHC have made more proactive efforts to secure such a State Council administrative determination when the novel coronavirus was officially identified and verified on January 8, rather than January 20, 2020? If the administrative decision had been made earlier, submission and public disclosure of cases, as well as the implementation of preventive measures, could have been accelerated based on the law. Unfortunately, no evidence indicates that such a proactive move was considered.

Third, the China CDC leadership dedicated significant resources to sampling the Huanan market and testing hundreds of collected samples for the presence of the novel coronavirus. However, as China CDC deputy director general Feng Zijian acknowledged, the senior leadership was considerably late in reviewing epidemiological data on cases admitted prior to January 3, 2020, and recognizing the importance of cases without exposure to the Huanan market. This substantial delay, regardless of its cause, reflects poorly on the quality of China's public health leadership, particularly the role of leading epidemiologists such as Feng who were also in important health leadership positions.

Fourth, although some clinicians and hospitals submitted new viral PUE cases that had no history of exposure to the Huanan market and highlighted evidence of human-to-human transmission in Wuhan, the case definition for novel coronavirus pneumonia was not expanded until cases without Huanan market exposure were confirmed outside China, and the WHO introduced a broader case definition. Epidemiologists like China CDC deputy director general Feng Zijian defended the initial emphasis on Huanan market exposure, but there is little justification for continuing to insist on the narrow definition when powerful new evidence emerged.

In a more open organizational and informational environment, the built-in ascertainment bias focusing on exposure to the Huanan market, as embodied in the original case definition, might have been corrected quickly. Both Chinese and international experts were concerned about viral spread from early on and would have spoken up to encourage inquiry when clinicians encountered cases that contradicted initial assumptions from very early on. However, due to the controls and prohibitions on health workers, hospitals, laboratories, and the media, abnormal information and alternative perspectives had no influence in Wuhan. As a result, while the NHC, China CDC leadership, and Wuhan/Hubei authorities diverted their attention to other matters or lost focus, the original ascertainment bias contributed greatly to community spread.[39]

Lastly, during the first half of January 2020, the NHC/China CDC/Hubei health authorities did not organize RT-PCR testing of suspected viral PUE cases without exposure to the Huanan market, which would have indicated viral spread. This failure resulted from a series of decisions in addition to the considerations enumerated above. Initially, NHC-imposed restrictions on laboratories limited testing capacity, making it nearly impossible for hospitals to use third-party commercial diagnostic laboratories as they had done in December 2019. Additionally, when the first test kits became available from the China CDC (Institute for Viral Disease Control and Prevention) and the Wuhan Institute of Virology, Hubei/Wuhan health authorities, likely under national guidance, opted to use the test kits to focus on testing existing viral PUE cases on January 6 and January 10, 2020. Furthermore, although Shenzhen in Guangdong began using the official test kit distributed by the China CDC on January 14, 2020, it is surprising that Wuhan officials, at the outbreak's epicenter, reported beginning to use the new test kits distributed under NHC auspices on January 16, 2020, not earlier.

Subsequently, Hubei and Wuhan officials repeatedly stated that testing was not conducted on suspected new cases because diagnostic test kits from the China CDC were not available in Wuhan until January 16, 2020. This excuse is, at best, unconvincing. If the NHC/China CDC and Hubei/Wuhan health leadership truly wanted to perform diagnostic tests on a modest number of newly suspected viral PUE cases, they could have secured the testing capacity. At that time, the China CDC was testing hundreds of environmental samples from Wuhan. The Hubei Provincial CDC, with its biosafety Level-3 lab, served as the validation laboratory for assessing novel coronavirus diagnostic test kits and was clearly capable of carrying out some tests. The Wuhan Institute of Virology, with top biosafety labs and leading coronavirus researchers, developed its own diagnostic test kits and had the capacity to perform PCR tests. Considering all these factors, the failure to officially conduct diagnostic testing of newly suspected viral PUE cases in Wuhan before January 16, 2020, is strong evidence of a failure in leadership.

Was the COVID-19 Pandemic Preventable?

The missteps and deficiencies in managing the responses to the Wuhan outbreak during the first half of January 2020 highlight the risks and weaknesses associated with relying on technocracy in a highly politicized institutional environment while excluding the public in addressing an infectious disease emergency. Strong clinical and scientific capacities are crucial, as are proactive leadership, effective information flows, and robust decision-making that counteracts cognitive biases. In the final analysis, it becomes clear that the characteristics of the Chinese political system, preoccupied with maintaining stability and quick to suppress unwelcome opinions and signals, were ill-suited for handling an outbreak that necessitated public involvement from the outset. No amount of investment, state-of-the-art equipment, or talent can make a meaningful difference in curbing the spread of a highly contagious virus if the public is kept uninformed about the dangers they face and if those with knowledge are not allowed to speak up or, if they do, are punished.

By examining the early history of China's outbreak response in Wuhan and the choices made by various leaders within the Chinese political-administrative hierarchy for health emergency response, the author's goal is to contribute to the informed discussion in the global community of concerned public health specialists and the public about pandemic prevention. Readers can then use the knowledge generated to reach their own conclusions on how to improve global public health and prevent future pandemics.

Studies of the coronavirus spread dynamics in and from Wuhan have confirmed that the Wuhan lockdown, coupled with nationwide human mobility curtailment during the Lunar New Year travel period, were crucial for China's eventual containment of COVID-19 in 2020.[40] It was estimated that, had the Wuhan lockdown and associated measures nationwide been delayed by 1 week, the number of COVID-19 cases nationwide would have doubled or tripled and would therefore have become much harder to contain within China.[41] Furthermore, Chinazzi et al. found that these measures, along with international travel restrictions, helped slow the pandemic's global spread until mid-February 2020.[42]

As mentioned in the introductory chapter, a small number of studies have also modeled how the outbreak might have unfolded had the public been warned earlier and asked to adopt preventive measures. The research team co-led by Dr. Zhong Nanshan found that implementing public epidemic control measures just 5 days earlier would have reduced China's total COVID-19 cases by two-thirds.[43] The international team led by Xu-Sheng Zhang of Public Health England concluded that, if the public epidemic control measures had been implemented 1, 2, or 3 weeks earlier in Wuhan, the number of confirmed cases (and deaths) in China would have been reduced by about 57%, 81%, and 93%, respectively.[44]

These findings have significant implications for understanding the pandemic's spillover outside China and raise further questions about what realistically could have been done to control the outbreak in Wuhan during the early weeks. One anonymous reviewer of the book manuscript posed a thought experiment for both author and reader to consider: "What would have happened (globally) had the virus emerged in another country with the same level of public health capacity and expertise as China but without censorship and limits on free flow of information?" In other words, with insights gained from examining the choices, missteps, and deficiencies in the initial outbreak response, was the COVID-19 pandemic preventable? How much difference would have been made had some of the missteps and deficiencies been avoided?

Given the magnitude of the COVID-19 pandemic and the millions of lives it has claimed, any evidence indicating a realistic chance of preventing the pandemic deserves attention and offers important lessons for global health as humanity faces potential new outbreaks, including those of coronaviruses. However, the reviewer's counterfactual question is challenging to answer because few countries possess China's size, scientific capabilities, bureaucratic capacity and complexity, and experiences that have included dealing with two novel coronavirus outbreaks 17 years apart. Thus, the question posed by the reviewer leads us back to Wuhan and how the Wuhan outbreak would have been handled had China possessed a generative rather than a bureaucratic-pathological organizational culture, "without censorship and limits on free flow of information."

A key consideration is that, at the end of December 2019 and early January 2020, Chinese authorities (both in Wuhan and nationally) had access to multiple genomic sequences and whole genomes of the SARS-like novel coronavirus, in addition to clusters of cases, suspected cases, and expert physicians' concerns that the viral pathogen causing the so-called PUE was contagious. Leaving aside the use of the national disease reporting system, the amount and quality of information available to Chinese health policymakers in late December 2019 were quite substantial from a disease prevention and control perspective.

With this consideration in mind and the modeling results by the Zhong Nanshan team and the Xu-Sheng Zhang team as reference, I believe there was a genuine and arguably considerable chance of containing the initial outbreak and preventing the pandemic from spiraling out of control if the decision makers had applied the lessons from the 2003 SARS coronavirus crisis and mobilized the health community and the public to join in a public health drive to control the novel coronavirus outbreak. This would have required disclosing the available information on the SARS-like coronavirus to the public and not punishing but allowing doctors, virologists, and public health experts to report on cases and to warn of the dangers of the SARS-like coronavirus. China's ability to contain the Wuhan epidemic by April 2020, after hundreds of thousands of individuals were infected, demonstrates that China possessed the capacity for doing so.

In interviews with Wuhan residents, I have learned that some members of the health community, and others who were well connected with the health community in Wuhan, discussed cordon sanitaire or sealing off the city as a possible option for responding to the outbreak as early as the end of December 2019 and the beginning of January 2020. To be sure, the existence of such an opinion among a small segment of the population does not make it reasonable or politically feasible to put a city of nearly 11 million people, like Wuhan, in lockdown at the end of December 2019 or the beginning of January 2020. However, I would suggest that, in a population that was highly sensitive to the dangers of a SARS-like coronavirus, it would not have been necessary to implement an immediate and complete lockdown as of January 1, 2020, or thereabouts, to contain the initial outbreak. Instead, alongside the honest sharing of epidemic information with the public, it would have been both advisable and feasible to encourage the public to wear facemasks, take preventive measures as indicated in the WMHC Update of December 31, 2019, as well as to apply targeted quarantine and control measures in sections of Wuhan with case clusters, along with vigorous contact tracing and quarantining of close contacts and of visitors to the Huanan Seafood Market and other possible sites of disease transmission.[45]

It should be noted that, if there had been no "censorship and limits on the free flow of information," the timeline for action would likely have been favorably altered. Individuals and organizations would have been much less inhibited from submitting SARS-like PUE cases via the NNDSS or associated programs. Hospitals, experts, and laboratories would have likely made more information available about the novel coronavirus and the disease it caused. Likewise, media reporting and public knowledge of such cases would likely have occurred significantly earlier. Respiratory doctors in Wuhan were known to discuss and inquire about the unusual pneumonia cases in mid-December 2019, so it is plausible that national health authorities could have learned about the situation in Wuhan by December 22–23, 2019, or about a week earlier than December 30, 2019, in the absence of the NNDSS. With the national disease reporting system in good working order for SARS-like PUE cases, national involvement would likely have been even earlier, providing health authorities and experts with more time to investigate the unusual pneumonia cases, conduct epidemiological and virological studies, and initiate preventive action.

The preexisting and strong public fear of a SARS-like disease could have been the best ally for health authorities, political leaders, and the public. Enlisting such fear, an open and transparent environment, as seen in Hong Kong and Taiwan, two societies that also had strong memories of SARS, could have mitigated or corrected most missteps and deficiencies in outbreak response by avoiding information-related crackdowns, encouraging information sharing and the consideration of alternatives in decision-making, trusting the public with epidemic information, and promoting proactive leadership in such situations. In other words, if the Chinese authorities had been transparent about the dangers of the novel coronavirus in December 2019 and allowed experts to speak out, laboratories to share results, and the media to report, the public in China and other countries would have been warned and strongly motivated to take precautions to avoid infection when the "wild-type" novel coronavirus was still significantly less contagious than its later variants. Thus, in the absence of "censorship and limits on the free flow of information," the probability of full containment in December 2019–2020 would have been greatly improved not only because prompt and public action could have occurred at the end of December 2019 or early January 2020 but also because the timing of national involvement and public action would likely have been even earlier as well as more vigorous.

The tragedy in the initial response to the Wuhan outbreak lies in the stark contrast between the WMHC's initial public advisory on December 31, 2019, and the subsequent actions taken. Without disclosing lab results showing a SARS-like coronavirus, the WMHC initially recommended precautionary measures to the public such as maintaining indoor air circulation; avoiding enclosed, poorly ventilated public places and crowded areas; and wearing facemasks when venturing outside.[46] In hindsight, these recommendations were remarkably good ones for mitigating the possibility of getting infected with the novel coronavirus.

Regrettably, propelled by political, organizational, and other considerations, actions taken over the following 3 weeks were diametrically opposite to these early recommendations. Instead, as we have learned, the bundle of official actions included the silencing of doctors and scientists, suppression of suspected case submissions, concealment of infections among medical staff, and discouragement of healthcare workers and other service personnel from wearing facemasks. This was a political and institutional environment that made it particularly difficult for leading experts and health leaders to overcome cognitive biases. The stark contrast between the initial advisory and subsequent actions in Wuhan is profoundly disturbing and the Chinese public clearly perceived it with their display of strong negative sentiments on January 18, 2020, when health authorities in Wuhan again began to disclose new confirmed novel coronavirus infections.[47]

The missteps and deficiencies in Wuhan underscore the pressing need for the WHO and national governments to strengthen health emergency regulations and protocols and accelerate the early detection, reporting, and disclosure of novel coronaviruses and other emerging pathogens. Drawing upon the lessons learned from the COVID-19 pandemic and other epidemic outbreaks, the enhancements in health emergency preparedness should aim to anticipate and mitigate both known and potential weaknesses, seek to avert costly delays, and encourage a more proactive and precautionary response to potential outbreaks.

APPENDIX 1

A Chronology of the COVID-19 Outbreak in Wuhan, China

Abbreviations used: CDC, Centers for Disease Control and Prevention; GISAID, Global Initiative on Sharing All Influenza Data; IVDC, Institute for Viral Disease Control and Prevention; NHC, National Health Commission; PHEIC, Public Health Emergency of International Concern; PUE, pneumonia of uncertain etiology; SARS, severe acute respiratory syndrome; TEM, transmission electron microscopy; WHO, World Health Organization; WMHC, Wuhan Municipal Health Commission

December 8, 2019

(Retrospective) First officially recorded COVID-19 case began to show pneumonia symptoms (disease onset); more (retrospective) cases visited different hospitals in the following days and weeks.

December 27, 2019

Clinicians and hospital administrators in several Wuhan hospitals are publicly known to have filed reports of PUE cases to local CDCs. Some of these reports were based on SARS-like clinical symptoms as well as knowledge of genomic diagnostic results that showed a SARS-like coronavirus as likely pathogen.

Vision Medicals (Guangzhou) identified novel coronavirus in a sample taken from a patient at Wuhan Central Hospital; the patient was transferred to Wuhan Tongji Hospital and put under the care of Dr. Zhao Jianping. Vision Medicals informed the clinicians of diagnostic results by phone.

Dr. Zhang Dingyu, president of Jinyintan Hospital, first learned of Vision Medicals' results and consulted Wuhan Institute of Virology researchers on the SARS-like coronavirus.

December 29, 2019

Dr. Zhang Jixian and the Hubei Provincial Hospital of Integrated Chinese and Western Medicine reported seven PUE cases to the Hubei Provincial Health Commission and WMHC. The first three were a family cluster with no known connection to the Huanan Seafood Market.

Wuhan Central Hospital reported PUE cases to WMHC and Wuhan CDC.

Vision Medicals' leadership reported novel coronavirus diagnostic results to WMHC/Wuhan CDC.

On the order of the Hubei Provincial Health Commission, WMHC arranged for transfer of unusual pneumonia patients from various hospitals to Wuhan Jinyintan Hospital, the designated infectious disease hospital.

A joint investigation team from the CDCs of Hubei Province, Wuhan municipality, and Wuhan districts started investigation of the unusual pneumonia cases.

December 30, 2019

The joint investigation team submitted its report on the outbreak of viral PUE cases. The report included the following case definition: "Individuals with exposure to the Huanan Seafood Market and their family members who have been diagnosed as pneumonia cases in hospitals since December 1, 2019."

WMHC issued emergency notices to major Wuhan hospitals asking for submission of PUE cases while demanding secrecy.

Dr. Ai Fen and Dr. Zhao Su of Wuhan Central Hospital received a patient's diagnostic results from CapitalBio (Beijing) that detected infection with a SARS-like coronavirus.

Twenty-eight leading experts in Hubei gathered at Jinyintan Hospital in the evening to consult on and treat the PUE patients transferred there. Dr. Zhao Jianping of Tongji Hospital: "28 experts went to Jinyintan to consult on 27 patients, of which 13 were critically or seriously ill."

China CDC director general (George) Gao Fu learned of the Wuhan outbreak from social media sources late in the evening and worked with the NHC leadership overnight to dispatch emergency response teams to Wuhan.

December 31, 2019, New Year's Eve

NHC and China CDC expert and emergency response teams in Wuhan.

Gao Fu reviewed novel coronavirus genomic sequence at a third-party entity in Beijing.

With national approval, WMHC issued the first official advisory on the outbreak and disclosed 27 viral PUE cases in the afternoon. No mention was made of novel coronavirus detection.

National, Hubei provincial, and Wuhan municipal experts and health leaders held an evening meeting in Wuhan to plan and organize disease prevention and control measures. The response plan was reported to and approved by the Hubei/Wuhan leadership overnight.

January 1, 2020, New Year's Day

Wuhan Huanan Seafood Market was shut down. China CDC emergency operations team led in the collection of samples.

NHC Leading Group on Epidemic Response and Handling was activated. Minister Ma Xiaowei led the group.

Wuhan Public Security (police) announced punishment of eight "rumormongers" for disseminating information saying pneumonia outbreak was caused by SARS or SARS-like coronavirus.

Dr. Ai Fen, director of Emergency Care of Wuhan Central Hospital, was reprimanded by Wuhan Central Hospital leadership for sharing patient diagnosis showing SARS-like coronavirus.

NHC official directed Wuhan Institute of Virology not to release "all testing and experimental data plus results and conclusions related to this outbreak."

NHC sent a vice minister to Wuhan to lead a front-line working team.

January 2, 2020

China Central Television broadcast punishment of "rumormongers" about the pneumonia outbreak in Wuhan.

Wuhan Institute of Virology became the first state research institution to obtain a whole genome of the novel coronavirus (SARS-CoV-2) from samples collected at Wuhan Jinyintan Hospital on December 30, 2019.

Wuhan University Zhongnan Hospital clinicians and laboratory staff identified two pneumonia patients infected with SARS-like coronavirus. One patient had no direct exposure to the Huanan Seafood Market. The cases were investigated by Wuhan CDC staff and transferred to Jinyintan Hospital.

January 3, 2020

Clinical experts led by Cao Bin and Li Xingwang collaborated with experts from Hubei to put together the "Diagnosis and Treatment Protocol for Viral Pneumonia of Unknown Etiology (trial)." This protocol was open to symptomatic individuals without exposure to the Huanan Seafood Market.

WMHC introduced restrictive "inclusion–exclusion criteria for viral pneumonia of unknown etiology (PUE)." This case definition required a direct or indirect link to the Huanan Seafood Market.

NHC "Communication No. 3" banned laboratories from investigating or testing samples of pneumonia patients in or from Wuhan without authorization. It also directed that non-designated organizations and individuals not keep relevant bio-samples and not release "information about the results of the pathogenic testing or experimental activities."

IVDC of China CDC became the second research institute to obtain the novel coronavirus whole genome.

Dr. Li Wenliang of Wuhan Central Hospital was administered stern admonition by Wuhan police.

Wuhan University Zhongnan Hospital clinicians and laboratory staff identified a family of three infected with SARS-like coronavirus. None of the three had been to the Huanan Seafood Market. These and other cases were reported to the Wuchang District Health Bureau and the district CDC and investigated.

January 4, 2020

WMHC conducted a training session for doctors and infection control specialists in Wuhan and distributed a handbook with a white cover containing 10 documents, including the WMHC inclusion–exclusion criteria.

The WMHC Command for Responding to PUE oversaw and managed the transfer of so-called viral PUE patients to the Wuhan Jinyintan Hospital for treatment. Only patients with a history of exposure to the Huanan Seafood Market were given permission for the transfer. Patients with similar clinical symptoms but no history of exposure to the Huanan market were excluded and left in the general hospitals.

January 5, 2020

WMHC disclosed there were 59 viral PUE cases, of which seven were announced as severe cases. "No clear evidence of human-to-human transmission."

Zhang Yongzhen's team at Shanghai Public Health Clinical Center obtained the whole genome of SARS-CoV-2 from a sample collected at Wuhan Central Hospital. Zhang submitted a report to the NHC to warn of danger from the novel coronavirus.

January 6, 2020

China CDC activated Level II emergency response (not publicly announced).

China CDC IVDC team took testing kit to Wuhan for training and testing.

The Wuhan municipal "two sessions" began: Wuhan People's Political Consultative Conference (January 6–10); Wuhan Municipal People's Congress (January 7–10).

Wuhan University Zhongnan Hospital admitted a severely ill PUE patient who came from the city of Huanggang.

January 7, 2020

General Secretary Xi Jinping made "requirements" on handling the outbreak in Wuhan at a Politburo Standing Committee meeting. (No details of the requirements have been made public.)

The IVDC team of China CDC observed the novel coronavirus with TEM and submitted the TEM image of the novel coronavirus to the NHC on January 8.

Dr. Lu Jun, a 31-year-old emergency medicine doctor at the Wuhan Tongji Hospital, was diagnosed. He began to show the so-called viral PUE symptoms on January 5 and was put into an isolation ward at the hospital on January 6.

A 67-year-old male patient died of suspected novel coronavirus infections at Jinyintan Hospital. An expert panel could only agree the deceased died of pneumonia but did not rule it a case of novel coronavirus infection in the absence of a diagnostic test. Officially, the first death (Mr. Zeng) from novel coronavirus infections occurred on January 9.

January 8, 2020

Second NHC expert team visited Wuhan during January 8–16.

January 9, 2020

NHC used a Xinhua interview with academician Xu Jianguo to make a low-key announcement that a novel coronavirus (then named "2019-nCoV") was identified as the causative pathogen of the PUE outbreak in Wuhan.

Zeng Guang, chief epidemiologist of China CDC, visited Wuhan and returned to Beijing on the same day.

Wuhan University Zhongnan Hospital (Medical Affairs Department) used the national disease reporting system to submit reports of two so-called viral PUE cases. The system indicated that the submission was successful, but the submitted cases were disappeared from the system. The city of Huanggang used the submitted information to conduct contact tracing.

January 10, 2020

Start of the Lunar New Year peak travel season.

An expert panel for the NHC conducted a blind test and evaluation of five polymerase chain reaction nucleic acid test kits for the novel coronavirus. The Hubei Provincial CDC laboratory served as the validation laboratory. The panel designated the China CDC IVDC

2019-nCov nucleic acid test reagent as the reagent used for testing in labs of the China CDC and of provincial/municipal CDCs.

Dr. Lu Jun of Wuhan Tongji Hospital was checked in as an inpatient to the respiratory ward of Tongji Hospital and put on supplemental oxygen and then on a ventilator. Dr. Zhao Jianping, leader of the Hubei provincial expert team, oversaw Dr. Lu's treatment.

Dr. Li Wenliang of Wuhan Central Hospital began to show symptoms of the so-called viral PUE.

Wuhan-area hospitals experienced major increases in the number of so-called viral PUE cases but were unsuccessful in having the cases accepted by the health authorities.

A suspected viral PUE patient was put in isolation in Jiangsu Province.

January 11, 2020

Dr. Wang Guangfa of Second NHC Expert Team said the outbreak was "preventable and controllable."

WMHC began to refer to pneumonia cases with novel coronavirus infections and announced 41 laboratory-confirmed cases as of January 10. WMHC stated that investigations by national, provincial, and municipal experts "have not found any newly infected patients after January 3, 2020" and "have not found clear evidence of human-to-human transmission."

The Hubei provincial "two sessions" began: Hubei Provincial People's Congress (January 12–17); Hubei Provincial Political Consultative Conference (January 11–15).

Zhang Yongzhen, via Eddie Holmes, released novel coronavirus genome on Virological.org.

WHO issued an interim guidance for surveillance to detect "any evidence of amplified or sustained human-to-human transmission." The WHO surveillance case definition included cases with a "history of travel to Wuhan, Hubei Province, China in the 14 days prior to symptom onset" as one consideration.

January 12, 2020

China CDC coordinated the release on GISAID of five novel coronavirus genomes plus the TEM image from IVDC of China CDC, Wuhan Institute of Virology, and Chinese Academy of Medical Sciences.

Dr. Li Wenliang was checked into Wuhan Central Hospital with symptoms of novel coronavirus infection.

The Beijing Municipal Health Commission arranged for the transfer of two suspected novel coronavirus cases, a husband and wife, to Beijing Ditan Hospital for treatment. The two patients had visited Wuhan for a wedding around January 7–9 but had no exposure to the Huanan Seafood Market.

Some members of an extended family in Shenzhen, Guangdong, tested positive for the novel coronavirus at the University of Hong Kong-Shenzhen Hospital using test kits developed in the lab of Professor Yuen Kwok-Yung.

Wuhan party secretary Ma Guoqiang later revealed on national television that he regretted not taking more decisive measures to control the outbreak on this date.

January 13, 2020

Premier Li Keqiang "set forth his requirements" for epidemic prevention and control of the outbreak in Wuhan during State Council Plenary Meeting.

NHC leadership convened a meeting to guide the Hubei and Wuhan authorities to "further strengthen control measures."

Thailand confirmed the first COVID-19 case outside China and notified WHO. The patient, a traveler from Wuhan, was first admitted to hospital with fever on January 8, 2020.

WHO stated that the case in Thailand confirmed its earlier concern that the novel coronavirus would spread beyond China. WHO director-general Dr. Tedros Adhanom Ghebreyesus consulted Emergency Committee members.

January 14, 2020

NHC leadership led by Ma Xiaowei convened a confidential national working teleconference on novel coronavirus pneumonia prevention and control (*fangkong*).

President Wang Xinghuan of Wuhan University Zhongnan Hospital pleaded with a Hubei provincial leader to act on the novel coronavirus infections.

Staff at the Shenzhen No. 3 People's Hospital, using self-developed test kits, also found members of the aforementioned extended family positive for the novel coronavirus. The Shenzhen Municipal CDC used newly received China CDC–allocated test kits to verify the diagnostic results later in the day. Guangdong Provincial CDC laboratory confirmed the results using genomic sequencing. A patient sample was dispatched the next day to China CDC for reconfirmation and final determination by an expert panel acting for the NHC

January 15, 2020

NHC confidentially distributed *fangkong* documents totaling 63 pages to provincial health authorities for immediate attention and action within 5 hours of reception. The case definition was broadened from strict emphasis on exposure to the Huanan Seafood Market. A patient may be considered a suspect or "observation case" for further diagnostic testing if the patient had the clinical expressions and if the patient had traveled to Wuhan within 2 weeks of disease onset or had direct or indirect exposure to Wuhan markets.

NHC/China CDC distributed diagnostic test kits. Note that Shenzhen used such test kits on January 14. Wuhan indicated use of such test kits beginning on January 16.

China CDC activated Level I emergency response (not publicly announced).

WMHC released a question-and-answer dated January 14: "No clear evidence of human-to-human transmission has been found; limited human-to-human transmission cannot be ruled out, but the risk of sustained human-to-human transmission is low." NHC provided the same information to WHO, which shared it with the rest of the world.

Word spread in Wuhan that doctors at Wuhan Union Hospital had contracted the unusual pneumonia from a January 11 operation on a patient who later tested positive for the novel coronavirus and was transferred to Wuhan Jinyintan Hospital on January 15.

January 17, 2020

Final session of the Hubei Provincial People's Congress.

Dr. Lu Jun of Wuhan Tongji Hospital was in critical condition and was transferred to Jinyintan Hospital in the evening.

Guangdong provincial health leadership accompanied Dr. Zhong Nanshan to visit the Shenzhen No. 3 People's Hospital to see patients with novel coronavirus infections. They concluded there was human-to-human transmission.

Guangdong Provincial CDC obtained the whole genome of the novel coronavirus.

Professor Yuen Kwok-yung of Hong Kong University sent *urgent* messages to China CDC director general Gao Fu and Guangdong Provincial CDC with supporting evidence for person-to-person transmission.

January 18, 2020

A week after announcing that 41 pneumonia cases with novel coronavirus infections were laboratory confirmed, WMHC disclosed four new confirmed cases (as of January 16) and one case each identified in Thailand and Japan.

NHC confidentially issued updated second edition of the *fangkong* documents, including updated Diagnosis and Treatment Protocol. NHC plainly stated that cases that lacked a history of exposure to the Huanan market were growing and essentially admitted that the outbreak was spreading. These documents were not disclosed to the public until January 22, 2020.

Baibuting Community of Wuhan held high-profile 40,000-Family Feast ahead of Lunar New Year.

NHC asked three of China's most prominent pulmonary and critical care medicine specialists—Du Bin, Tong Zhaohui, Qiu Haibo—to go to Wuhan to provide help and clinical leadership.

NHC organized six-member Senior Advisory Panel (Highly-ranked Experts Mission) led by 83-year-old Dr. Zhong Nanshan to visit Wuhan and assess the epidemic situation.

January 19, 2020

Ahead of visit by Senior Advisory Panel, Wuhan released interviews with Vice Mayor Chen Xiexin; Wuhan CDC director Li Gang; and Dr. Huang Chaolin of Jinyintan Hospital to defend its record on outbreak response. Li Gang reiterated that "the risk of sustained human-to-human transmission is low."

Senior Advisory Panel visited Wuhan. Upon questioning, Dr. Zhong Nanshan was told there were already 198 confirmed cases, including 13 medical staff infections in the Neurosurgery Department of Union Hospital.

NHC issued a statement on its website enumerating its efforts in responding to the outbreak but called attention to the principle of "territorial responsibility" for health emergency response.

January 20, 2020

Premier Li Keqiang convened State Council Executive Meeting on the Wuhan epidemic. Zhong Nanshan and Li Lanjuan attended as invited experts.

State Council Executive Meeting authorized NHC to classify novel coronavirus pneumonia as a Class II infectious disease but regulated using Class I prevention and control measures.

Vice Premier Sun Chunlan activated the State Council Joint Prevention and Control Mechanism involving 32 central government ministries and administrations. NHC minister Ma Xiaowei was made lead coordinator.

Dr. Zhong Nanshan appeared on China Central Television in the evening to inform the public of novel coronavirus human-to-human transmission, including 14 medical staff infections.

January 21, 2020

Hubei Province activated Level II Emergency Response for novel coronavirus pneumonia.
Hubei leaders attended Lunar New Year gala.
General Secretary and President Xi Jinping returned to Beijing from visit to Myanmar (January 17–18) and tour of Yunnan Province.

January 22, 2020

In the afternoon, Xi Jinping approved "the strict closure of exit channels," or cordon sanitaire, for Wuhan and the rest of Hubei Province.
Vice Premier Sun Chunlan arrived in Wuhan to superintend the local authorities on behalf of the central leadership.

January 23, 2020

At about 2:30 AM, the Wuhan Municipal leadership, in the name of the Wuhan Municipal Command for the Prevention and Control of Novel Coronavirus Pneumonia, announced the cordon sanitaire would be in effect at 10 AM. About 500,000 people were able to leave Wuhan between this announcement and 10 AM.
Wuhan was "sealed off" from the rest of China at 10 AM.
A few hours later, the WHO secretary general reconvened its Emergency Committee to study the information from China about the outbreak and the containment measures taken. The committee finished the meeting at 15:10 Geneva time (9:10 PM in Beijing). It set down seven stipulations addressed to China but did not declare the novel coronavirus outbreak a PHEIC then. WHO made the PHEIC declaration a week later, on January 30, 2020.
Guangdong, Hunan, and Zhejiang activated Level I Public Health Emergency Response.

January 24, 2020

Hubei raised its emergency response to Level I.
With the approval of Xi Jinping, Chairman of the Central Military Commission, three military medical teams of 150 each, organized by the Army, Navy, and Air Force Medical Universities and their affiliated hospitals, reached Wuhan.

January 25, 2020, Lunar New Year's Day

General Secretary Xi Jinping convened the Politburo Standing Committee on the epidemic and declared that the epidemic posed an existential threat to "the whole picture" and vowed to "win the epidemic *fangkong* battle."
Central Leading Group for Epidemic Response was established. Premier Li Keqiang was made head of this group. A Central Steering Group led by Vice Premier and Politburo member Sun Chunlan represented. The Central Leading Group in Wuhan/Hubei. Sun also oversaw the State Council Joint Prevention and Control Mechanism.
Led by the national leadership, China mobilized a total of 344 medical teams from the armed forces and every provincial unit to offer medical assistance to Wuhan/Hubei. This national

campaign, with more than 44,000 health workers, was the largest ever medical assistance mission in China's history.

All provincial units in China (except for Tibet) declared Level I emergency response.

January 29, 2020

The novel coronavirus was detected in all provincial units in China. Tibet declared Level I emergency response.

January 30, 2020

WHO declared the coronavirus outbreak that started in Wuhan a PHEIC.

February 4, 2020

NHC released the fifth edition of the Diagnosis and Treatment Protocol, which acknowledged the possibility of asymptomatic transmission.

The emergency Fire God Mountain Hospital went into operation.

February 5, 2020

The 1,600-bed Jianghan Fangcang Hospital (located in the Wuhan International Convention Center) and the 800-bed Wuchang Fangcang Hospital (housed in the Hongshan Sports Stadium) became the first *fangcang* Shelter hospitals for treating patients with milder symptoms.

February 6, 2020

Dr. Li Wenliang died of novel coronavirus infection in the evening. He was officially pronounced dead on February 7, 2020.

February 8, 2020

The emergency Thunder God Mountain Hospital went into operation.

February 10, 2020

General Secretary Xi Jinping made his first public appearance since the Wuhan lockdown, visiting the Anhuali community in Chaoyang District, Ditan Hospital, and the Chaoyang District CDC in Beijing.

Wang Hesheng, NHC vice minister and Central Steering Group member, was made both party secretary and director general of the Hubei Provincial Health Commission, replacing Zhang Jin and Liu Yingzi.

February 11, 2020

The International Committee on Taxonomy of Viruses named the novel coronavirus SARS-CoV-2 and WHO named the disease COVID-19 (coronavirus disease 2019).

As of February 11, Wuhan had 1,103 infected healthcare workers confirmed, while the rest of Hubei had another 400.

February 13, 2020

Jiang Chaoliang and Ma Guoqiang were replaced as the party secretaries of Hubei and Wuhan, respectively.

March 11, 2020

WHO declared COVID-19 a pandemic.

April 8, 2020

The lockdown in Wuhan was successfully lifted following a 2-week period during which no new COVID-19 cases were reported.

September 8, 2020

The Chinese leadership convened a nationally televised Grand Commendation Ceremony in the Great Hall of the People to recognize organizations and individuals that made distinguished contributions to the fight against COVID-19. Xi Jinping presented Dr. Zhong Nanshan with the Medal of the Republic, China's highest civilian honor. Dr. Zhang Boli, Dr. Zhang Dingyu, and Major General Chen Wei were honored as "People's Heroes." Hubei Province held its own ceremony at the Wuhan International Expo Center—which was converted into a *fangcang* hospital—on September 21, 2020.

Much of the rest of the world continued to scramble to cope with the rapidly spreading COVID-19 pandemic, while China pursued a zero-COVID strategy with tightly sealed borders and stringent control measures.

Winter 2022–2023 China exited zero COVID in December 2022. In the ensuing viral wave that swept across China in December 2022 and January 2023, about 80% of the Chinese population were infected.

May 5, 2023 On the advice of the International Health Regulations Emergency Committee, the WHO secretary general determined that COVID-19 was an established and ongoing health issue and no longer a PHEIC.

APPENDIX 2

Notable Officials during and after the Wuhan Outbreak

Hubei Provincial Leaders

Hubei Party Secretary

Jiang Chaoliang (蒋超良, born 1957) was the party secretary of Hubei Province (2016–2020) and chair of the Hubei Provincial People's Congress (January 2017–March 2020). One of the preeminent bankers of his generation, he transitioned from banking to political governance as the governor of Jilin in 2014 and subsequently was appointed party secretary of Hubei in 2016. Earlier in his career, between September 2002 and May 2004, he served as a vice governor in Hubei on a secondment, during which time he participated in managing Hubei's response to the 2003 SARS crisis.

Jiang faced criticism for his conspicuous absence during the initial response to the outbreak in Wuhan. He was relieved of his duties as Hubei party secretary on February 13, 2020, although he retained his status as a member of the Chinese Communist Party (CCP) Central Committee until 2022.

After being sidelined, Jiang resurfaced as vice chair of the Agriculture and Rural Committee of the National People's Congress in August 2021. Such a role is typically given to individuals retiring from provincial leadership positions.

Jiang's replacement as Hubei party secretary was Ying Yong (应勇), formerly deputy secretary and mayor of Shanghai. After serving as Hubei party secretary until 2022, Ying was thought to have retired but was then given a promotion to the role of prosecutor general of the Supreme People's Procuratorate in 2023.

Hubei Deputy Secretary and Governor

Wang Xiaodong (王晓东, born 1960) was reassigned to Hubei in 2011 and ascended to the position of provincial governor in January 2017. In the interim, he served in various capacities, including deputy governor, deputy party secretary, and secretary of the Provincial Political and Legal Affairs Commission. As governor, Wang assumed a secondary role to the provincial party secretary, Jiang Chaoliang; and his influence in Wuhan, the provincial capital, was limited. Ma Guoqiang, the Wuhan party secretary, was considered his peer as they both held the role of provincial deputy party secretary.

When the cordon sanitaire was imposed in Wuhan, Wang asserted that Hubei was well equipped to handle the epidemic, a claim that was called into question as hospitals urgently appealed for medical supplies, particularly personal protective equipment. Despite the criticism, Governor Wang diligently led the COVID-19 prevention and control efforts outside of Wuhan in Hubei Province. Interviewees highlighted his effectiveness in collaborating with local authorities to enforce lockdown measures. In late September 2020, Wang was reportedly hospitalized for a stroke, but he resumed his duties by November of the same year.[1]

Wang was retired from the governorship in May 2021 and made a vice chair of the Agriculture and Rural Affairs Committee of the advisory Chinese People's Political Consultative Conference. His successor as governor was Wang Zhonglin.

Secretary General of the Hubei Provincial Party Committee

Liang Weinian (梁伟年, born 1959) was the secretary general of the Hubei Provincial Communist Party Committee from April 2017 to January 2020. Concurrently, from December 2018 to January 2020, he served as the secretary and director of the provincial party committee National Security Office. In his capacity as secretary general, Liang was the principal coordinator for the Hubei Communist Party leadership during the first weeks of the Wuhan outbreak. Before becoming secretary general, he held the position of Hubei Provincial Propaganda Department chief.

In January 2020, Liang was at a major inflection point in his career and on the way out from his position as secretary general. He was appointed as the vice chair of the Standing Committee of the Hubei Provincial People's Congress on January 16, 2020, and subsequently assumed the position of its deputy party group secretary.

Propaganda Department Director

Wang Yanling (王艳玲, born 1962) was named director of the Hubei Provincial Party Propaganda Department in March 2017, following her service as a vice governor of Henan Province from 2013 to 2017. She became a Central Committee alternate member later in 2017. Wang thus played an instrumental role in managing or limiting public access to epidemic information during the Wuhan outbreak and the ensuing lockdown.

Following the Wuhan lockdown, Wang was appointed secretary of the provincial Political and Legal Affairs Commission (July 2020–June 2022). In January 2022, she became the vice chair of the Standing Committee of the Hubei Provincial People's Congress and, in January 2023, its Party group secretary. Ma Guoqiang, who outranked her prior to the outbreak, was the deputy party group secretary.[2]

Provincial Political and Legal Affairs Commission Secretary

Luo Yonggang (罗永纲, born 1966) served in this role in Hubei from April 2019 to October 2020, having previously served in the same capacity for the Inner Mongolia Region prior to his reassignment to Hubei. He was thus instrumental in coordinating the police actions on the silencing of doctors, among other things. After his stint in Hubei, Luo was posted as a deputy director in the central government liaison offices for Macau and Hong Kong.

Vice Governor with the Health Portfolio

Yang Yunyan (杨云彦, born1963) was the vice governor, responsible for the health portfolio, from January 2018 to 2021. A specialist in human migration and the economy, he had previously served as the director general of the Hubei Provincial Health and Family Planning Commission from 2008 to 2018. Notably, Yang is not a member of the CCP. In January 2023, Yang Yunyan was appointed as a vice chair of the Standing Committee of the Hubei Provincial People's Congress.

Hubei Provincial Health Commission

Party Group Secretary

Zhang Jin (张晋, born 1965) served as the Hubei Provincial Health Commission (HPHC) party secretary from March 2016 until he was sacked in February 2020. He was deputy director general and deputy party secretary of the commission from 2012 to 2016. Zhang majored in medicine in college but thrived as a Communist Youth League officer and in a variety of roles in college and university administration, rising to become vice president and deputy party secretary of Huazhong University of Science and Technology (HUST) between 2008 and 2012.

With strong networking and organizational abilities, Zhang was the most influential leader in Hubei's health policy arena, partly because Vice Governor Yang Yunyan with the health portfolio was not a CCP member and partly because Director General Liu Yingzi was a newcomer with little health background.

After Zhang was replaced on February 10, 2020, amid public outrage over the shortcomings of the official outbreak response in Wuhan, he retained a membership on the Standing Committee of the Hubei Provincial People's Political Consultative Conference. In October 2021, he was transferred to the Provincial People's Congress and has since served as the vice chair of the Education, Science, Culture, and Health Committee of the Provincial People's Congress Standing Committee.

Director General of the HPHC

Liu Yingzi (刘英姿, born 1965) became HPHC director general in March 2016 and held this position until February 2020. Prior to this role, Liu had served as a vice mayor in Wuhan. Liu's professional background was in computer graphics and management. She was a faculty member in the HUST School of Management until she moved into government service in 2004.

With no professional background in health and medicine, Liu's appointment as the director general of the HPHC highlighted the gender-based stereotyping of health administration prevalent among provincial authorities.

After she was relieved of her duties alongside Zhang Jin following public criticism surrounding the handling of the outbreak, Liu disappeared from public view for an extended period. In October 2021, Liu was appointed vice chair of the Culture, History, and Study Committee of the Hubei Provincial People's Political Consultative Conference, signaling her transition into semi-retirement from official duties.

Hubei Provincial Centers for Disease Control and Prevention

Party Secretary

Liu Jiafa (刘家发, born 1961), a decorated career public health specialist, served as the Hubei Provincial Centers for Disease Control and Prevention (Hubei CDC) director general for the maximum two terms (2009–2019). He was then made the party secretary and deputy director general in September 2019. His successor as director general was Yang Bo (杨波, born 1975), a bureaucrat with no background in public health or medical practice.

Following the Wuhan lockdown, Liu Jiafa was promoted to deputy director general of the HPHC in October 2020 and retired in 2021 upon reaching retirement age. Yang Bo was transferred to the Hubei University of Chinese Medicine to serve as a vice president in July 2020. Interviewees in Hubei noted that this was a belated response to Yang's sub-par performance during the outbreak and recognition of his poor qualifications for the CDC role.

Wuhan Municipal Leaders

Party Secretary

Ma Guoqiang (马国强, born 1963) was appointed deputy party secretary of Hubei Province and party secretary of Wuhan in 2018, following a distinguished corporate career that led him to the position of chair of China Baowu Steel Group, one of the world's largest steel makers. Additionally, he was chair of the Standing Committee of the Wuhan Municipal People's Congress from September 2017 to January 6, 2020.

Ma, known for his zeal to enhance Wuhan's business environment, faced criticism for his inadequate leadership during the outbreak. Notably, he didn't assume the co-chair position of the Wuhan Command for Epidemic Prevention and Control until the day before the imposition of the cordon sanitaire in Wuhan.

On February 13, 2013, Ma Guoqiang was dismissed from his role as party secretary of Wuhan. His successor was Wang Zhonglin, formerly the party secretary of Jinan in Shandong Province. Wang, along with other leaders, implemented aggressive measures to enforce the lockdown and break the chains of virus transmission. With the successful conclusion of the lockdown, Wang was promoted to the positions of deputy party secretary of Hubei and governor in April–May 2021. He also became a member of the Central Committee in 2022.

After a period of political limbo, Ma Guoqiang re-emerged in August 2021 as a member of the Party Group of the Standing Committee of the Hubei Provincial People's Congress. In January 2023, he was appointed vice chair and deputy party group secretary of the Hubei Provincial People's Congress, a position that placed him under Wang Yanling, who had ranked below Ma prior to the Wuhan outbreak.

During the Twentieth Party Congress in October 2022, Ma, then an alternate member of the CCP Central Committee, was elevated to fill a vacancy on the committee for the remainder of the meeting period, serving as a full Central Committee member for 10 days. However, he was not re-elected, a clear indication that his previously soaring political career had come to an end.

Mayor and Deputy Party Secretary of Wuhan

Zhou Xianwang (周先旺, born 1962) served as mayor and deputy party secretary of Wuhan from May 2018 to January 2021. A native of Hubei and a member of the Tujia ethnic group, Zhou advanced from grassroots roles to become a versatile leader in several cities, as well as in the Commerce Bureau of Hubei. He was appointed vice governor of Hubei in spring 2017 and assumed the role of mayor of Wuhan in September 2018.

After the epidemic became public, Mayor Zhou emerged as the most eloquent spokesperson for Wuhan. He acknowledged shortcomings in the disclosure of epidemic information but attributed the delay to the superior levels of authorities. Subsequently, he led and received commendation for efforts to secure hospital and quarantine facilities, especially the transformation of public facilities into *fangcang* shelter hospitals.

Zhou fulfilled his term as mayor and stepped down in January 2021. Following this, he was appointed as a vice chair of the Hubei Provincial People's Political Consultative Conference.

Vice Mayor with the Health Portfolio

Chen Xiexin (陈邂馨, born 1961) held the position of vice mayor of Wuhan with a focus on health from April 2019 to July 2020. Prior to this, Chen gained experience in urban construction, serving in several roles within the Wuhan municipal government. These included director of the Culture Bureau and Dongxihu District party secretary before his appointment as vice mayor. In July 2020, he was moved from the vice mayorship and assigned to the Wuhan People's Political Consultative Conference. He assumed the role of vice chair of the conference in January 2021.

Wuhan Municipal Health Commission

Zhang Hongxing (张红星, born 1971) held the position of party secretary and director of the Wuhan Municipal Health Commission (WMHC) from September 2018 until May 2022. A native of Hubei, Zhang has a medical background and boasts a wealth of experience in municipal health bureaucracy as well as hospital administration. He served as president of Wuhan No. 1 Hospital prior to his appointment as the WMHC director.

Following the Wuhan lockdown, Zhang retained his position as the WMHC leader and played a crucial role in securing substantially increased resources for the Wuhan municipal CDC. In May 2022, he was transferred out of the health sector and appointed as a vice president of Jianghan University.

Wuhan Municipal CDC

Li Gang (李刚, n.a.), trained in preventive medicine at the HUST Tongji Medical School, served as the party secretary and director of the Wuhan Municipal CDC. He also functioned as the de facto official spokesperson during the Wuhan outbreak. His public downplaying of the outbreak's severity during the early weeks of the outbreak drew substantial criticism. Despite the controversy, he remained in his positions throughout the duration of the Wuhan lockdown. During his tenure, he oversaw the construction of a major new laboratory building, which included a P3 (BSL3) biosafety lab and an animal toxicology laboratory.

Li Gang stepped down from his leadership roles at the Wuhan CDC in mid-2022. Both official and unofficial media in China maintained a strict silence regarding the change of leadership at the Wuhan CDC and Li Gang's subsequent roles. In addition to his government roles, Li Gang served as vice president and secretary general of the Wuhan Preventive Medicine Society.

National Leaders

The State Council

Li Keqiang (李克强, born 1955) was premier and a member of the Politburo Standing Committee of the CCP Central Committee. He headed the Central Leading Group on Responding to the Novel Coronavirus Disease Outbreak from January 25, 2020, to October 2022.

In the period following the Wuhan lockdown, General Secretary Xi Jinping stood firm as a staunch advocate for the zero-COVID strategy. Conversely, Li Keqiang's efforts tended to be focused on mitigating the severe impact of these rigorous zero-COVID measures on the economy and society. Li Keqiang's tenure as premier concluded in March 2023, after China had shifted away from the zero-COVID policy in the winter of 2022–2023.

Sun Chunlan (孙春兰, born 1950), vice premier and member of the Politburo of the CCP Central Committee, oversaw education and health from 2018 to 2023. She represented the national leadership in superintending the lockdown in Wuhan. After the Wuhan lockdown was lifted, Sun emerged as the leading national figure in implementing China's zero-COVID strategy. She retired from the Politburo in October 2022 and concluded her tenure as vice premier in March 2023, after China's exit from the zero-COVID strategy.

National Health Commission

The leadership of the National Health Commission (NHC) has demonstrated impressive stability since the end of 2019. As of Fall 2023, Minister Ma Xiaowei and the four vice ministers—Wang Hesheng, Li Bin, Zeng Yixin, and Yu Xuejun—who were appointed prior to the Wuhan outbreak, continue in their roles. They are joined by two additional vice ministers, who were appointed in 2020 and 2022.

During the lockdown, China's national leadership orchestrated for Vice Minister Wang Hesheng to assume the dual roles of party secretary and director general of the HPHC. Concurrently, Wang was also appointed as a member of the CCP's Hubei Provincial Standing Committee. He relinquished his dual roles at the HPHC in July 2020 and May 2021, respectively, while concurrently taking on the leadership of the newly established National Administration of Disease Prevention and Control (NADPC).

As China pursued the zero-COVID strategy from 2020 to 2022, the NHC amassed significant power and resources, including the establishment of the NADPC. Several mid-ranking officials in the NHC received promotions following the Wuhan lockdown, notably Jiao Yahui (焦雅辉, born 1973), deputy director general of the Department of Medical Administration, who became director general in May 2020.

Liang Wannian (梁万年, born 1961), director general of the Health System Reform Department of the NHC, retired from the commission in 2020. Despite his retirement, Liang has chaired the NHC Expert Team on COVID-19 Response and led the Chinese expert team for the China–World Health Organization SARS-CoV-2 origins investigation. As one of the architects of the zero-COVID strategy, he frequently serves as the designated official expert on the COVID-19 situation. Despite regulations prohibiting senior government officials from taking up post-retirement appointments in government-funded universities, Liang has been appointed as the Vanke Chair Professor and executive vice-dean of the newly established Vanke School of Public Health at Qinghua (Tsinghua) University.

China CDC

Gao Fu (George, 高福, born 1961), a virologist and immunologist, is an academician of the Chinese Academy of Sciences. Gao was appointed deputy director of the China CDC in April 2011 and director general in August 2017. He stepped down from the position of director general in July 2022 upon reaching retirement age.

With the establishment of the NADPC, a vice-ministerial agency under the NHC, the administrative reporting line of the China CDC shifted from the NHC to the lower-ranked NADPC. Simultaneously, the leadership composition of the China CDC experienced a significant overhaul that has led to the diminishment of internally promoted specialist leaders. As of Fall 2023, the top six of the eight leaders in the China CDC were appointees who had built their careers outside the organization.

Notes

Chapter 1

1. “新冠肺炎‘吹哨人’李文亮: 真相最重要,” 财新网, 2020-02-07, https://china.caixin.com/2020-02-07/101509761.html.
2. “白岩松八问钟南山: 新型冠状病毒肺炎, 情况到底如何?” 央视新闻客户端, 2020-01-21, http://m.news.cctv.com/2020/01/20/ARTIpzG9gFnLXsE7amZvU9MY200120.shtml.
3. “中央广播电视总台: 全媒矩阵发力, 凝聚强大正能量,” 人民网, 2020-02-25, https://k.sina.cn/article_6456450127_180d59c4f02000wd5t.html.
4. Alexander E. Gorbalenya et al., “Severe Acute Respiratory Syndrome–Related Coronavirus: The Species and Its Viruses—A Statement of the Coronavirus Study Group,” bioRxiv, 2020-02-11, https://www.biorxiv.org/content/10.1101/2020.02.07.937862v1.
5. World Health Organization, “Global Excess Deaths Associated with COVID-19, January 2020–December 2021,” 2022-05, https://www.who.int/data/stories/global-excess-deaths-associated-with-covid-19-january-2020-december-2021. For an update to these estimates, see Richard Van Noorden, “COVID Death Tolls: Scientists Acknowledge Errors in WHO Estimates,” *Nature*, 2022-06-01, https://www.nature.com/articles/d41586-022-01526-0.
6. Maya Prabhu and Jessica Gergen, “History’s Seven Deadliest Plagues,” VaccinesWork, 2021-11-15, https://www.gavi.org/vaccineswork/historys-seven-deadliest-plagues.
7. Dali Yang, “Will China’s Leaders Rise to the SARS Challenge?,” *South China Morning Post*, 2003-04-19, A11.
8. Karl Taro Greenfeld, *China Syndrome: The True Story of the 21st Century’s First Great Epidemic* (New York: HarperCollins, 2006).
9. Joseph S. M. Peiris, Yi Guan, and Kwok-yung Yuen, “Severe Acute Respiratory Syndrome,” *Nature Medicine* 10, no. 12 (2004): S88–S97.
10. 杨洋, “黄永: 非典危机时,” 中国周刊, 2013-04-09, last accessed 2020-06-24, http://chinaweekly.blog.sohu.com/261115080.html; John Pomfret, “Beijing Told Doctors to Hide SARS Victims,” *Washington Post*, 2003-04-20, https://www.washingtonpost.com/archive/politics/2003/04/20/beijing-told-doctors-to-hide-sars-victims/3eb7d1aa-d2ff-477b-bc15-d0164377b123/.
11. “Hu on SARS: My Heart Was on Fire,” *China Daily*, 2003-10-22, https://www.chinadaily.com.cn/en/doc/2003-10/22/content_274175.htm.
12. Yanzhong Huang, “The SARS Epidemic and Its Aftermath in China: A Political Perspective,” in *Learning from SARS: Preparing for the Next Disease Outbreak: Workshop Summary*, ed. Stacey Knobler et al. (Washington, DC: National Academies Press, 2004), 116–136, https://www.ncbi.nlm.nih.gov/books/NBK92479/; Dali Yang, *Remaking the Chinese Leviathan: Market Transition and the Politics of Governance in China* (Palo Alto, CA: Stanford University Press, 2004); Patricia Thornton, “Crisis and Governance: SARS and the Resilience of the Chinese Body Politic,” *The China Journal* 61 (2009): 23–48.
13. Dali L. Yang @Dali_Yang, 8:50 PM, 2019-12-30, https://twitter.com/Dali_Yang/status/1211842156345856000.

14. Dali L. Yang @Dali_Yang, 10:30 PM, 2019-12-30, https://twitter.com/Dali_Yang/status/1211867272589041664.
15. "人民日报 2019-12-31 11:56," https://weibo.com/2803301701/IniAErTYL.
16. "老炭头," 2019-12-31, https://weibo.com/2803301701/IniAErTYL?type=repost#_rnd1656111367453.
17. Dali L. Yang @Dali_Yang, 10:36 PM. 2019-12-30, https://twitter.com/Dali_Yang/status/1211868611800907777.
18. Dali L. Yang @Dali_Yang 10:42 PM, 2019-12-30, https://twitter.com/Dali_Yang/status/1211870217523154944.
19. See, especially, Dali Yang, *Calamity and Reform in China: State, Rural Society, and Institutional Change since the Great Leap Famine* (Palo Alto, CA: Stanford University Press, 1996).
20. Dali Yang, "Wuhan Officials Tried to Cover up Covid-19—And Sent It Careening Outward," *Washington Post*, 2020-03-10, https://www.washingtonpost.com/politics/2020/03/10/wuhan-officials-tried-cover-up-covid-19-sent-it-careening-outward/.
21. Dali L. Yang, "China's Early Warning System Didn't Work on COVID-19. Here's the Story," *Washington Post*, 2020-02-24, https://www.washingtonpost.com/politics/2020/02/24/chinas-early-warning-system-didnt-work-covid-19-heres-story/.
22. Dali Yang, "China's Zero-COVID Campaign and the Body Politic," *Current History* 121, no. 836 (2022): 203–210.
23. William Sewell, "Historical Events as Transformations of Structures: Inventing Revolution at the Bastille," *Theory and Society* 25, no. 6 (1996): 841–881.
24. Quoted in 丰西西, "全国政协委员高福: 要对中国疫苗有信心, 出现问题要倒逼解决," 金羊网, 2019-03-05, https://www.sohu.com/a/299089554_119778.
25. Todd LaPorte and Paula Consolini, "Working in Practice but not in Theory: Theoretical Challenges of 'High-Reliability Organizations,'" *Journal of Public Administration Research and Theory* 1, no. 1 (1991): 19–48; Karl Weick and Kathleen Sutcliffe, *Managing the Unexpected: Resilient Performance in An Age of Uncertainty* (Hoboken, NJ: John Wiley & Sons, 2011); Stephanie Veazie, Kim Peterson, and Donald Bourne, "Evidence Brief: Implementation of High Reliability Organization Principles," US Department of Veterans Affairs, 2019.
26. Charles Perrow, *Normal Accidents: Living with High-Risk Technologies* (Princeton, NJ: Princeton University Press, 1999); Scott Sagan, *The Limits of Safety* (Princeton, NJ: Princeton University Press, 2020).
27. Diane Vaughan, *The Challenger Launch Decision: Risky Technology, Culture, and Deviance at NASA*, Enlarged Edition (Chicago: University of Chicago Press, 2016).
28. Diane Vaughan, "NASA Revisited: Theory, Analogy, and Public Sociology," *American Journal of Sociology* 112, no. 2 (2006): 353–393.
29. Samir Shrivastava, Karan Sonpar, and Federica Pazzaglia, "Normal Accident Theory Versus High Reliability Theory: A Resolution and Call for an Open Systems View of Accidents," *Human Relations* 62, no. 9 (2009): 1357–1390.
30. State Council Information Office, "Fighting COVID-19: China in Action," 2020-06-07, http://english.scio.gov.cn/whitepapers/2020-06/07/content_76135269.htm; Alex Jingwei He, Yuda Shi, and Hongdou Liu, "Crisis Governance, Chinese Style: Distinctive Features of China's Response to the Covid-19 Pandemic," *Policy Design and Practice* 3, no. 3 (2020): 242–258; Ehtisham Ahmad, "Multilevel Responses to Risks, Shocks and

Pandemics: Lessons from the Evolving Chinese Governance Model," *Journal of Chinese Governance* 7, no. 2 (2022): 291–319.

31. Clare Wenham et al., "Preparing for the Next Pandemic," *BMJ* 373 (2021): 1295; Bill Gates, "I Worry We're Making the Same Mistakes Again," *New York Times*, 2023-03-19, https://www.nytimes.com/2023/03/19/opinion/bill-gates-pandemic-preparedness-covid.html.
32. 习近平, "在中央政治局常委会会议研究应对新型冠状病毒肺炎疫情工作时的讲话," 求是, no. 4 (2020), 2020-02-15, http://www.qstheory.cn/dukan/qs/2020-02/15/c_1125572832.htm.
33. Dake Kang, Maria Cheng, and Sam McNeil, "China Clamps Down in Hidden Hunt for Coronavirus Origins," Associated Press, 2020-12-30, https://apnews.com/article/united-nations-coronavirus-pandemic-china-only-on-ap-bats-24fbadc58cee3a40bca2ddf7a14d2955.
34. 习近平,"在中央政治局常委会会议研究应对新型冠状病毒肺炎疫情工作时的讲话"; and see, especially, Lei Zhou et al., "One Hundred Days of Coronavirus Disease 2019 Prevention and Control in China," *Clinical Infectious Diseases* 72, no. 2 (2021): 332–339.
35. Amartya Sen, *Development as Freedom* (Oxford: Oxford University Press, 1999).
36. Matthew Kavanagh, "Authoritarianism, Outbreaks, and Information Politic," *Lancet Public Health* 5, no. 3 (2020): e135–e136.
37. Barry Turner and Nick F. Pidgeon, *Man-Made Disasters* (Oxford: Butterworth-Heinemann, 1997).
38. Ron Westrum, "The Study of Information Flow: A Personal Journey," *Safety Science* 67 (2014): 58–63.
39. Nick Pidgeon and Mike O'Leary, "Man-Made Disasters: Why Technology and Organizations (Sometimes) Fail," *Safety Science* 34, no. 1–3 (2000): 15–30, at 16. Emphasis in original.
40. Edgar Schein, *Organizational Culture and Leadership*, 4th ed. (Hoboken, NJ: John Wiley & Sons, 2010).
41. James Reason, *Managing the Risks of Organizational Accidents* (Abingdon, UK: Routledge, 2016).
42. Ron Westrum, "A Typology of Organizational Cultures," Suppl., *BMJ Quality & Safety* 13, no. 2 (2004): ii22–ii27.
43. Westrum, "Typology of Organizational Cultures," ii23.
44. James Reason, *Human Error* (Cambridge: Cambridge University Press, 1990).
45. Howard Aldrich and Jeffrey Pfeffer, "Environments of Organizations," *Annual Review of Sociology* 2 (1976): 79–105; John Child, "Strategic Choice in the Analysis of Action, Structure, Organizations and Environment," *Organization Studies* 18, no. 1 (1997): 43–76.
46. Patricia Yancey Martin and Barry A. Turner, "Grounded Theory and Organizational Research," *Journal of Applied Behavioral Science* 22, no. 2 (1986): 141–157.
47. Barry Turner, *Man-Made Disasters* (London: Wykeham Publications, 1987), 180.
48. Robert Hogan and Robert B. Kaiser, "What We Know about Leadership," *Review of General Psychology* 9, no. 2 (2005): 169–180.
49. Barry Naughton, "Inside and Outside: The Modernized Hierarchy That Runs China," *Journal of Comparative Economics* 44, no. 2 (2016): 404–415.
50. Martin Dimitrov, "The Political Logic of Media Control in China," *Problems of Post-Communism* 64, nos. 3–4 (2017): 121–127; Jeremy Wallace, *Seeking Truth and Hiding Facts: Information, Ideology, and Authoritarianism in China* (New York: Oxford University Press, 2022).

51. Amos Tversky and Daniel Kahneman, "Judgment under Uncertainty: Heuristics and Biases," *Science* 185, no. 4157 (1974): 1124–1131; Daniel Kahneman, *Thinking, Fast and Slow* (New York: Farrar, Straus and Giroux, 2011).
52. Turner and Pidgeon, *Man-Made Disasters*.
53. Barry Turner, "The Organization and Inter-Organizational Development of Disasters," *Administrative Science Quarterly* 21, no. 3 (1976): 378–397, at 382.
54. Scott Halpern, Robert Truog, and Franklin Miller, "Cognitive Bias and Public Health Policy during the COVID-19 Pandemic," *JAMA* 324, no. 4 (2020): 337–338.
55. Gilberto Montibeller and Detlof Von Winterfeldt, "Cognitive and Motivational Biases in Decision and Risk Analysis," *Risk Analysis* 35, no. 7 (2015): 1230–1251.
56. State Council Information Office, "Fighting COVID-19."
57. Peter Baldwin, *Fighting the First Wave: Why the Coronavirus Was Tackled so Differently across the Globe* (Cambridge: Cambridge University Press, 2021).
58. To be more specific, I would include both the announcement by Dr. Zhong of human-to-human transmission on January 20, 2020, and the imposition of the cordon sanitaire on Wuhan on January 23, 2020, as the two key components of this milestone.
59. Yang, "China's Zero-COVID Campaign and the Body Politic."
60. 杨维中(编), 中国卫生应急十年*(2003-2013)* (北京: 人民卫生出版社, 2014).
61. Turner, *Man-Made Disasters*, 180; Dali Yang, "China's Troubled Quest for Order: Leadership, Organization and the Contradictions of the Stability Maintenance Regime," *Journal of Contemporary China* 26, no. 103 (2017): 35–53; Jianrong Yu, "Rigid Stability: An Explanatory Framework for China's Social Situation," *Contemporary Chinese Thought* 46, no. 1 (2014): 72–84.
62. Sarah Biddulph, *The Stability Imperative: Human Rights and Law in China* (Vancouver, Canada: UBC Press, 2015); Yanhua Deng and Kevin J. O'Brien, "Relational Repression in China: Using Social Ties to Demobilize Protesters," *China Quarterly* 215 (2013): 533–552; Ching Kwan Lee and Yonghong Zhang, "The Power of Instability: Unraveling the Microfoundations of Bargained Authoritarianism in China," *American Journal of Sociology* 118, no. 6 (2013): 1475–1508.
63. Turner, *Man-Made Disasters*, 180
64. John M. Barry, *The Great Influenza: The Epic Story of the Deadliest Plague in History* (New York: Viking, 2004), 461.
65. Dake Kang, "In Xi's China, Even Internal Reports Fall Prey to Censorship," AP, 2022-10-31, https://apnews.com/article/health-china-beijing-covid-wuhan-3c199e3f1a084013da18fc9e6061e775.
66. Albert Camus, *The Plague*, trans. Stuart Gilbert (New York: Modern Library, 1948), pt. 1.
67. Vaughan, *Challenger Launch Decision*, 394.
68. Emily Feng, "Angry Chinese Ask Why Their Government Waited so Long to Act on Coronavirus," NPR, 2020-01-29, https://www.npr.org/2020/01/29/800938047/angry-chinese-ask-why-their-government-waited-so-long-to-act-on-coronavirus.
69. Zifeng Yang et al., "Modified SEIR and AI Prediction of the Epidemics Trend of COVID-19 in China under Public Health Interventions," *Journal of Thoracic Disease* 12, no. 3 (2020): 165–174.
70. Xu-Sheng Zhang et al., "Transmission Dynamics and Control Measures of COVID-19 Outbreak in China," *Scientific Reports* 11, no. 1 (2021): 2652.

Chapter 2

1. Andrew Price-Smith, *Contagion and Chaos: Disease, Ecology, and National Security in the Era of Globalization* (Cambridge, MA: MIT Press, 2008).
2. "中共中央关于坚持和完善中国特色社会主义制度　推进国家治理体系和治理能力现代化若干重大问题的决定 (2019-10-31)," 新华社, 2019-11-05, http://www.gov.cn/zhengce/2019-11/05/content_5449023.htm.
3. Dali Yang, "China's Developmental Authoritarianism: Dynamics and Pitfalls," *Taiwan Journal of Democracy* 12, no. 1 (2016): 100–123.
4. Kenneth Lieberthal and David Lampton, eds., *Bureaucracy, Politics, and Decision Making in Post-Mao China* (Berkeley: University of California Press, 1992); Andrew Mertha, "Fragmented Authoritarianism 2.0: Political Pluralization in the Chinese Policy Process," *China Quarterly* 200 (2009): 995–1012.
5. Jing Vivian Zhan and Shuang Qin, "The Art of Political Ambiguity: Top–Down Intergovernmental Information Asymmetry in China," *Journal of Chinese Governance* 2, no. 2 (2017): 149–168.
6. Jiying Jiang, "Leading Small Groups, Agency Coordination, and Policy Making in China," *China Journal* 89, no. 1 (2023): 95–120.
7. Frank Pieke, *The Good Communist: Elite Training and State Building in Today's China* (Cambridge: Cambridge University Press, 2009); Tony Saich, *From Rebel to Ruler: One Hundred Years of the Chinese Communist Party* (Cambridge, MA: Harvard University Press, 2021).
8. 习近平, 论坚持党对一切工作的领导 (北京: 中央文献出版社, 2019).
9. Deng Xiaoping, *Selected Works of Deng Xiaoping: 1975–1982* (Beijing: Foreign Languages Press, 1996).
10. 邓小平, 邓小平文选 (第三卷) (北京: 人民出版社, 1993).
11. Yang, "China's Developmental Authoritarianism."
12. Gabriella Montinola, Yingyi Qian, and Barry R. Weingast, "Federalism, Chinese Style: The Political Basis for Economic Success in China," *World Politics* 48, no. 1 (1995): 50–81.
13. Fubing Su, Ran Tao, and Dali Yang, "Rethinking the Institutional Foundations of China's Hyper Growth: Official Incentives, Institutional Constraints, and Local Developmentalism," in *The Oxford Handbook of the Politics of Development*, ed. Carol Lancaster and Nicolas Van de Walle (Oxford: Oxford University Press, 2018), 626–651.
14. Barry Naughton, "Inside and Outside: The Modernized Hierarchy That Runs China," *Journal of Comparative Economics* 44, no. 2 (2016): 404–415.
15. Ling Li, "Politics of Anticorruption in China: Paradigm Change of the Party's Disciplinary Regime 2012–2017," *Journal of Contemporary China* 28, no. 115 (2019): 47–63; "Visualizing China's Anti-Corruption Campaign," China File, 2018-08-15, https://www.chinafile.com/infographics/visualizing-chinas-anti-corruption-campaign.
16. Hua Gao, *How the Red Sun Rose: The Origin and Development of the Yan'an Rectification Movement, 1930–1945* (Hong Kong: The Chinese University of Hong Kong Press, 2018); 袁倩, "中国共产党党内集中教育的历史进程、基本特征和当代启示," 求实, 6 (2021), https://www.dswxyjy.org.cn/n1/2021/1111/c428053-32279478.html.
17. Cheng Li, *Chinese Politics in the Xi Jinping Era: Reassessing Collective Leadership* (Washington, DC: Brookings Institution Press, 2016).

18. Xuezhi Guo, *The Politics of the Core Leader in China: Culture, Institution, Legitimacy, and Power* (Cambridge: Cambridge University Press, 2019).
19. Josh Chin, "Xi Jinping's Leadership Style: Micromanagement That Leaves Underlings Scrambling," *Wall Street Journal*, 2021-12-15, https://www.wsj.com/articles/xi-jinpings-leadership-style-micromanagement-that-leaves-underlings-scrambling-11639582426.
20. Baogang Guo, "A Partocracy with Chinese Characteristics: Governance System Reform under Xi Jinping," *Journal of Contemporary China* 29, no. 126 (2020): 809–823.
21. "中国共产党重大事项请示报告条例," 新华社, 2019-02-28, http://www.gov.cn/zhengce/2019-02/28/content_5369363.htm.
22. "中国共产党重大事项请示报告条例."
23. Lieberthal and Lampton, *Bureaucracy, Politics, and Decision Making*; Kjeld Erik Brødsgaard, *Chinese Politics as Fragmented Authoritarianism* (New York: Routledge, 2017); Mertha, "Fragmented Authoritarianism 2.0."
24. Andrew Mertha, "China's 'Soft' Centralization: Shifting Tiao/Kuai Authority Relations," *China Quarterly* 184 (2005): 791–810; Dali Yang, *Remaking the Chinese Leviathan: Market Transition and the Politics of Governance in China* (Palo Alto, CA: Stanford University Press, 2004), chaps. 2–3.
25. Yang, "China's Developmental Authoritarianism."
26. Ernan Cui, Ran Tao, Travis Warner, and Dali Yang, "How Do Land Takings Affect Political Trust in Rural China?" *Political Studies* 63, no. S1 (2015): 91–109.
27. Yuhua Wang and Carl Minzner, "The Rise of the Chinese Security State," *China Quarterly* 222 (June 2015): 339–359.
28. Peter Sandby-Thomas, *Legitimating the Chinese Communist Party since Tiananmen: A Critical Analysis of the Stability Discourse* (Abingdon, UK: Routledge, 2010).
29. Mary Gallagher, "China in 2004: Stability above All," *Asian Survey* 45, no. 1 (2005): 21–32; Yongshun Cai, *Collective Resistance in China* (Palo Alto, CA: Stanford University Press, 2010).
30. Xie Yue, "The Political Logic of Weiwen in Contemporary China," *Issues & Studies* 48, no. 3 (September 2012): 1–41, at 19.
31. Jonathan Benney, "Weiwen at the Grassroots: China's Stability Maintenance Apparatus as a Means of Conflict Resolution," *Journal of Contemporary China* 25, no. 99 (2016): 389–405; Sandby-Thomas, *Legitimating the Chinese Communist Party*; Xiaojun Yan, "Patrolling Harmony: Pre-emptive Authoritarianism and the Preservation of Stability in W County," *Journal of Contemporary China* 25, no. 99 (2016): 406–421.
32. The December 1991 documents are "关于社会治安综合治理工作实行属地管理原则的规定" and "关于实行社会治安综合治理一票否决权制的规定."
33. 沈岿, "疫情资讯发布的法治难题," 铭传大学法学论丛 no. 34 (2021-02): 71–101.
34. Yanhua Deng and Kevin J. O'Brien, "Relational Repression in China: Using Social Ties to Demobilize Protesters," *China Quarterly* 215 (2013): 533–552; Jennifer Pan, *Welfare for Autocrats: How Social Assistance in China Cares for Its Rulers* (Oxford: Oxford University Press, 2020); Wang and Minzner, "Rise of the Chinese Security State"; 肖唐镖, "当代中国的维稳政治：沿革与特点—以抗争政治中的政府回应为视角," 学海, no. 1 (2015): 138–152.
35. Jérôme Doyon, "Local Governments under Pressure: The Commodification of Stability Maintenance," *China Perspectives* 2012, no. 3 (2012): 80–82; Carl Minzner, "China's Turn against Law," *American Journal of Comparative Law* 59, no. 4 (2011): 935–984; Yue, "Political Logic of Weiwen"; Dali Yang, "China's Troubled Quest for Order: Leadership,

Organization and the Contradictions of the Stability Maintenance Regime," *Journal of Contemporary China* 26, no. 103 (2017): 35–53.

36. Florian Schneider, *Staging China: The Politics of Mass Spectacle* (Leiden: Leiden University Press, 2019).
37. "习近平考察奥运安保: '没有平安奥运, 一切无从谈起,'" 新华网, 2008-07-22, https://news.ifeng.com/mainland/200807/0722_17_668636.shtml.
38. Wang and Minzner, "Rise of the Chinese Security State."
39. 陈红梅, "东城奥运场馆引入网格化管理, 发现问题第一时间上报," 北京日报, 2007-08-02, http://2008.sina.com.cn/hd/other/2007-08-02/092920821.shtml.
40. 贺勇, "网格化探索的北京经验," 人民日报, 2016-05-16, http://cssn.cn/mkszy/rd/201605/t20160517_3013313.shtml; Huirong Chen and Sheena Chestnut Greitens, "Information Capacity and Social Order: The Local Politics of Information Integration in China," *Governance* 35, no. 2 (2022): 497–523.
41. 贺勇, "网格化探索的北京经验"; Pan, *Welfare for Autocrats*.
42. Rory Truex, "Focal Points, Dissident Calendars, and Preemptive Repression," *Journal of Conflict Resolution* 63, no. 4 (2019): 1032–1052.
43. 习近平, 关于防范风险挑战、应对突发事件论述摘编 (北京: 中央文献出版社, 2020).
44. David Lampton, "Xi Jinping and the National Security Commission," *Journal of Contemporary China* 24 (2015): 759–777.
45. "中国共产党政法工作条例," 新华网, 2019-01-18, http://www.xinhuanet.com/politics/2019-01/18/c_1124011592.htm.
46. "习近平对政法工作作出重要指示," 新华网, 2018-01-22, http://www.xinhuanet.com/politics/2018-01/22/c_1122296147.htm.
47. 陈训秋, "推进立体化社会治安防控体系创新," 中国长安网, 2013-11-11, http://www.chinapeace.gov.cn/2013-12/11/content_9779691.htm.
48. "2019年平安建设(综治工作)考核评价工作会议在京召开," 正义网, 2019-12-25, https://news.sina.cn/gn/2019-12-25/detail-iihnzhfz8121262.d.html.
49. Yanzhong Huang, *Governing Health in Contemporary China* (Abingdon, UK: Routledge, 2015).
50. "中共中央、国务院关于卫生改革与发展的决定," 1997-01-15, http://pkulaw.cn/fulltext_form.aspx?Db=chl&Gid=2992e0a0ea173673bdfb.
51. 规划发展与信息化司, "2020年我国卫生健康事业发展统计公报," 国家卫生健康委员会, 2021-07-13, http://www.nhc.gov.cn/guihuaxxs/s10743/202107/af8a9c98453c4d9593e07895ae0493c8.shtml.
52. Jeremy Page, Wenxin Fan, and Natasha Khan, "How It All Started: China's Early Coronavirus Missteps," *Wall Street Journal*, 2020-03-06, https://www.wsj.com/articles/how-it-all-started-chinas-early-coronavirus-missteps-11583508932.
53. Ji You, "How Xi Jinping Dominates Elite Party Politics: A Case Study of Civil–Military Leadership Formation," *China Journal* 84, no. 1 (2020): 1–28.
54. Li, "Politics of Anticorruption in China"; Susan Shirk, "China in Xi's 'New Era': The Return to Personalistic Rule," *Journal of Democracy* 29, no. 2 (2018): 22–36; Suisheng Zhao, "The Ideological Campaign in Xi's China: Rebuilding Regime Legitimacy," *Asian Survey* 56, no. 6 (2016): 1168–1193.
55. Zhengxu Wang and Jinghan Zeng, "Xi Jinping: The Game Changer of Chinese Elite Politics?," *Contemporary Politics* 22, no. 4 (2016): 469–486; David Kelly, "Risk Aversion in Domestic Chinese Politics," *The Interpreter*, 2017-12-01, https://www.lowyinstitute.org/the-interpreter/risk-aversion-domestic-chinese-politics.

56. 习近平, 关于全面从严治党论述摘编 (北京: 中央文献出版社, 2021), 153.
57. "中央不忘初心、牢记使命主题教育领导小组印发'关于开展第二批不忘初心、牢记使命主题教育的指导意见,'" 新华网, 2019-09-05, http://www.xinhuanet.com/politics/2019-09/05/c_1124965727.htm.
58. "关于成立'不忘初心.牢记使命'主题教育领导小组的通知," 湖北省卫生计生委综合监督局, 2019-07-06, http://wjw.hubei.gov.cn/hbwsjd/ztzl/wqzl_wjwzhjdj/bwcxljsmztjy/202009/t20200908_2897714.shtml.
59. "凝心聚力, 推动公立医院党的建设," 湖北省卫生健康委员会, 2019-09-18, http://wjw.hubei.gov.cn/fbjd/dtyw/201910/t20191031_170940.shtml.
60. "全国公立医院党建工作研讨会在我委召开," 湖北省卫生健康委员会, 2019-09-18, http://wjw.hubei.gov.cn/bmdt/dtyw/201910/t20191031_170940.shtml.
61. "中央不忘初心、牢记使命主题教育领导小组印发'关于开展第二批不忘初心、牢记使命主题教育的指导意见.'"
62. See, for example, in the city of Xiaogan in Hubei: 方敏, "市中心医院稳定推进'不忘初心牢记使命'主题教育活动," 孝感市卫生健康委员会, 2019-11-13, http://wjw.xiaogan.gov.cn/lxyz/372390.jhtml.
63. 高翔, "摘口罩行动拉近医患距离," 健康报网, 2019-11-11, http://health.people.com.cn/n1/2019/1111/c14739-31447862.html.
64. Quoted in 樊巍, "武汉市中心医院医护人员吐真情: 疫情是面照妖镜," 环球时报, 2002-03-17, www.medsci.cn/article/show_article.do?id=2f19190169f7.
65. World Health Organization Western Pacific Region, *SARS: How a Global Epidemic Was Stopped* (Geneva: World Health Organization, 2006).
66. "张文康不认为香港的非典型肺炎一定由内地传入," 中新社, 2003-03-22, http://www.chinanews.com/n/2003-03-22/26/285935.html.
67. David Fidler, *SARS, Governance and the Globalization of Disease* (London: Palgrave Macmillan, 2004), chap. 5.
68. "China under Fire for Virus Spread," BBC News, 2003-04-06, http://news.bbc.co.uk/2/hi/health/2922993.stm.
69. "卫生部关于将传染性非典型肺炎（严重急性呼吸道综合征）列入法定管理传染病的通知," 卫生部, 2003-04-08.
70. 杨洋, "黄永: 非典危机时," 中国周刊, 2013-04-09, http://chinaweekly.blog.sohu.com/261115080.html; John Pomfret, "Beijing Told Doctors to Hide SARS Victims," *Washington Post*, 2003-04-20, https://www.washingtonpost.com/archive/politics/2003/04/20/beijing-told-doctors-to-hide-sars-victims/3eb7d1aa-d2ff-477b-bc15-d0164377b123/; Kristen Lundberg, "Credible Voices: WHO-Beijing and the SARS Crisis," Mailman School of Public Health Case Consortium @Columbia, 2013-02, https://ccnmtl.columbia.edu/projects/caseconsortium/casestudies/112/casestudy/www/layout/case_id_112.html.
71. Alan Schnur, "The Role of the World Health Organization in Combating SARS, Focusing on the Efforts in China," in *SARS in China: Prelude to Pandemic?*, ed. Arthur Kleinman and James Watson (Palo Alto, CA: Stanford University Press, 2006), 31–52; 卫毅, "蒋彦永: 真话的力量," 南方人物周刊, 2013-03-11, https://www.haodf.com/zhuanjiaguandian/kim123_935116759.htm.
72. David Heymann, "How SARS Was Contained," *New York Times*, 2013-03-14, https://www.nytimes.com/2013/03/15/opinion/global/how-sars-was-contained.html.
73. "Summary of Probable SARS Cases with Onset of Illness from 1 November 2002 to 31 July 2003," World Health Organization, 2015-07-24, https://www.who.int/publicati

ons/m/item/summary-of-probable-sars-cases-with-onset-of-illness-from-1-november-2002-to-31-july-2003.

74. 慧聪, "SARS考验传染病防治法," *21*世纪经济报道, 2003-05-10, http://finance.sina.com.cn/roll/20030510/2132338916.shtml.
75. Longde Wang et al., "Emergence and Control of Infectious Diseases in China," *The Lancet* 372, no. 9649 (2008): 1598–1605.
76. "传染性非典型肺炎防治管理办法," 中国政府门户网站, 2005-08-01, http://www.gov.cn/banshi/2005-08/01/content_19099.htm.
77. "突发公共卫生事件应急条例," 中央政府门户网站, 2003-05-09, http://www.gov.cn/zwgk/2005-05/20/content_145.htm.
78. 高强, "关于中华人民共和国传染病防治法(修订草案)的说明," 中国人大网, 2004-04-30, http://www.npc.gov.cn/zgrdw/npc/ztxw/crbfz/2004-04/30/content_1804038.htm.
79. Yanzhong Huang, "The SARS Epidemic and Its Aftermath in China: A Political Perspective," in *Learning from SARS: Preparing for the Next Disease Outbreak: Workshop Summary* (Washington, DC: National Academies Press, 2004), https://www.ncbi.nlm.nih.gov/books/NBK92479/; Karl Taro Greenfeld, *China Syndrome: The True Story of the 21st Century's First Great Epidemic* (New York: HarperCollins, 2006).
80. "关于疾病预防控制体系建设的若干规定," 国务院公报, 28 (2005), http://www.gov.cn/gongbao/content/2005/content_75219.htm.
81. 中华人民共和国卫生部, "关于疾病预防控制体系建设的若干规定," 国务院公报 28 (2005), http://www.gov.cn/gongbao/content/2005/content_75219.htm.
82. Yang, *Remaking the Chinese Leviathan*, 169–171.
83. "国家公共卫生信息系统建设方案(草案)," 国家卫生部, 2003-09-12, http://www.nhc.gov.cn/wsb/pzcjd/200804/23617.shtml; "中国疫情网络直报系统开通 建公卫信息网络平台," 中国新闻网, 2004-01-02, https://news.sohu.com/2004/01/02/45/news217744513.shtml.
84. The key supporting document is "突发公共卫生事件与传染病疫情监测信息报告管理办法," first issued as MOH Order 37 in November 2003 and revised in 2006.
85. 洪荣涛, 欧剑鸣, 章灿明, "福建省2004年传染病监测时效性分析," 中华流行病学杂志 26, no. 9 (2005): 694–697.
86. Liping Wang et al., "Systematic Review: National Notifiable Infectious Disease Surveillance System in China," *Online Journal of Public Health Informatics* 11, no. 1 (2019): e414.
87. 赵自雄, 赵嘉,马家奇, "我国传染病监测信息系统发展与整合建设构想," 疾病监测 33, no. 5 (2018): 423–427.
88. "全国不明原因肺炎病例监测实施方案(试行)公布," 卫生部, 2004-08-04, http://www.nhc.gov.cn/wsb/pzcjd/200804/21317.shtml.
89. Wang et al., "Emergence and Control of Infectious Diseases in China."
90. David Fidler and Lawrence Gostin, "The New International Health Regulations," *Journal of Law, Medicine & Ethics* 34, no. 1 (2006): 85–94.
91. Wang et al., "Emergence and Control of Infectious Diseases in China."
92. "全国不明原因肺炎病例监测、排查和管理方案," 卫生部, 2007-08-06, www.nhc.gov.cn/bgt/pw10708/200708/4455f46a2f5e4908a8561c079ecbcf0e.shtml.
93. 王宇, "不明原因肺炎监测系统评价," 中国疾病预防控制中心, 2017.
94. 舒跃龙, "流感监测的发展历史及思考," 中华流行病学杂志 32, no. 4 (2011): 334–336.
95. Yuelong Shu et al., "A Ten-Year China–US Laboratory Collaboration: Improving Response to Influenza Threats in China and the World, 2004–2014," *BMC Public Health* 19, no. 3 (2019): 1–8.

96. Weijuan Huang et al., "Epidemiological and Virological Surveillance of Seasonal Influenza Viruses—China, 2020–2021," *China CDC Weekly* 3, no. 44 (2021): 918–922; Xiaoting Yang et al., "Comparing the Similarity and Difference of Three Influenza Surveillance Systems in China," *Scientific Reports* 8, no. 1 (2018): 1–7.
97. 张兆慧, "2019版流感方案公布 新添医院感染控制措施," 新京报, 2019-11-14, https://www.sohu.com/a/353829317_114988.
98. Min Xu and Shi-Xue Li, "Analysis of Good Practice of Public Health Emergency Operations Centers," *Asian Pacific Journal of Tropical Medicine* 8, no. 8 (2015): 677–682; Fan Ding, Qun Li, and Lian-Mei Jin, "Experience and Practice of the Emergency Operations Center, Chinese Center for Disease Control and Prevention: A Case Study of Response to the H7N9 Outbreak," *Infectious Diseases of Poverty* 10, no. 1 (2021): 87–94.
99. "国家突发公共卫生事件应急预案," 2006-02-26, http://www.gov.cn/yjgl/2006-02/26/content_211654.htm.
100. "湖北省突发公共卫生事件应急预案," 湖北省人民政府, 2011-02-11, http://www.hubei.gov.cn/zhuanti/2018zt/xfxcy/201811/t20181106_1365438.shtml.
101. "湖北省突发事件医疗卫生救援应急预案," 湖北省人民政府, 2011-05-10, http://www.hubei.gov.cn/zhuanti/2018zt/xfxcy/201811/t20181106_1365439_2.shtml.
102. 张洪伟, 李香蕊, 王瑞夏, 王亚东, "突发公共卫生事件应急条例修订必要性、可行性分析," 中国卫生事业管理 2011 (10): 768–770.
103. 李洪雷, 张亮, "论地方政府在应对突发公共卫生事件中的发布预警职责," 中国社会科学院研究生院学报 4 (2021), http://iolaw.cssn.cn/zxzp/202111/t20211110_5373408.shtml.
104. "卫生部关于印发《卫生部法定传染病疫情和突发公共卫生事件信息发布方案》的通知," 国家卫生和计划生育委员会, 2006-03-20, http://www.nhc.gov.cn/zwgkzt/wsbysj/200902/39121.shtml#.
105. Yan-Ling Wu et al., "Preliminary Success in the Characterization and Management of a Sudden Breakout of a Novel H7N9 Influenza A Virus," *International Journal of Biological Sciences* 10, no. 1 (2014): 109; Qun Li et al., "Epidemiology of Human Infections with Avian Influenza A (H7N9) Virus in China," *New England Journal of Medicine* 370, no. 6 (2014): 520–532; Chengjun Li and Hualan Chen, "H7N9 Influenza Virus in China," *Cold Spring Harbor Perspectives in Medicine* 11, no. 8 (2021): a038349.
106. George Fu Gao and Yong Feng, "On the Ground in Sierra Leone," *Science* 346, no. 6209 (2014): 666; Hui-Jun Lu et al., "Ebola Virus Outbreak Investigation, Sierra Leone, September 28–November 11, 2014," *Emerging Infectious Diseases* 21, no. 11 (2015): 1921–1927; Yi-Gang Tong et al., "Genetic Diversity and Evolutionary Dynamics of Ebola Virus in Sierra Leone," *Nature* 524, no. 7563 (2015): 93–96; Chang-Qing Bai et al., "Clinical and Virological Characteristics of Ebola Virus Disease Patients Treated with Favipiravir (T-705)—Sierra Leone, 2014," *Clinical Infectious Diseases* 63, no. 10 (2016): 1288–1294.
107. 何建明, 死亡征战, 天地出版社, 2018.
108. Angus Liu, "China Approves Domestic Ebola Vaccine Developed from Recent Outbreak," FiercePharma, 2017-10-24, https://www.fiercepharma.com/vaccines/china-approves-self-developed-ebola-vaccine-from-2014-outbreak-virus-type.
109. Ben Hu et al., "Discovery of a Rich Gene Pool of Bat SARS-Related Coronaviruses Provides New Insights into the Origin of SARS Coronavirus," *PLoS Pathogens* 13, no. 11 (2017): e1006698; Wendong Li et al., "Bats Are Natural Reservoirs of SARS-Like Coronaviruses," *Science* 310, no. 5748 (2005): 676–679; Jamal Sabir et al., "Co-circulation of Three Camel Coronavirus Species and Recombination of MERS-CoVs in Saudi Arabia," *Science* 351, no. 6268 (2016): 81–84.

110. Huang, *Governing Health in Contemporary China*, 95–100.
111. Wuqi Qiu, Cordia Chu, Ayan Mao, and Jing Wu, "The Impacts on Health, Society, and Economy of SARS and H7N9 Outbreaks in China," *Journal of Environmental and Public Health* (2018): 2710185.
112. Yanzhong Huang, "Pursuing Health as Foreign Policy: The Case of China," *Indiana Journal of Global Legal Studies* 17, no. 1 (2010): 105–146.
113. Huang, *Governing Health in Contemporary China*, 105.
114. Huang, *Governing Health in Contemporary China*, 107–108.
115. "钟南山质疑国内甲流死亡数据," 荆楚网-楚天都市报, 2009-11-20, http://news.sina.com.cn/o/2009-11-20/061516637769s.shtml.
116. Quoted in "曾光: 没有血的教训, 疫情瞒报问题解决不了!" 中国县域卫生, 2020-03-29, https://www.sohu.com/na/384066376_456029.
117. Even a member of the founding generation of leaders of the NNDSS I spoke with was not fully aware of the potential impact of this difference in legal status.
118. "传染病信息报告管理规范(2015)," 疾病预防控制局, 2015-11-11, http://www.nhc.gov.cn/jkj/s3577/201511/f5d2ab9a5e104481939981c92cb18a54.shtml.
119. "关于加强卫生应急工作规范化建设的指导意见," 卫生应急办公室, 2016-12-15, www.nhc.gov.cn/yjb/s7859/201612/3a3b5ce97fa940c58a64ff1892f4b3e1.shtml.
120. "习近平在学习贯彻党的十九大精神研讨班开班式上发表重要讲话," 新华社, 2018-01-05, http://www.gov.cn/zhuanti/2018-01/05/content_5253681.htm.
121. 冯子健, "流感, 禽流感和流感大流行: 我们准备好了吗?" 中华流行病学杂志 39, no. 8 (2018): 1017–1020.
122. 许雯, "后SARS时代, 上演最大规模应急演练," 新京报, 2019-08-04, http://epaper.bjnews.com.cn/html/2019-08/04/content_761598.htm.
123. 艾红霞, 陈力玲, 袁剑, "军运会航空口岸专用通道开通测试," 湖北日报, 2019-09-26, http://m.xinhuanet.com/hb/2019-09/26/c_1125040756.htm.
124. Details of this event and its recommendations are found at https://www.centerforhealthsecurity.org/event201/about and https://www.centerforhealthsecurity.org/event201/scenario.html.
125. Qiurong Cai and Jihong Ye, "Is China's Emergency Management System Resilient against the COVID-19 Pandemic?," *Management and Organization Review* 16, no. 5 (2020): 991–995.
126. Quoted in 丰西西, "全国政协委员高福: 要对中国疫苗有信心, 出现问题要倒逼解决," 金羊网, 2019-03-05, https://www.sohu.com/a/299089554_119778.
127. World Health Organization, "A Strategic Framework for Emergency Preparedness," World Health Organization, 2017, https://www.who.int/publications/i/item/a-strategic-framework-for-emergency-preparedness.

Chapter 3

1. 谢海涛, 张颖钰, "与新冠病毒搏斗的民营诊所医生," 财新网, 2020-04-07, http://china.caixin.com/2020-04-07/101539697.html.
2. 黄霁洁, 明鹊, 朱莹, 温潇潇, 葛明宁, 张小莲, 张卓, 沈青青, 陈媛媛, 蓝泽齐, "被新冠击中的医护们: 1716例感染缘何发生," 澎湃新闻, 2020-02-18, https://www.thepaper.cn/newsDetail_forward_6041568.
3. Interview of Walter Ian Lipkin by the Committee on Oversight and Accountability, Select Committee on the Coronavirus Pandemic, U.S. House of Representatives, Washington,

D.C., 2023-04-06, https://oversight.house.gov/wp-content/uploads/2023/07/2023.04.06-Lipkin-Transcript.pdf.

4. Andy Kroll, "Why Respectable Doctors Choose to Mix with Cranks and Quacks on Fox News," *Rolling Stone*, 2020-04-15, https://www.rollingstone.com/politics/politics-features/trump-fox-news-doctors-lipkin-coronavirus-lou-dobbs-hannity-983859/; Eddie Holmes @edwardcholmes 2023-07-17, https://twitter.com/edwardcholmes/status/1681096858989633536.
5. 王嘉兴, "在钟南山之前，她向附近学校发出疫情警报," 中国青年报客户端, 2020-01-28, https://shareapp.cyol.com/cmsfile/News/202001/28/toutiao320881.html.
6. State Council Information Office, "Fighting COVID-19: China in Action," 2020-06-07, http://english.scio.gov.cn/whitepapers/2020-06/07/content_76135269.htm.
7. 上海广播电视台, 湖北广播电视台, "一级响应," 2021-04-08 to 2021-04-10, episode 1. Documentary Series.
8. 田巧萍, "最早上报疫情的她，怎样发现这种不一样的肺炎?," 长江日报, 2020-02-02, https://weibo.com/ttarticle/p/show?id=2309404467421229482021.
9. 王一苇, "一年前的今天：武汉张继先医生看到第一例新冠病人," 知识分子, 2020-12-26, http://www.zhishifenzi.com/depth/character/10623.html. This interview provides finer details of Dr. Zhang's thoughts and actions.
10. 上海广播电视台, 湖北广播电视台, "一级响应."
11. "全国不明原因肺炎病例监测、排查和管理方案 (卫应急发[2007]158 号)," 2007.
12. 王一苇, "一年前的今天."
13. 吴尊友, "新冠疫情形势与防控策略," 财经年会2021: 预测与战略, 2020-11-25，http://economy.caijing.com.cn/20201125/4717538.shtml. Full transcript at https://finance.sina.com.cn/meeting/2020-11-25/doc-iiznctke3179937.shtml.
14. 赵雯, "张继先：拉响'警报'只是开始," 党员生活, 2020年2期, 2020-04-17, https://m.fx361.com/news/2020/0417/6576039.html.
15. 田巧萍, "最早上报疫情的她，怎样发现这种不一样的肺炎?"
16. 王一苇, "一年前的今天."
17. Interview with Zhang Jixian in "中国战疫录," 中国新闻网, 2020-04-02, video, https://www.youtube.com/watch?v=MMm27Mj12x8.
18. An Changqing (安长青), the president of the hospital, was a pediatrician by specialty and did not figure in this unfolding story.
19. 上海广播电视台, 湖北广播电视台, "一级响应."
20. 田巧萍, "最早上报疫情的她，怎样发现这种不一样的肺炎?"
21. 田巧萍, "最早上报疫情的她，怎样发现这种不一样的肺炎?"
22. 上海广播电视台, 湖北广播电视台, "一级响应."
23. 田巧萍, "最早上报疫情的她, 怎样发现这种不一样的肺炎?"
24. "关于给予张定宇和张继先同志记大功奖励的决定," 湖北省人民政府, 2020-02-06, https://www.hubei.gov.cn/hbfb/bmdt/202002/t20200206_2020365.shtml.
25. 信娜, 王小, 孙爱民, "谁是第一个基因检测出的新冠肺炎患者?," 财经, 2020-02-19, https://finance.sina.com.cn/china/gncj/2020-02-19/doc-iimxxstf2808664.shtml.
26. 杜玮, "亲历者讲述: 武汉市中心医院医护人员被感染始末," 中国新闻周刊, 2020-02-17, https://mp.weixin.qq.com/s/1zNY2YXy75snzwX3Tg09Cg.
27. "武汉市中心医院呼吸与危重症医学科: 支气管镜'梦之队'炼成记," 医师报社, 2021-01-04, https://k.sina.cn/article_2637767371_9d3922cb01900y16u.html.
28. 高昱 et al., "新冠病毒基因测序溯源: 警报是何时拉响的," 财新网, 2020-02-26, accessed 2020-02-26, china.caixin.com/2020-02-26/101520972.html. Article has been removed.

29. 信娜, 王小, 孙爱民, "谁是第一个基因检测出的新冠肺炎患者?"
30. 赵天宇 et al., "我丈夫感染了新型冠状病毒，治愈了," 财经杂志, 2020-01-22, https://mp.weixin.qq.com/s/zy0Pj-9CGT5rDC3j5ULnJg.
31. Quoted in 雷宇, 童萱, "赵建平是如何率先发现新型肺炎疫情的," 中国青年报客户端, 2020-02-03, https://shareapp.cyol.com/cmsfile/News/202002/03/toutiao323374.html; 柳洁 et al., "赵建平: 从组长叔叔到专家爷爷 平'疫'战士逆行17年," 经济日报, 2020-02-01, https://www.sohu.com/a/369971419_118392. The last byline in these two reports is a pseudonym representing Tongji Hospital.
32. "武汉市防痨学会副理事长赵建平: 时刻谨记'无症状也能人传人,' 它比SARS判断难很多, 这些细节会铸成大错……," 武汉市科协, 2020-02-03, www.whkx.org.cn/news_show.aspx?id=45249.
33. "武汉市防痨学会副理事长赵建平."
34. 雷宇, 童萱, "赵建平是如何率先发现新型肺炎疫情的."
35. WeChat message in circulation as seen by the author.
36. "张定宇: 我在'风暴之眼,'" in 中央广播电视总台, 武汉*!* 武汉*!: 2020*战疫口述实录 (北京: 现代出版社, 2020), 3; 刘志勇, "生死金银潭," 健康报, 2020-03-09, http://www.nhc.gov.cn/xcs/fkdt/202003/9502b2d78ea94ea9a43e855ca9e0a5e2.shtml.
37. "张定宇."
38. "张定宇."
39. "张定宇."
40. "小山狗", "记录一下首次发现新型冠状病毒的经历," 2020-01-30, https://matters.news/@2020Era/记录一下首次发现新型冠状病毒的经历-zdpuB2EXfBsBL9a9bzTn1tSGZw1D6MHV9cN3GfizJ2xvceyJn. I note that, after I had written on the role of Vision Medicals, the *Washington Post* published a special opinion piece on it in Editorial Board, "As the Pandemic Exploded, a Researcher Saw the Danger, China's Leaders Kept Silent," *Washington Post*, 2022-04-22, https://www.washingtonpost.com/opinions/interactive/2022/china-researcher-covid-19-coverup/.
41. "小山狗", "记录一下首次发现新型冠状病毒的经历."
42. 龚菁琦, "发哨子的人," 人物, 2020-03-10, https://www.weibo.com/ttarticle/p/show?id=2309404480863474679890.
43. "同叙科技战疫情谊, 共话生命健康发展—武汉市金银潭医院与武汉病毒所召开弘扬伟大抗疫精神座谈会," 武汉病毒所, 2020-12-24, http://www.whiov.cas.cn/xwdt_160278/zhxw2019/202012/t20201224_5840967.html.
44. "张定宇."
45. "张定宇."
46. 信娜, 王小, 孙爱民, "谁是第一个基因检测出的新冠肺炎患者?"
47. This and the next two paragraphs are based on "小山狗," "记录一下首次发现新型冠状病毒的经历."
48. "小山狗," "记录一下首次发现新型冠状病毒的经历."
49. "小山狗," "记录一下首次发现新型冠状病毒的经历."
50. 高昱, 彭岩锋, 杨睿, 冯禹丁, 马丹萌, "新冠病毒基因测序溯源: 警报是何时拉响的."
51. 上海广播电视台, 湖北广播电视台, "一级响应."
52. 李想俣, "金银潭副院长黄朝林病愈隔离, 自述被传染和当'试药人'内情," 中国新闻周刊, 2020-02-14, https://mp.weixin.qq.com/s/qpztvhmnkNTtHQZi_e5PNw.
53. 张定宇," 4; 刘晨玮, 赵子晗, "官旭华：把好疫情防控第一道关口责任重大," 长江网, 2020-08-19, http://news.cnhubei.com/content/2020-08/19/content_13281727.html.

54. Dr. Zhang Jixian and Dr. Zhang Dingyu mention that experts from the provincial CDC were present as well those from the the Wuhan CDC and the Jianghan District CDC. 王一苇, “一年前的今天”; “张定宇,” 4.
55. 王一苇, “一年前的今天.”
56. 李想俣, “金银潭副院长黄朝林病愈隔离，自述被传染和当‘试药人’内情.”
57. 刘志勇, “生死金银潭.”
58. “张定宇.”
59. 李想俣, “金银潭副院长黄朝林病愈隔离，自述被传染和当‘试药人’内情.”
60. 警报是这样拉响的——对话疫情上报第一人张继先,” 瞭望, 2020-04-20, http://www.xinhuanet.com/politics/2020-04/20/c_1125878293.htm.
61. 吴 君, “湖北省疾控中心传染病防治研究所所长官旭华—‘疫情就是考验，我必须冲锋在前,’” 人民日报, 2020-03-02, http://cpc.people.com.cn/n1/2020/0302/c64387-31611693.html.
62. 王唱, “我有一个心愿: 当好抗疫战斗的前哨,” 湖北省疾控中心, 2020-03-08, https://www.hbcdc.com/jkjy/jkzd/xgft/fkdt/6929.htm.
63. 省市区疾控中心联合调查组, “关于医院报告华南海鲜市场多例肺炎病例情况的调查处置报告,” 2019-12-30.
64. Gérard Krause et al., “Reliability of Case Definitions for Public Health Surveillance Assessed by Round-Robin Test Methodology,” *BMC Public Health* 6, no. 1 (2006): 1–10.
65. 杜玮, “亲历者讲述.”
66. At the time of investigation, the 20 patients were being treated in Jinyintan Hospital (4), Wuhan Central Hospital Houhu Branch (7), Tongji Hospital (8), and residence (1).
67. “张定宇,” 5; 李春雷，“铁人张定宇,” 人民日报, 2020-04-01, 20.
68. “张定宇,” 5.
69. “张定宇,” 6.
70. “张定宇,” 5.
71. “张定宇,” 5–6; 张定宇, “在战斗最早打响的地方—对话武汉市金银潭医院院长张定宇,” 瞭望, 2020-04-20, http://www.xinhuanet.com/politics/2020-04/20/c_1125878292.htm.
72. 上海广播电视台, 湖北广播电视台, “一级响应.”
73. Jane Qiu, “How China's ‘Bat Woman’ Hunted Down Viruses from SARS to the New Coronavirus,” *Scientific American*, 2020-03-11 (updated 2020-06-01), https://www.scientificamerican.com/article/how-chinas-bat-woman-hunted-down-viruses-from-sars-to-the-new-coronavirus1. Whereas the Wuhan CDC had received the Vision Medicals sequencing results, Qiu's original language said the Wuhan CDC “had detected a novel coronavirus in two hospital patients with atypical pneumonia.”
74. “市卫生健康委关于报送不明原因肺炎救治情况的紧急通知,” 2019-12-30; “关于做好不明原因肺炎救治工作的紧急通知,” 2019-12-30. The notices said that they were prepared by the WMHC Medical Administration Division.
75. “市卫生健康委关于报送不明原因肺炎救治情况的紧急通知.”
76. “关于做好不明原因肺炎救治工作的紧急通知.”
77. 信娜, 王小, 孙爱民, “谁是第一个基因检测出的新冠肺炎患者?”; on the transfer, see also 赵天宇 et al., “我丈夫感染了新型冠状病毒, 治愈了,” 财经, 2020-01-22, https://finance.sina.com.cn/wm/2020-01-22/doc-iihnzhha4186239.shtml.
78. 杨楠, 张明萌, 雷寒冰, “专访湖北专家组组长赵建平: 约有五分之一的患者会由轻症转为重症,” 南方人物周刊, 2020-02-20, https://www.infzm.com/contents/177141.
79. “中国战疫录,” 中国新闻网, 2020-04-02, video, , episode 1, https://www.youtube.com/watch?v=MMm27Mj12x8; 杨程晨, “专访金银潭医院医生张丽：率先吁建隔离病区、

负责域内大多病患在好转," 中国新闻网, 2020-01-29, http://www.chinanews.com/sh/2020/01-29/9072709.shtml.

80. 温如军, "武汉医生回述: 发现疑似病例之后," 中国慈善家, 2020-02-05, https://k.sina.com.cn/article_2015391145_78206da901900tiwt.html; "金银潭战疫故事: 结婚纪念日终于可以回家了," 中国慈善家, 2020-01-30 (2020-03-13), https://www.sohu.com/a/379944003_120521421.
81. 杨楠, 何沛芸, "重组金银潭 : 疫情暴风眼的秘密," 南方周末, 2020-03-05 , http://www.infzm.com/contents/178385.
82. 上海广播电视台, 湖北广播电视台, "一级响应."
83. 温如军, "武汉医生回述."
84. 温如军, "武汉医生回述."
85. "17例死亡病例病情介绍," 国家卫生健康委卫生应急办公室, 2020-01-23 , http://www.nhc.gov.cn/yjb/s3578/202001/5d19a4f6d3154b9fae328918ed2e3c8a.shtml. The date of ECMO use is given as January 2 in Li-Li Ren et al., "Identification of a Novel Coronavirus Causing Severe Pneumonia in Human: A Descriptive Study," *Chinese Medical Journal* 133, no. 9 (2020): 1015–1024.
86. Nanshan Chen et al., "Epidemiological and Clinical Characteristics of 99 Cases of 2019 Novel Coronavirus Pneumonia in Wuhan, China: A Descriptive Study," *The Lancet* 395, no. 10223 (2020): 507–513.
87. 温如军, "武汉医生回述."
88. Dali L. Yang, "China's Early Warning System Didn't Work on Covid-19. Here's the Story," *Washington Post*, 2020-02-24, https://www.washingtonpost.com/politics/2020/02/24/chinas-early-warning-system-didnt-work-covid-19-heres-story/.
89. 杨晰, 刘健, "凤凰专访中疾控主任高福 : 疫情初期, 情况未上报国家层面," 凤凰新闻, 2021-03-19, https://ishare.ifeng.com/c/s/v004lx6IlT-_2rVEoO1jBoBL5kWo5urKp-_gsJYy-_ujNCUfO4.

Chapter 4

1. 刘荒, "武汉市中心医院一位护士长战疫亲历," 新华每日电讯, 2020-04-13, http://www.xinhuanet.com/politics/2020-04/13/c_1125847161.htm.
2. 龚菁琦, "发哨子的人," 人物, 2020-03-10, https://www.weibo.com/ttarticle/p/show?id=2309404480863474679890. Dr. Ai Fen graduated from the Huazhong University of Science and Technology's Tongji Medical School and has worked at Wuhan Central Hospital since 1997. She was in the cardiovascular section before becoming chief of Emergency Care.
3. 龚菁琦, "发哨子的人."
4. "亲历者讲述 : 武汉市中心医院医护人员被感染始末," 中国新闻周刊, 2020-02-17, https://news.sina.com.cn/c/2020-02-17/doc-iimxyqvz3653366.shtml.
5. WeChat screen captures in 毛淑杰, "被训诫的武汉医生李文亮," 南方都市报, 2020-01-30, https://new.qq.com/omn/20200130/20200130A0JX7G00.html.
6. 吴尊友, "新冠疫情形势与防控策略," 财经年会2021: 预测与战略, 2020-11-25, http://economy.caijing.com.cn/20201125/4717538.shtml.
7. Interviews with NHC sources. An official report on the outbreak states that "on December 30, health authorities from Hubei Province reported this cluster to China CDC" but neglected to mention that Hubei made the report only after the China CDC leadership had asked about the outbreak in Wuhan. 2019-nCoV Outbreak Joint Field Epidemiology

Investigation Team and Qun Li, "An Outbreak of NCIP (2019-nCoV) Infection in China—Wuhan, Hubei Province, 2019–2020," *China CDC Weekly* 2, no. 5 (2020-01-31): 79–80. Submitted 2020-01-20.

8. "疫线疾控人: 6, 使命与担当," 健康报, 2020, available at bilibili.com or https://mp.weixin.qq.com/s/HjMBvIWcZHeSKHhlERAcpw.
9. 华生, "如果群殴高福是搞错了对象," Weibo blog, 2020-02-16, https://www.weibo.com/ttarticle/p/show?id=2309404472629854601490. Some international press such as the *Wall Street Journal* reported incorrectly that the Wuhan CDC reported cases to the "national CDC headquarters" on December 30, 2019, and that China reported to the WHO the next day. Jeremy Page, Wenxin Fan, and Natasha Khan, "How It All Started: China's Early Coronavirus Missteps," *Wall Street Journal*, 2020-03-06, https://www.wsj.com/articles/how-it-all-started-chinas-early-coronavirus-missteps-11583508932.
10. 信娜, "高福：疫情防控我给自己打满分," 财经, 2021-01-12, https://www.dazuig.com/caij/cj/677252.html.
11. 杨晰, 刘健, "凤凰专访中疾控主任高福: 疫情初期, 情况未上报国家层面," 凤凰新闻, 2021-03-19, https://ishare.ifeng.com/c/s/v004lx6IlT-_2rVEoO1jBoBL5kWo5urKp-_gsJYy-_ujNCUfO4__?spss=np; "疫线疾控人."
12. Edward Warner, "Present Conditions under the NRA," *American Marketing Journal* 1 (1934): 12.
13. 国家突发公共卫生事件专家咨询委员会. The only published membership was from 2011 ("关于成立突发事件卫生应急专家咨询委员会的通知," 卫生应急办公室, 2011-03-21, http://www.nhc.gov.cn/yjb/s7859/201103/8f99ac98fa7641cebeb5a882cf751a52.shtml). It is likely that this list had been updated with additional members such as Cao Bin. Xu Shuqiang, the director general of the NHC Health Emergency Response Center, was a vice president at the Sino-Japanese Friendship Hospital during the SARS crisis and asked Cao Bin to go to Wuhan for this emergency trip.
14. 信娜, "高福."
15. 吴尊友, "新冠疫情形势与防控策略."
16. 吴尊友, "新冠疫情形势与防控策略."
17. 曹彬, 王一民, "关于瑞德西韦, 试验负责人曹彬首次透露重要信息," 呼吸界, 2020-03-09, https://shareapp.cyol.com/cmsfile/News/202003/08/toutiao345833.html. According to Wu Zunyou, the key members of the epidemiology team arrived by the first flight from Beijing to Wuhan in the morning of December 31. 吴尊友, "新冠疫情形势与防控策略."
18. 曹彬, 王一民, "关于瑞德西韦, 试验负责人曹彬首次透露重要信息."
19. "疫线疾控人."
20. 周琦, 高亮, "探访涉多例病毒性肺炎的武汉华南海鲜城: 有的摊位垃圾遍地," 澎湃新闻, 2019-12-31, https://www.thepaper.cn/newsDetail_forward_5391375; "不明原因肺炎出现地: 商户戴口罩做生意," 澎湃新闻, 2019-12-31, video (14:29), https://www.thepaper.cn/newsDetail_forward_5391299.
21. "张定宇: 我在'风暴之眼,'" 中央广播电视总台, 武汉! 武汉!: *2020*战疫口述实录 (北京: 现代出版社, 2020), 5–6.
22. 国务院新闻办公室, "国务院新闻办公室2020年1月22日新闻发布会文字实录," 国家卫生健康委员会宣传司, 2020-01-22, http://www.nhc.gov.cn/xcs/ptpxw/202001/61add0d230e047eaab777d062920d8a8.shtml.
23. "武汉市卫健委关于当前我市肺炎疫情的情况通报," 武汉市卫生健康委员会, 2019-12-31, wjw.wuhan.gov.cn/front/web/showDetail/2019123108989.

24. 杨楠, 张明萌, 雷寒冰, “专访湖北专家组组长赵建平: 约有五分之一的患者会由轻症转为重症,” 南方人物周刊, 2020-02-20, https://www.infzm.com/contents/177141.
25. “武汉市卫健委关于当前我市肺炎疫情的情况通报.”
26. Zhengli Shi, “Reply to Science Magazine,” link in Jon Cohen, “Trump ‘Owes Us an Apology.’ Chinese Scientist at the Center of COVID-19 Origin Theories Speaks Out,” *Science*, 2020-07-24, https://www.sciencemag.org/news/2020/07/trump-owes-us-apology-chinese-scientist-center-covid-19-origin-theories-speaks-out.
27. “张定宇,” 5.
28. 高昱 et al., “新冠病毒基因测序溯源: 警报是何时拉响的,” 财新网, 2020-02-26, china.caixin.com/2020-02-26/101520972.html.
29. 高昱 et al., “新冠病毒基因测序溯源.”
30. 信娜, “高福.”
31. In 2008, Gao Fu became vice president of the Chinese Academy of Sciences’ Beijing Institutes of Life Science, which have strong historical ties to BGI. Gao also knows BGI chair Wang Jian well.
32. Quoted from Interview of Walter Ian Lipkin by the Committee on Oversight and Accountability, Select Committee on the Coronavirus Pandemic, U.S. House Of Representatives, Washington, D.C., 2023-04-06, https://oversight.house.gov/wp-content/uploads/2023/07/2023.04.06-Lipkin-Transcript.pdf. First reported in Jane McMullen, “Covid-19: Five Days That Shaped the Outbreak,” BBC News, 2020-01-26, https://www.bbc.com/news/world-55756452. Lipkin later disclosed that he thought Gao was “just wrong” about the transmissibility, given the number of people already infected.
33. It is generally reported that this meeting took place in the 10th Floor Meeting Room of the Wuhan Municipal Health Commission. However, Dr. Zhang Dingyu mentioned in an interview that the expert team met at the Wuhan Jinyintan Hospital that evening. 张定宇, “在战斗最早打响的地方—对话武汉市金银潭医院院长张定宇,” 瞭望, 2020-04-20, http://www.xinhuanet.com/politics/2020-04/20/c_1125878292.htm.
34. One source described Dr. Zhao’s role as that of a keynote speaker (主讲人).
35. 曹彬、王一民, “关于瑞德西韦，试验负责人曹彬首次透露重要信息.”
36. Chaolin Huang et al., “Clinical Features of Patients Infected with 2019 Novel Coronavirus in Wuhan, China,” *The Lancet* 395, no. 10223 (2020): 501.
37. When interviewed later, some clinicians in Wuhan with good knowledge of the leading research hospitals told me that they believed the Chinese government should have publicly treated the outbreak as a SARS or at least SARS-like outbreak.
38. Rui-Heng Xu et al., “Epidemiologic Clues to SARS Origin in China,” *Emerging Infectious Diseases* 10, no. 6 (2004): 1030–1037; Ben Hu et al., “Discovery of a Rich Gene Pool of Bat SARS-Related Coronaviruses Provides New Insights into the Origin of SARS Coronavirus,” *PLoS Pathogens* 13, no. 11 (2017): e1006698.
39. Yongzhen Zhang and Edward C. Holmes, “A Genomic Perspective on the Origin and Emergence of SARS-CoV-2,” *Cell* 181, no. 2 (2020): 223–227.
40. Sarah Newey, “Wuhan Officials Identified Huanan Market as a Pandemic Risk at Least Five Years before Covid Emerged,” *The Telegraph*, 2021-04-18, https://www.telegraph.co.uk/global-health/science-and-disease/wuhan-officials-identified-huanan-market-pandemic-risk-least/.
41. “湖北推进‘昆仑5号’行动，打击破坏野生动植物资源违法犯罪，” 湖北省人民政府门户网站，2019-09-06，http://www.hubei.gov.cn/hbfb/bmdt/201909/t20190909_1517060.shtml.

42. 游天燚 et al.，“聚焦武汉肺炎疫情: ‘大众畜牧野味’确实存在, 市场休市后才闭店,” 新京报, 2020-01-21, https://m.bjnews.com.cn/detail/157961554615693.html; 邓琦 et al., “失控的野味,” 新京报，2020-01-22，https://www.cenews.com.cn/legal/fzyw/202001/t20200122_926388.html.
43. “绿会政研室收到武汉华南市场大众畜牧野味的相关回复，” 中国绿发会，2020-05-31，https://www.sohu.com/a/398873203_100001695.
44. “2019年行政处罚，” 武汉市园林和林业局，2019-05-30，http://ylj.wuhan.gov.cn/zwgk/zwxxgkzl_12298/cfqz/xzcf/202011/t20201110_1499879.shtml. This notice has been removed from the WLFB website but is archived at https://archive.md/Qo8H3.
45. Xiao Xiao et al., "Animal Sales from Wuhan Wet Markets Immediately Prior to the COVID-19 Pandemic," *Scientific Reports* 11, no. 1 (2021): 1–7.
46. 魏凡，“重回华南海鲜市场，” 澎湃新闻，2020-02-23，https://www.thepaper.cn/newsDetail_forward_6078874.
47. Jeremy Page and Natasha Khan, "On the Ground in Wuhan, Signs of China Stalling Probe of Coronavirus Origins," *Wall Street Journal*, 2020-05-12, https://www.wsj.com/articles/china-stalls-global-search-for-coronavirus-origins-wuhan-markets-investigation-11589300842.
48. William Jun Liu et al., "Surveillance of SARS-CoV-2 at the Huanan Seafood Market," *Nature* (forthcoming), https://doi.org/10.1038/s41586-023-06043-2. China CDC Director General George F. Gao (Gao Fu) was one of three corresponding authors.
49. Alex Crits-Christoph et al., "Genetic Evidence of Susceptible Wildlife in SARS-Cov-2 Positive Samples at the Huanan Wholesale Seafood Market, Wuhan: Analysis and Interpretation of Data Released by the Chinese Center for Disease Control," 2023-03-20, https://zenodo.org/record/7754299#.ZC0emHbMJD8 .
50. “官旭华: 传染病防控战线的尖兵,” 湖北疾控健康教育, 2018-12-25, https://www.sohu.com/a/284445723_456084.
51. 许雯, “中疾控独家回应: ‘人传人’早有推论，保守下结论有原因,” 新京报, 2020-01-31, http://www.bjnews.com.cn/news/2020/01/31/682224.html.
52. "Exclusive Interview with Chinese CDC Director Gao Fu," World Insight with Tian Wei, CGTN, 2020-04-21, video, https://www.youtube.com/watch?v=q2PmAGvTCEQ.
53. Jon Cohen, "Not Wearing Masks to Protect against Coronavirus is a 'Big Mistake,' Top Chinese Scientist Says," *Science*, 2020-03-27, https://www.science.org/content/article/not-wearing-masks-protect-against-coronavirus-big-mistake-top-chinese-scientist-says.
54. Roujian Lu et al., "Genomic Characterisation and Epidemiology of 2019 Novel Coronavirus," *The Lancet* 395, no. 10224 (2020): 565–574.
55. Quoted in McMullen, "Covid-19."
56. 吴尊友, “新冠疫情形势与防控策略.”
57. 2019-nCoV Outbreak Joint Field Epidemiology Investigation Team and Qun Li, "An Outbreak of NCIP (2019-nCoV) Infection in China—Wuhan, Hubei Province, 2019–2020," *China CDC Weekly*, 2020-01-31, 2, no. 5, 79–80.
58. 吴尊友, “新冠疫情形势与防控策略.”
59. 吴尊友, “新冠疫情形势与防控策略.”
60. 吴尊友, “新冠疫情形势与防控策略.”
61. “武汉市卫健委关于当前我市肺炎疫情的情况通报.”
62. 不明原因的病毒性肺炎诊疗方案(试行). On file.
63. Huang et al., "Clinical Features of Patients."
64. 吴尊友, “新冠疫情形势与防控策略.”

65. “中国战疫录,” 中国新闻网, 2020-04-02, video, episode 1, https://www.youtube.com/watch?v=MMm27Mj12x8; 上海广播电视台, 湖北广播电视台, “一级响应,” 2021, episode 1.
66. 吴娇颖, 许雯, “武汉华南海鲜市场仍休市, 商户退租金领万元补贴,” 新京报, 2020-01-21, https://news.sina.com.cn/c/2020-01-21/doc-iihnzhha3884839.shtml.
67. 吴尊友, “新冠疫情形势与防控策略.”
68. 国家卫生健康委党组, “在战疫中把人民生命安全和身体健康摆在最高位置,” 旗帜网, 2020-03-19, http://dangjian.people.com.cn/n1/2020/0319/c117092-31639856.html. On January 9, 2020, the Hubei Health Commission revealed that Li Bin made a visit to a department in the Hubei Health Commission on January 4, 2020: “国家卫健委李斌副主任来我局调研指导,” 湖北省卫生计生委综合监督局, 2020-01-09, http://wjw.hubei.gov.cn/hbwsjd/xwzx/szgz/202009/t20200905_2888874.shtml.
69. “于学军,” 国家卫生健康委员会, last accessed 2021-05-04, www.nhc.gov.cn/wjw/wld/201901/eaadb69f10cc4d25ad9db6b5884b0300.shtml.Copy on file.
70. 国家卫生健康委党组, “在战疫中把人民生命安全和身体健康摆在最高位置,” 旗帜网, 2020-03-19, http://dangjian.people.com.cn/n1/2020/0319/c117092-31639856.html.
71. Vice Minister Li Bin's statement in 国务院新闻办公室, “国务院新闻办公室2020年1月22日新闻发布会文字实录,” 国家卫生健康委员会宣传司, 2020-01-22, http://www.nhc.gov.cn/xcs/ptpxw/202001/61add0d230e047eaab777d062920d8a8.shtml.
72. “不明原因的病毒性肺炎防控‘三早’方案.”
73. “人感染H7N9禽流感疫情防控方案,” 2013-04-08, http://www.gov.cn/govweb/fwxx/jk/2013-04/08/content_2372214.htm.
74. Shibo Jiang et al., “A Distinct Name Is Needed for the New Coronavirus,” *The Lancet* 395, no. 10228 (2020): 949; Guizhen Wu, Jianwei Wang, and Jianqing Xu, “Voice from China: Nomenclature of the Novel Coronavirus and Related Diseases,” *Chinese Medical Journal* 133, no. 09 (2020): 1012–1014.
75. 武汉市不明原因的病毒性肺炎应急监测方案, 武汉市不明原因的病毒性肺炎密切接触者管理方案, “湖北疾控传防所: 战疫一线担起中流砥柱,” 健康报, 2020-03-09, http://wjw.hubei.gov.cn/bmdt/ztzl/fkxxgzbdgrfyyq/yxdx/202003/t20200309_2176448.shtml; 王唱, “我有一个心愿: 当好抗疫战斗的前哨,” 湖北省疾控中心, 2020-03-08, https://www.hbcdc.com/jkjy/jkzd/xgft/fkdt/6929.htm.
76. “守护人民健康和生命安全的疾控人—李群,” 保健时报, 2022-05-31, https://www.toutiao.com/article/7103564060053996068/. This standard is publicly available on local government websites. See, for example, the Hangzhou website: “杭州市人民政府办公厅转发市卫生局关于传染性非典型肺炎密切接触者留验工作补充意见的通知,” 2019-07-30, http://www.hangzhou.gov.cn/art/2019/7/30/art_1671578_6157.html.
77. “在一线，疾控勇士与新型冠状病毒赛跑,” China CDC, 2020-02-01, http://www.chinacdc.cn/yw_9324/202002/t20200201_212137.html.
78. 刘志勇, “生死金银潭,” 健康报, 2020-03-09, https://news.sina.cn/gn/2020-03-09/detail-iimxxstf7499522.d.html.
79. Bin Cao et al., “Diagnosis and Treatment of Community-Acquired Pneumonia in Adults: 2016 Clinical Practice Guidelines by the Chinese Thoracic Society, Chinese Medical Association,” *The Clinical Respiratory Journal* 12, no. 4 (2018): 1320–1360; “曹彬,” 首都医科大学, https://www.ccmu.edu.cn/rczy_6468/jcrc_13876/gjjrcxm_7903/gjjcqnjj_7913/cb12/index.htm.
80. 曹彬, 王一民, “关于瑞德西韦，试验负责人曹彬首次透露重要信息.”
81. 曹彬, 王一民, “关于瑞德西韦，试验负责人曹彬首次透露重要信息.”

82. “武汉不明原因的病毒性肺炎诊疗方案(试行)”; 刘志勇, “生死金银潭.”
83. 温潇潇, 孟津津, “一家没有传染病隔离硬件的武汉定点医院, 最早让全院戴上口罩,” 澎湃新闻, 2020-05-14, https://www.thepaper.cn/newsDetail_forward_7378109.
84. “新闻1+1：新型冠状病毒肺炎疫情，防控进行时!” 央视网, 2020-01-15, http://tv.cctv.com/2020/01/15/VIDEVPaxZBFtDLGUA6mk5PW2200115.shtml.
85. 温潇潇, 孟津津, “一家没有传染病隔离硬件的武汉定点医院, 最早让全院戴上口罩”; 张赫, “武汉市肺科医院院长: 我们从未缺过物资,” 健康时报, 2020-04-06, https://new.qq.com/omn/20200406/20200406A0OIZK00.html.
86. 王晓东, “新型冠状病毒溯源取得阶段性进展,” 中国日报网, 2020-01-26, https://cn.chinadaily.com.cn/a/202001/26/WS5e2d2cfba3107bb6b579b9bd.html.
87. Liu served as the deputy head of the Gao Fu lab and was a member of the Gao team that won a major award for research on the origins and transmission of the H7N9 and H5N1 avian influenzas. They also worked together on the Ebola mission to Sierra Leone in 2014. “高福院士领导的流感等重要病原致病机制与防控团队获得2019年度求是杰出科技成就集体奖,” 中国疾病预防控制中心病毒病预防控制所, 2019-09-23, http://ivdc.chinacdc.cn/kjgz/kxyj/202001/t20200129_211992.htm.
88. 高宏明, “中国疾病预防控制中心病毒病预防控制所荣获全国卫生健康系统新冠肺炎疫情防控工作先进集体称号,” 中国疾病预防控制中心, 2020-03-12, http://www.chinacdc.cn/yw_9324/202003/t20200312_214348.html. For a video report of the sampling effort, see “2020春天纪事,” CCTV记录, 2020-09-08, episode 2, https://tv.cctv.com/2020/09/04/VIDA2RwP6u7FU6RPgDzr2wG8200904.shtml.
89. WHO, “Timeline: WHO’s COVID-19 Response,” https://www.who.int/emergencies/diseases/novel-coronavirus-2019/interactive-timeline.
90. Bob Woodward, *Rage* (New York: Simon & Schuster, 2020), 215.
91. “The Virus—What Went Wrong?” *Frontline*, 2020-06-16, video, https://www.pbs.org/wgbh/frontline/film/the-virus/; also Lawrence Wright, *The Plague Year: America in the Time of Covid* (New York: Aldred Knopf, 2021), 11–12.
92. “The Virus—What Went Wrong?”
93. 周琳, “专家：汉港病例未见直接关係,” 大公报, 2020-01-05, http://www.takungpao.com/news/232108/2020/0105/400593.html.
94. 周琳, “专家.”
95. Nils Chr. Stenseth et al., “Lessons Learnt from the COVID-19 Pandemic,” *Frontiers in Public Health* 9 (2021): 694705.
96. 许雯, “中疾控独家回应.”

Chapter 5

1. Dali Yang, *Beyond Beijing: Liberalization and the Regions in China* (Abingdon, UK: Routledge, 1997).
2. “中共中央、国务院关于促进中部地区崛起的若干意见,” 2006-04-15, http://www.reformdata.org/2006/0415/5002.shtml.
3. “武汉天河国际机场,” accessed 2020-05-20, https://zh.wikipedia.org/wiki/武汉天河国际机场.
4. “自称铁路枢纽的城市遍地都是，但真正称得上铁路枢纽的却没几个,” 山川网 2017-10-31, https://mp.weixin.qq.com/s/plC-Yyi9RRz45tXsQNHdrQ?.
5. 贺斌, “疫情后, 武汉还能否稳居中部C位?,” 中国新闻周刊, 2020-04-20, https://page.om.qq.com/page/OHrImYhC8orFVvYr04Zr2u3Q0.

6. The ranking is made using the Human Development Indices at the Global Data Lab (globaldatalab.org).
7. Kevin Yao and Benjamin Kang Lim, "China Banking Regulator, Hubei Chief Front Runners to Head Central Bank: Sources," Reuters, 2017-10-13, https://www.reuters.com/article/us-china-economy-pboc/china-banking-regulator-hubei-chief-front-runners-to-head-central-bank-sources-idUSKBN1CI0X5.
8. For discussion of the patterns of provincial party secretaries transitioning to the National People's Congress, see王姝, "高龄省委书记的下一站," 新京报, 2016-09-04, http://www.bjnews.com.cn/news/2016/09/04/415765.html.
9. 郑汝可, 王雪, "为了这件事, 武汉市委书记坐镇, 4位副市长上台承诺!," 长江日报, 2019-03-15, http://www.app.dawuhanapp.com/p/82585.html.
10. "从营商环境优化, 至四大中心建设, 武汉如何布局未来?," 荆楚连线, 2019-09-26, https://www.sohu.com/a/343489837_100210959.
11. "展现中国速度, 搭好军运大舞台," 新华每日电讯, 2019-10-16, http://www.xinhuanet.com/politics/2019-10/16/c_1125109219.htm.
12. Marcel at large, "知情者口述: 盛会, 病人, 难以逾越的冬天," 荷戟周戡, 2020-03-01, https://mp.weixin.qq.com/s/k0HELMTysMTZyF7ECuDKSA.
13. "马国强辞去武汉市人大常委会主任职务," 长江网, 2020-01-06, http://www.xinhuanet.com/2020-01/06/c_1125428166.htm.
14. "省委专职副书记, 从哪里来, 到哪里去?," 深圳评论, 2021-06-23, https://www.163.com/dy/article/GD6I8IKH05529EMB.html.
15. Dahai Yue et al., "Impact of the China Healthy Cities Initiative on Urban Environment," *Journal of Urban Health* 94, no. 2 (2017): 149–157; Ding Li et al., "Impact of Performance Contest on Local Transformation and Development in China: Empirical Study of the National Civilized City Program," *Growth and Change* 53, no. 2 (2022): 559–592; Chi Zhang et al., "The Impact of Government Intervention on Corporate Environmental Performance: Evidence from China's National Civilized City Award," *Finance Research Letters* 39 (2021): 101624.
16. "国家卫生城市标准(2014版)," 全国爱国卫生运动委员会, 2014-05-16, http://www.nhc.gov.cn/jkj/s5898/201405/a8ce63259ee640729671917865467a88.shtml.
17. "武汉全面启动国家卫生城市创建, 现已达到8项指标," 湖北省人民政府门户网站, 2013-03-26, http://www.hubei.gov.cn/hbfb/szsm/201303/t20130326_1538393.shtml.
18. "武汉梦圆'国家卫生城市,' 咸宁仙桃襄阳亦获此殊荣"楚天金报, 2015-03-25, http://news.cnhubei.com/xw/wuhan/201503/t3214923.shtml.
19. "住房城乡建设部关于印发国家园林城市系列标准及申报评审管理办法的通知," 中华人民共和国住房和城乡建设部, 2016-10-28, baike.baidu.com/item/国家园林城市系列标准/20187700.
20. "2019年12月31日武汉市政府常务会议," 长江日报, 2020-01-04, http://cjw.wuhan.gov.cn/zwgk_11915/jgxx_11916/qtzdgknr/zfhy/202010/t20201022_1471083.html.
21. "曾光: 没有血的教训, 疫情瞒报问题解决不了!," 中国县域卫生, 2020-03-29, https://www.sohu.com/na/384066376_456029. See also "中国疾病预防控制中心流行病学首席科学家曾光: 公共卫生首先要姓公," 瞭望, 2020-05-11, http://www.xinhuanet.com/local/2020-05/11/c_1125967825.htm.
22. 汤琪, 廖艳, "专访武汉肺科医院院长: 危重病例救治仍在高峰期," 澎湃新闻, 2020-03-25, https://m.thepaper.cn/newsDetail_forward_6679129.
23. 张赫, "武汉市肺科医院院长：我们从未缺过物资," 健康时报, 2020-04-06, https://new.qq.com/omn/20200406/20200406A0OIZK00.html.

24. 王多龙, “我省在2020年全国卫生健康工作会议上交流健康湖北经验,” 湖北省卫生健康委员会, 2020-01-10, http://wjw.hubei.gov.cn/bmdt/dtyw/202001/t20200116_1913865.shtml.
25. Francesca Cavallo, *Doctor Li and the Crown Wearing Virus* (Los Angeles: Undercats, 2020); Alicia Lee, “New Children's Book Tells the Story of Dr. Li Wenliang, Who Sounded the Alarm on Coronavirus,” CNN, 2020-04-15, https://www.cnn.com/2020/04/15/world/coronavirus-doctor-li-francesca-cavallo-book-trnd/index.html.
26. Stephen Roach and Weijian Shan, “The Fable of the Chinese Whistleblower,” Project Syndicate, 2020-05-18, https://www.project-syndicate.org/commentary/trump-charges-against-china-covid19-alternative-facts-by-stephen-s-roach-and-weijian-shan-2020-05.
27. 国家监委调查组, “关于群众反映的涉及李文亮医生有关情况调查的通报,” 新华网 2020-03-19, http://www.nhc.gov.cn/xcs/fkdt/202003/0afc839b55904f8e9a750e4f86868fb0.shtml.
28. 信娜 et al., “李文亮生前所在医院之痛,” 财经, 2020-03-13, https://finance.sina.com.cn/wm/2020-03-13/doc-iimxxstf8783232.shtml.
29. 韩谦, “受训诫的武汉医生: 11天后被病人传染住进隔离病房,” 北青深一度, 2020-01-27, https://chinadigitaltimes.net/chinese/633323.html.
30. 韩谦, “受训诫的武汉医生.”
31. A copy of Dr. Li's self-criticism is later made available as “Dr. Li's Apology Letter,” *New York Times*, 2022-10-05, https://www.nytimes.com/interactive/2022/10/05/world/asia/li-wenliang-letter.html.
32. 韩谦, “受训诫的武汉医生.”
33. 张玥 et al., “四人殉职，四人濒危-武汉中心医院‘至暗时刻,’” 南方周末, 2020-03-11, https://www.infzm.com/content/178912.
34. 杜玮, “亲历者讲述：武汉市中心医院医护人员被感染始末,” 中国新闻周刊, 2020-02-17, https://mp.weixin.qq.com/s/1zNY2YXy75snzwX3Tg09Cg.
35. 杜玮, “亲历者讲述.”
36. 龚菁琦, “发哨子的人,” 人物, 2020-03-10, https://www.weibo.com/ttarticle/p/show?id=2309404480863474679890 .
37. This quote was made available on social media by a reporter with *Southern Weekend*.
38. 龚菁琦, “发哨子的人.”
39. 龚菁琦, “发哨子的人.”
40. For a perspective on the political psychology of leaders like Cai Li, see “蔡莉不撤 民怨难平,” 法制洋葱头, 2020-03-17, https://mp.weixin.qq.com/s/Fs40QSBX9DryHqlwHnD2rA.
41. 龚菁琦, “发哨子的人.”
42. According to a doctor on Weibo, the three WeChat groups were for Wuhan University Medical School Clinical '04, Union Red Cross Society Hospital Neurology Section, and (Union Hospital) Cancer Center.
43. “武汉相关人士打来电话，和胡锡进亲口说了内情!,” 环球时报, 2020-01-21, https://finance.sina.com.cn/wm/2020-01-21/doc-iihnzhha4011476.shtml.
44. Central South Road police station of the Wuchang District Public Security Bureau.
45. 国家监委调查组, “关于群众反映的涉及李文亮医生有关情况调查的通报.”
46. 中华人民共和国治安管理处罚法; “Public Security Administration Punishment Law of the People's Republic of China,” https://www.cecc.gov/resources/legal-provisions/public-security-administration-punishment-law-chinese-text.

47. The police action against "rumormongers" was announced on January 1, but Dr. Li was not given admonishment until January 3. Hence, there is the possibility that Dr. Li was not one of the eight people who were initially targeted by police but was added later. However, a Weibo post by Wuhan police on January 29, 2020, appeared to indirectly confirm that Dr. Li Wenliang was among the eight "netizens" subjected to punishment. 覃建行, 高昱, 包志明, 丁刚, "新冠肺炎'吹哨人'李文亮: 真相最重要," 财新网, 2020-04-07, https://china.caixin.com/2020-02-07/101509761.html.
48. 覃建行, 王颜玉, "第三名吹哨人现身," 财新网, 2020-02-07, https://china.caixin.com/2020-02-07/101512901.html.
49. 覃建行, 王颜玉, "第三名吹哨人现身"; 张晓晖, "专访武汉'造谣'者之一谢琳卡医生," 经济观察网, 2020-02-01, www.eeo.com.cn/2020/0201/375357.shtml.
50. "武汉相关人士打来电话, 和胡锡进亲口说了内情!"
51. 王一苇, 汤佩兰, "改变新冠诊断标准的女医生张笑春," 知识分子, 2020-09-21, http://zhishifenzi.com/depth/depth/10030.html.
52. "武汉市委书记自责：早采取严厉管控措施会比现在好," 央视新闻, 2020-02-01, https://shareapp.cyol.com/cmsfile/News/202002/01/share322383.html .
53. "梁伟年," 百度百科, 2020-10-02, https://baike.baidu.com/item/梁伟年/11024175.
54. Jennifer Pan and Kaiping Chen, "Concealing Corruption: How Chinese Officials Distort Upward Reporting of Online Grievances," *American Political Science Review* 112, no. 3 (2018): 602–620; Qiuqing Tai, "China's Media Censorship: A Dynamic and Diversified Regime," *Journal of East Asian Studies* 14, no. 2 (2014): 185–209.
55. "突发! 武汉发现不明原因肺炎，这些谣言别信!," 澎湃政务, 2019-12-31，https://m.thepaper.cn/baijiahao_5405745.
56. Quote from 平安武汉 on Weibo.com, 2020-01-01, copy of original on file.
57. For a video of the China Central Television broadcast, see "8名散布谣言者被查处," 2020-01-28, https://www.youtube.com/watch?v=Xn3RPjXutes&feature=youtu.be.
58. Chun Han Wong, "China's Glowing Coronavirus-Response Coverage Triggers Anger at State Media," *Wall Street Journal*, 2020-03-18, https://www.wsj.com/articles/chinas-glowing-coronavirus-response-coverage-triggers-anger-at-state-media-11584529203.
59. Haifeng Huang, "The Pathology of Hard Propaganda," *Journal of Politics* 80, no. 3 (2018): 1034–1038.
60. Quoted in 黄霁洁 et al., "被新冠击中的医护们: 1716例感染缘何发生," 澎湃新闻, 2020-02-18, https://www.thepaper.cn/newsDetail_forward_6041568. Parenthesis was in original.
61. David Kirton, "Coronavirus Outbreak May Be over in China by April—Expert," Reuters, 2020-02-11, https://www.reuters.com/article/us-china-health-doctor-exclusive-idUSKBN2050VF.
62. "还原 '超级传播者'传染路径; 武汉医生: 疫情刚开始'整个不让说,'" 中国新闻周刊, 2020-01-25, https://new.qq.com/omn/20200125/20200125A07TT200.html.
63. "还原'超级传播者'传染路径; 武汉医生: 疫情刚开始'整个不让说.'"
64. 高昱 et al., "现场篇：武汉围城," 财新周刊, 2020-02-03, https://weekly.caixin.com/2020-02-01/101510145_1.html.
65. 张玥 et al., "四人殉职，四人濒危-武汉中心医院'至暗时刻.'"
66. 吴靖, 王晨, "武汉社区告急: 领导干部亲自搬遗体, 基层防疫压力巨大," 八点健闻, 2020-02-02, https://mp.weixin.qq.com/s/T9PNlc7BNJUypPk7ffwGnw.
67. "白衣山猫" (aka Wang Guobao of Zhejiang Province), Weibo, 2020-01-29.

68. An example of the social media criticism she received is 东八线, "廖记者，您的人血馒头掉了," 2020-03-14, WeChat essay on file.
69. "人民日报 2019-12-31 11:56," https://weibo.com/2803301701/IniAErTYL.
70. Chinese netizens collated these front pages and shared them widely on social media. See, for example, "全是铁证据！谁在隐瞒真相?," 2020-04-22, https://mp.weixin.qq.com/s/b4Il8Tqr9lhrwY5_Gm5ZEg. Archived copy at https://archive.li/fy6LL.
71. "中国战疫录," 中国新闻网, 2020-04-02, video, episode 1, https://www.youtube.com/watch?v=MMm27Mj12x8.
72. Guobin Yang, *The Wuhan Lockdown* (New York: Columbia University Press, 2022).
73. Screen captures from 雯_雯小妖 are available at "武汉网友爆2位家人患不明肺炎 器官衰竭," 澳洲新闻网, 2020-01-07, https://www.huaglad.com/lovecn/20200107/373297.html.
74. "武汉肺炎暗与明," bit.ly/anyuming, 2020-01-22, https://telegra.ph/武汉肺炎暗与明-01-22.
75. World Health Organization, "Summary of Probable SARS Cases with Onset of Illness from 1 November 2002 to 31 July 2003," 2015-07-24, https://www.who.int/publications/m/item/summary-of-probable-sars-cases-with-onset-of-illness-from-1-november-2002-to-31-july-2003.
76. Lee Shiu Hung, "The SARS Epidemic in Hong Kong: What Lessons Have We Learned?," *Journal of the Royal Society of Medicine* 96, no. 8 (2003): 374–378; Terry T. F. Leung and Hung Wong, "Community Reactions to the SARS Crisis in Hong Kong: Analysis of a Time-Limited Counseling Hotline," *Journal of Human Behavior in the Social Environment* 12, no. 1 (2005): 1–22; Christine Loh, ed., *At the Epicenter: Hong Kong and the SARS Outbreak* (Hong Kong: Hong Kong University Press, 2004), 2.
77. Elizabeth Cheung, "Hong Kong Activates 'Serious Response Level' for Infectious Diseases as Wuhan Pneumonia Outbreak Escalates," *South China Morning Post*, 2020-01-04, https://www.scmp.com/news/hong-kong/health-environment/article/3044654/hong-kong-activates-serious-response-level.
78. There are three response levels: alert, serious, and emergency. Government of the Hong Kong Special Administrative Region, "Government Launches Preparedness and Response Plan for Novel Infectious Disease of Public Health Significance," press release, 2020-01-04, https://www.info.gov.hk/gia/general/202001/04/P2020010400179.htm.
79. "44 Wuhan-Related Cases Detected," News.gov.hk, 2020-01-03, https://www.news.gov.hk/eng/2020/01/20200103/20200103_193832_067.html.
80. 李明子, "'超级传播者': 他转移4次病房, 传染了14名医护人员," 中国新闻周刊, 2020-01-25, https://mp.weixin.qq.com/s/Z8JSBuK_-hEweM_yG9KbBQ.
81. Laurie Chen et al., "China Pneumonia Outbreak Raises Specter of SARS as Number Infected Jumps to 44," *South China Morning Post*, 2020-01-03, https://www.scmp.com/news/china/society/article/3044535/wuhan-pneumonia-dramatic-rise-cases-44-11-serious.
82. Karen Zhang, "Supplies of N95 Mask Running Low in Hong Kong as Wuhan Virus Scare Sparks Panic Buying and Marked-Up Prices," *South China Morning Post*, 2020-01-07, https://www.scmp.com/news/hong-kong/health-environment/article/3044906/supplies-n95-mask-running-low-hong-kong-wuhan.
83. Hong Kong Department of Health data: "Data in Coronavirus Disease (COVID-19)," accessed 2023-04-30, https://data.gov.hk/en-data/dataset/hk-dh-chpsebcddr-novel-infectious-agent.

84. 泉野, "从庙堂到江湖 谁该为肺炎集体恐慌潮负责?," 香港01, 2020-02-10, https://www.hk01.com/深度報道/432342/武漢肺炎-从庙堂到江湖谁该为肺炎集体恐慌潮负责.
85. While this is my own assessment, various interviewees I have spoken to who are familiar with Weibo shared this view.
86. 唐兴华, "治理有关新型肺炎的谣言问题, 这篇文章说清楚了!," @最高人民法院, 2020-01-27 , https://weibo.com/ttarticle/p/show?id=2309404465698775629865.

Chapter 6

1. 杨维中(主编), 中国卫生应急十年 *2003–2013* (北京 : 人民卫生出版社, 2014).
2. Ling Lan, "Open Government and Transparent Policy: China's Experience with SARs," *International Public Management Review* 6, no. 1 (2005): 60–75.
3. Hitoshi Oshitani, "Lessons Learned from International Responses to Severe Acute Respiratory Syndrome (SARS)," *Environmental Health and Preventive Medicine* 10, no. 5 (2005): 251–254; Yu-Chen Hsu et al., "Risk and Outbreak Communication: Lessons from Taiwan's Experiences in the Post-SARS Era," *Health Security* 15, no. 2 (2017): 165–169.
4. Erik Baekkeskov and Olivier Rubin, "Information Dilemmas and Blame-Avoidance Strategies: From Secrecy to Lightning Rods in Chinese Health Crises," *Governance* 30, no. 3 (2017): 425–443.
5. Yanzhong Huang, *Governing Health in Contemporary China* (Abingdon, UK: Routledge, 2015), chap. 4.
6. 吴尊友, "新冠疫情形势与防控策略," 财经年会2021: 预测与战略, 2020-11-25 , http://economy.caijing.com.cn/20201125/4717538.shtml, transcript at https://finance.sina.com.cn/meeting/2020-11-25/doc-iiznctke3179937.shtml.
7. 国务院新闻办公室, "国务院新闻办公室2020年1月22日新闻发布会文字实录," 国家卫生健康委员会宣传司, 2020-01-22, http://www.nhc.gov.cn/xcs/ptpxw/202001/61add0d230e047eaab777d062920d8a8.shtml.
8. 曾光, "中国疾控系统如何改革?," 腾讯视频, 2020-09-26, video, https://v.qq.com/x/cover/mzc0020010fs5mi/c3156i1hneq.html. Video.
9. 许雯, "中疾控独家回应: '人传人'早有推论 , 保守下结论有原因," 新京报, 2020-01-31, http://www.bjnews.com.cn/news/2020/01/31/682224.html.
10. 柠檬木聚糖. Comments at post of Feng Zijian interview, 2020-1-31, 19:41, https://weibo.com/5247938240/Is3SMemCn.
11. 高昱 et al., "新冠病毒基因测序溯源: 警报是何时拉响的," 财新网, 2020-02-26, http://china.caixin.com/2020-02-26/101520972.html; 包志明 et al., "武汉中心医院为何医护人员伤亡惨重|疫情回眸," 财新网, 2020-03-10 , http://china.caixin.com/2020-03-10/101526309.html. The first article has been censored but is archived at https://archive.ph/YylMt.
12. 王延轶/Yan-Yi Wang email message, 2020-01-02, 10:28, circulated on social media.
13. "国家卫生健康委办公厅关于在重大突发传染病防控工作中加强生物样本资源及相关科研活动管理工作的通知," 国家卫生健康委办公厅, 2020-01-03, https://zh.wikisource.org/wiki/国家卫生健康委办公厅关于重大突发传染病防控工作中加强生物样本资源及相关科研活动管理工作的通知 (国卫科教函[2020]3号).
14. "国家卫生健康委关于同意湖北省疾病预防控制中心生物安全三级实验室临时开展不明原因的肺炎病毒实验活动的批复,"国家卫生健康委办公厅, 2020-01-03. (国卫科教函[2020]4号). Copy on file.

15. "Xinhua Hospital," in *WHO-Convened Global Study of Origins of SARS-CoV-2: China Part, Joint WHO–China Study, 14 January–10 February 2021* (Geneva: World Health Organization, 2021), annex D1, https://apps.who.int/gb/COVID-19/pdf_files/2021/28_03/20210328-%20Full%20report.pdf.
16. Cong Cao, "SARS: 'Waterloo' of Chinese Science," *China: An International Journal* 2, no. 2 (2004): 262–286.
17. "国家卫生健康委积极开展新型冠状病毒感染的肺炎疫情防控工作," 国家卫生健康委员会, 2020-01-19, http://www.nhc.gov.cn/xcs/xxgzbd/202001/de5f07afe8054af3ab2a25a61d19ac70.shtml.
18. 信娜, "高福：疫情防控我给自己打满分," 财经, 2021-01-12, https://www.dazuig.com/caij/cj/677252.html. Sometimes Chinese authors, including Gao Fu, omitted mention of the Academy of Military Medical Sciences from the line-up; see, for example, Nils Chr. Stenseth et al., "Lessons Learnt from the COVID-19 Pandemic," *Frontiers in Public Health* 9 (2021): 694705.
19. Zhengli Shi, "Reply to Science Magazine," link in Jon Cohen, "Wuhan Coronavirus Hunter Shi Zhengli Speaks Out," *Science*, 2020-07-24, https://www.sciencemag.org/news/2020/07/trump-owes-us-apology-chinese-scientist-center-covid-19-origin-theories-speaks-out; "武汉病毒所全力开展新型冠状病毒肺炎科研攻关," 中国科学院武汉病毒研究所, 2020-01-29, http://www.whiov.cas.cn/xwdt_160278/zhxw2019/202005/t20200511_5577853.html.
20. Jane Qiu, "How China's 'Bat Woman' Hunted Down Viruses from SARS to the New Coronavirus," *Scientific American*, 2020-03-11, https://www.scientificamerican.com/article/how-chinas-bat-woman-hunted-down-viruses-from-sars-to-the-new-coronavirus1; Chao Shan et al., "Infection with Novel Coronavirus (SARS-Cov-2) Causes Pneumonia in Rhesus Macaques," *Cell Research* 30, no. 8 (2020): 670–677.
21. Wenjie Tan, Xiang Zhao, Xuejun Ma, Wenling Wang, Peihua Niu, Wenbo Xu, George F. Gao, and Guizhen Wu, "A Novel Coronavirus Genome Identified in a Cluster of Pneumonia Cases—Wuhan, China 2019–2020," *China CDC Weekly* 2, no. 4 (2020): 61–62; Qiang Wei, Yanhai Wang, Juncai Ma, Jun Han, Mengnan Jiang, Li Zhao, Fei Ye, Jingdong Song, Bo Liu, Linhuan Wu, Wenjie Tan, Guizhen Wu, George F. Gao, and Jianjun Liu, "Description of the First Strain of 2019-nCoV, C-Tan-nCoV Wuhan Strain—National Pathogen Resource Center, China, 2020," *China CDC Weekly* 2, no. 6 (2020): 81–82. I include all names of the authors for discerning readers.
22. "在一线，疾控勇士与新型冠状病毒赛跑," China CDC, 2020-02-01, http://www.chinacdc.cn/yw_9324/202002/t20200201_212137.html; "疫线疾控人: 6, 使命与担当," 健康报, 2020, available at bilibili.com or https://mp.weixin.qq.com/s/HjMBvIWcZHeSKHhlERAcpw.
23. "在一线，疾控勇士与新型冠状病毒赛跑".
24. Wuhan Institute of Biological Products is a subsidiary of Sinopharm's subsidiary company China National Biotec Group. 张驰, 黄秋霞, "和病毒赛跑: 记'中国青年五四奖章'获得者、国药集团中国生物武汉生物制品研究所," 中央纪委国家监委网站, 2021-05-31, https://www.ccdi.gov.cn/yaowen/202105/t20210531_242899.html; 赵倩, 吴阳, "中国生物高层揭秘全球首个新冠灭活疫苗," 红星新闻, 2020-04-16, https://news.sina.cn/gn/2020-04-16/detail-iirczymi6573081.d.html; "武汉病毒所2020年度十大重要事件揭晓," 武汉病毒所, 2021-02-07, www.whiov.cas.cn/xwdt_160278/zhxw2019/202102/t20210207_5890528.html.
25. 王振雅, "首个国产抗新冠口服药研发的背后故事," 健康时报, 2022-08-07, http://www.jksb.com.cn/html/xinwen/2022/0807/177604.html; Jin-Lan Zhang et al., "Azvudine

Is a Thymus-Homing Anti-SARS-Cov-2 Drug Effective in Treating COVID-19 Patients," *Signal Transduction and Targeted Therapy* 6, no. 1 (2021): 1–15.

26. "专家称系新型冠状病毒, 武汉不明原因的病毒性肺炎疫情病原学鉴定取得初步进展," 新华网, 2020-01-09, http://www.xinhuanet.com/politics/2020-01/09/c_1125438971.htm.
27. Dennis Normile, "Mystery Virus Found in Wuhan Resembles Bat Viruses but not SARS, Chinese Scientist Says," *Science*, 2020-01-10, https://www.science.org/content/article/mystery-virus-found-wuhan-resembles-bat-viruses-not-sars-chinese-scientist-says.
28. The military's Academy of Military Medical Sciences simply stayed away from this assessment and later used the reagent it developed to partner with a company (Sansure Biotech).
29. "中国疾病预防控制中心病毒病预防控制所荣获全国卫生健康系统新冠肺炎疫情防控工作先进集体称号," China CDC, 2020-03-12, http://www.chinacdc.cn/yw_9324/202003/t20200312_214348.html.
30. The technical standards are set out in a two-page document, "武汉新型冠状病毒核酸检测试剂盒评价技术方案." Written interview with a China CDC researcher.
31. 张磊, "新病毒是如何发现的? 检测试剂盒使用如何? 听中疾控专家详解!," 澎湃新闻, 2020-01-26, http://m.thepaper.cn/rss_newsDetail_5642258.
32. Dake Kang, "China Testing Blunders Stemmed from Secret Deals with Firms," Associated Press, 2020-12-03, https://apnews.com/article/china-virus-testing-secret-deals-firms-312f4a953e0264a3645219a08c62a0ad.
33. 谢欣, "三家生物科技公司确定成为多地疾控新型冠状肺炎病毒核酸检测试剂盒供应方," 界面新闻, 2020-01-20, https://www.jiemian.com/article/3896699.html.
34. Liangjun Chen et al., "RNA Based mNGS Approach Identifies a Novel Human Coronavirus from Two Individual Pneumonia Cases in 2019 Wuhan Outbreak," *Emerging Microbes & Infections*, 9, no. 1 (2020), 313–319; for details on Zhongnan Hospital, I have relied on the extraordinary reporting by 萧辉, 包志明, 高昱, "武汉疫情中的中南医院: 他们打满全场," 财新周刊, no. 14, 2020-04-13, weekly.caixin.com/2020-04-10/101540932.html, archived at https://archive.ph/vmPbn.
35. 李晨, "武汉检验科博士: 我们3通宵自测病毒序列, 看到结果即感不妙," 科学网微信, 2020-02-03, http://news.sciencenet.cn/htmlnews/2020/2/435360.shtm.
36. Chen et al., "RNA Based mNGS Approach."
37. Xin-Cheng Qin et al., "A Tick-Borne Segmented RNA Virus Contains Genome Segments Derived from Unsegmented Viral Ancestors," *Proceedings of the National Academy of Sciences of the United States of America* 111, no. 18 (2014): 6744–6749.
38. Yongzhen Zhang, "Breaking the Wall to Redefine the RNA Virosphere," Falling Walls and Berlin Science Week: World Science Summit 2020, 2020-09-24, video, https://www.youtube.com/watch?v=bNp5pwnrzis.
39. Mang Shi et al., "Redefining the Invertebrate RNA Virosphere," *Nature* 540, no. 7634 (2016): 539–543; Yong-Zhen Zhang et al., "Expanding the RNA Virosphere by Unbiased Metagenomics," *Annual Review of Virology* 6 (2019): 119–139.
40. 全国创新争先奖.
41. 王丽颖, "与'瘟神'生死赛跑——专访上海市公共卫生临床中心主任朱同玉教授," 国际金融报, 2020-05-08, https://finance.sina.com.cn/wm/2020-05-08/doc-iirczymk0568054.shtml.
42. "Full Talk by Dr. Yongzhen Zhang from the BGI GigaScience Awards at ICG-15," Annual Meeting of the International Conference on Genomics, Wuhan, 2020-10-26, video, https://www.youtube.com/watch?v=SCSnfRaw5_0.
43. 高昱, et al., "新冠病毒基因测序溯源: 警报是何时拉响的."

44. "Full Talk by Dr. Yongzhen Zhang."
45. Detractors of Zhang argue that the Wuhan CDC researchers should not have shipped the sample with a dangerous pathogen by courier and that the SPHCC had worked on the novel coronavirus without obtaining NHC authorization. Song, however, recalled that he did not know they were handling a sample with coronavirus. He also stated that the P3 Lab was used because the P2 Lab was under renovation. 瞿依贤, "P3实验室建设的背后：需求、成本和热潮," 经济观察网, 2020-07-03, http://www.eeo.com.cn/2020/0703/388662.shtml.
46. Wen Wang et al., "Discovery of a Highly Divergent Coronavirus in the Asian House Shrew from China Illuminates the Origin of the Alphacoronaviruses," *Journal of Virology* 91, no. 17 (2017): e00764-17; "Full Talk by Dr. Yongzhen Zhang."
47. 明来, "张永振: '土得掉渣'的中国科学家和他的病毒探险之旅," 科技工作者之家, 2021-05-21, https://www.scimall.org.cn/article/detail?id=5514841.
48. "Full Talk by Dr. Yongzhen Zhang."
49. "Full Talk by Dr. Yongzhen Zhang."
50. "复旦大学附属上海市公共卫生临床中心卢洪洲教授来校作讲座," 华东政法大学新闻网, 2020-09-27, https://news.ecupl.edu.cn/2020/0927/c672a171497/page.htm.
51. 杜雯雯, 金钱熠, "公卫专家: 1月5日提交正式报告, 直报系统有需改进地方," 新京报, 2020-02-25, http://www.bjnews.com.cn/feature/2020/02/25/695000.html.
52. Zhang Yongzhen, as interviewed by Amy Qin et al., "Voices from China's Covid-19 Crisis: 'If I Survive This, What Will I Do?,'" *New York Times*, 2021-01-22, https://www.nytimes.com/2021/01/22/world/asia/wuhan-coronavirus.html.
53. "Full Talk by Dr. Yongzhen Zhang."
54. "Full Talk by Dr. Yongzhen Zhang."
55. 信娜, "高福：疫情防控我给自己打满分," 财经, 2021-01-12, https://www.dazuig.com/caij/cj/677252.html.
56. Copy of email communication between Wang Dayan of IVDC and GISAID dated 2020-01-12, 04:29, as seen by author.
57. "Full Talk by Dr. Yongzhen Zhang"; David Cyranoski, "Zhang Yongzhen: Genome Sharer," *Nature*, 2020-12-14, https://www.nature.com/immersive/d41586-020-03435-6/index.html.
58. State Council Information Office, "Fighting COVID-19: China in Action," 2020-06-07, http://english.scio.gov.cn/whitepapers/2020-06/07/content_76135269.htm.
59. 信娜, "高福."
60. "WHO Official Says Countries Must Rely on Speed, not Perfection in Response," Globalnews.ca, 2020-03-13, https://globalnews.ca/video/6673069/coronavirus-outbreak-who-official-says-countries-must-rely-on-speed-not-perfection-in-response.
61. Zijian Feng, Wenkai Li, and Jay K. Varma, "Gaps Remain in China's Ability to Detect Emerging Infectious Diseases Despite Advances Since the Onset of SARS and Avian Flu," *Health Affairs* 30, no. 1 (2011): 127–135.
62. Yi Jiang et al., "Epidemiological Characteristics and Trends of Notifiable Infectious Diseases in China from 1986 to 2016," *Journal of Global Health* 10, no. 2 (2020); A. Hansen et al., "Experts' Perceptions on China's Capacity to Manage Emerging and Re-emerging Zoonotic Diseases in an Era of Climate Change," *Zoonoses and Public Health* 64, no. 7 (2017): 527–536.
63. Jason Gale, "Early Coronavirus Genetic Data May Have Forewarned Outbreak," Bloomberg, 2020-02-11, https://www.bloomberg.com/news/articles/2020-02-12/early-coronavi

rus-data-was-available-weeks-before-public-release; membership of the COVID-19 IHR Emergency Committee is located at https://www.who.int/groups/covid-19-ihr-emergency-committee.

64. Screen capture—ERAUTZ3UAAATzPB.jpg, on file with author.
65. "China Delayed Releasing Coronavirus Info, Frustrating WHO," Associated Press, 2020-06-01, https://apnews.com/article/3c061794970661042b18d5aeaaed9fae.
66. Edward Gu and Lantian Li, "Crippled Community Governance and Suppressed Scientific/Professional Communities: A Critical Assessment of Failed Early Warning for the COVID-19 Outbreak in China," *Journal of Chinese Governance* 5, no. 2 (2020): 160–177.
67. Dennis Normile, Jon Cohen, and Kai Kupferschmidt, "Scientists Urge China to Quickly Share Data on Virus Linked to Pneumonia Outbreak," *Science*, 2020-01-09, https://www.sciencemag.org/news/2020/01/scientists-urge-china-quickly-share-data-virus-linked-pneumonia-outbreak.
68. 包志明 et al., "武汉中心医院为何医护人员伤亡惨重," 财新网, 2020-03-10, http://china.caixin.com/2020-03-10/101526309.html.

Chapter 7

1. Sonja Rasmussen and Richard A. Goodman, eds., *The CDC Field Epidemiology Manual* (Oxford: Oxford University Press, 2018), 5.
2. "Patricia Buffler Gives Opening Address at North American Congress of Epidemiology," *The Epidemiology Monitor*, 2011-07/08, http://www.epimonitor.net/Buffler_Speech.htm.
3. 许雯, "中疾控独家回应:'人传人'早有推论，保守下结论有原因," 新京报, 2020-01-31, http://www.bjnews.com.cn/news/2020/01/31/682224.html.
4. 许雯, "中疾控独家回应."
5. Chaolin Huang et al., "Clinical Features of Patients Infected with 2019 Novel Coronavirus in Wuhan, China," *The Lancet* 395, no. 10223 (2020): 497–506; Qun Li et al., "Early Transmission Dynamics in Wuhan, China, of Novel Coronavirus-Infected Pneumonia," *New England Journal of Medicine* 382 (2020): 1199–1207. The date of release was January 29, 2020.
6. In invoking the concept of epidemiological imagination, I have benefited from John Ashton, ed., *The Epidemiological Imagination: A Reader* (New York: McGraw-Hill Education, 1994).
7. 信娜, "高福：疫情防控我给自己打满分," 财经, 2021-01-12, https://www.dazuig.com/caij/cj/677252.html.
8. Fan Ding, Qun Li, and Lian-Mei Jin, "Experience and Practice of the Emergency Operations Center, Chinese Center for Disease Control and Prevention: A Case Study of Response to the H7N9 Outbreak," *Infectious Diseases of Poverty* 10, no. 1 (2021): 87–94.
9. "2020年全国卫生健康工作会议在北京召开," 国家卫生健康委员会, 2020-01-07, http://www.nhc.gov.cn/bgt/jdt/202001/85ab864836ac46ef9d9c4b657f6f04ee.shtml.
10. State Council Information Office, "Fighting COVID-19: China in Action," 2020-06-07, http://english.scio.gov.cn/whitepapers/2020-06/07/content_76135269.htm .
11. "中共中央政治局常务委员会召开会议, 习近平主持," 新华网, 2020-01-07, http://jhsjk.people.cn/article/31538441.
12. 习近平, "在中央政治局常委会会议研究应对新型冠状病毒肺炎疫情工作时的讲话(2020-02-03)," 求是, no. 4 (2020), 2020-02-15, http://www.qstheory.cn/dukan/qs/2020-02/15/c_1125572832.htm.

13. "新闻1+1：新型冠状病毒肺炎疫情，防控进行时!," 央视网, 2020-01-15, http://tv.cctv.com/2020/01/15/VIDEVPaxZBFtDLGUA6mk5PW2200115.shtml.
14. "在一线，疾控勇士与新型冠状病毒赛跑," China CDC, 2020-02-01, http://www.chinacdc.cn/yw_9324/202002/t20200201_212137.html.
15. 2019-nCoV Outbreak Joint Field Epidemiology Investigation Team and Qun Li, "An Outbreak of NCIP (2019-nCoV) Infection in China—Wuhan, Hubei Province, 2019–2020," *China CDC Weekly*, 2020-01-31, 2, no. 5, 79–80.
16. 2019-nCoV Outbreak Joint Field Epidemiology Investigation Team and Li, "Outbreak of NCIP (2019-nCoV) Infection in China."
17. 许雯, "中疾控独家回应."
18. Li et al., "Early Transmission Dynamics in Wuhan."
19. 陈鑫, "疾控中心争议论文作者谈'人传人12月已出现,'" 界面新闻, 2020-01-31, https://news.sina.cn/gn/2020-01-31/detail-iimxxste7917239.d.html.
20. 丁蕾 et al., "新型冠状病毒感染疫情下的思考," 中国科学: 生命科学, 50, no. 3 (2020): 247–257.
21. Jon Cohen, "Not Wearing Masks to Protect against Coronavirus Is a 'Big Mistake,' Top Chinese Scientist Says," *Science*, 2020-03-27, https://www.science.org/content/article/not-wearing-masks-protect-against-coronavirus-big-mistake-top-chinese-scientist-says.
22. Cohen, "Not Wearing Masks."
23. 俞琴, 黎诗韵, "专访卫健委派武汉第二批专家: 为何没发现人传人?," 财经E法, 2020-02-26, https://news.caijingmobile.com/article/detail/412839.
24. 俞琴, 黎诗韵, "专访卫健委派武汉第二批专家"; 王广发, "卫健委专家组成员王广发出院了, 回答了我们8个问题," 中国青年报-冰点周刊, 2020-02-02, https://mp.weixin.qq.com/s/DWcRVz10zps27VIrml_Khg.
25. ITV, "Outbreak—The Virus that Shook the World," 2021-01-19, accessed 2021-01-22, video, https://www.youtube.com/watch?v=cjdpImcPVc8.
26. Nicola Smith, "'They Wanted to Take Us Sightseeing. I Stayed in the Hotel,' Says First Foreign Official to Enter Wuhan," *The Telegraph*, 2020-05-06, https://www.telegraph.co.uk/global-health/science-and-disease/wanted-take-us-sight-seeing-stayed-hotel-says-first-foreign/.
27. Smith, "'They Wanted to Take Us Sightseeing'"; ITV, "Outbreak." The interview referred to an NHC official, but it was likely a China CDC official such as Feng Zijian, who was also an NHC expert.
28. Erin Hale, "COVID 'Could Have Been Contained': Taiwan's Ex-Health Minister," Aljazeera, 2021-01-22, https://www.aljazeera.com/news/2021/1/22/prompt-action-in-wuhan-who-involvement-could-have-stopped-covid.
29. Smith, "'They Wanted to Take Us Sightseeing.'"
30. Smith, "'They Wanted to Take Us Sightseeing.'"
31. Dennis Xie, "CDC Announces Travel Alert for Wuhan," *Taipei Times*, 2020-01-17, https://www.taipeitimes.com/News/front/archives/2020/01/17/2003729386.
32. Xie, "CDC Announces Travel Alert for Wuhan."
33. 魏铭言, "卫计委: 不排除H7N9有限'人传人,'" 新京报, 2013-04-18, http://epaper.bjnews.com.cn/html/2013-04/18/content_427477.htm.
34. "2020春天纪事," CCTV记录, 2020-09-08, episode 2, https://tv.cctv.com/2020/09/04/VIDA2RwP6u7FU6RPgDzr2wG8200904.shtml.
35. "国家卫健委高级别专家组就新型冠状病毒肺炎答记者问," 央视新闻客户端, 2020-01-20, http://m.news.cctv.com/2020/01/20/ARTIF4Fl7LEu8TRqIsnde93B200120.shtml;

"高福: 武汉华南海鲜市场或为受害单位, 动物样本中未提取到病毒," 观察者网, 2020-05-25, https://news.sina.com.cn/c/2020-05-26/doc-iircuyvi5002958.shtml; "2020春天纪事."

36. "国家卫健委高级别专家组就新型冠状病毒肺炎答记者问."
37. "国家卫健委高级别专家组就新型冠状病毒肺炎答记者问."
38. "卫健委专家高福院士: 疫区'口罩文化'至关重要," 新京报, 2020-01-24, https://finance.sina.com.cn/china/2020-01-24/doc-iihnzahk6095278.shtml. Note also Xu Wenbo, director of the IVDC: "It is highly suspected that the epidemic outbreak is related to wildlife trade." Quoted in 张磊, "新病毒是如何发现的?," 澎湃新闻, 2020-01-26, http://m.thepaper.cn/rss_newsDetail_5642258.
39. Edward C. Holmes et al., "The Origins of SARS-CoV-2: A Critical Review," *Cell* 184, no. 19 (2021): 4848–4856; Jacques van Helden et al., "An Appeal for an Objective, Open, and Transparent Scientific Debate about the Origin of SARS-CoV-2," *The Lancet* 398, no. 10309 (2021): 1402–1404.
40. Jeremy Page and Natasha Khan, "On the Ground in Wuhan, Signs of China Stalling Probe of Coronavirus Origins," *Wall Street Journal*, 2020-05-12, https://www.wsj.com/articles/china-stalls-global-search-for-coronavirus-origins-wuhan-markets-investigation-11589300842.
41. William J. Liu, et al. "Surveillance of SARS-CoV-2 at the Huanan Seafood Market," *Nature* (2023). https://doi.org/10.1038/s41586-023-06043-2.
42. Jonathan Pekar et al., "The Molecular Epidemiology of Multiple Zoonotic Origins of SARS-CoV-2," *Science* 377, no. 6609 (2022): 960–966; Michael Worobey et al., "The Huanan Seafood Wholesale Market in Wuhan Was the Early Epicenter of the COVID-19 Pandemic," *Science* 377, no. 6609 (2022): 951–959.
43. Jon Cohen, "Wuhan Seafood Market May Not Be Source of Novel Virus Spreading Globally," *Science* 10, 2020-01-26, https://www.sciencemag.org/news/2020/01/wuhan-seafood-market-may-not-be-source-novel-virus-spreading-globally.
44. CGTN, "Exclusive Interview with Chinese CDC Director Gao Fu," World Insight with Tian Wei, 2020-04-21, video, https://www.youtube.com/watch?v=q2PmAGvTCEQ.
45. CGTN, "Exclusive Interview with Chinese CDC Director Gao Fu."
46. Blakeley McShane and David Gal, "Blinding Us to the Obvious? The Effect of Statistical Training on the Evaluation of Evidence," *Management Science* 62, no. 6 (2016): 1707–1718; Blakeley McShane et al., "Abandon Statistical Significance," Suppl., *The American Statistician* 73, no. S1 (2019): 235–245.
47. "凤凰记者对话高福: 武汉动物样本无病毒 华南海鲜市场或为受害者," 凤凰卫视, 2020-05-25, https://www.sohu.com/a/397506382_120640988.
48. Hongxuan He, "Surveillance of SARS-CoV-2 in Wild Animals," in *WHO-Convened Global Study of Origins of SARS-CoV-2: China Part. Joint WHO–China Study: 14 January–10 February 2021* (Geneva: World Health Organization, 2021), annex C6, https://www.who.int/publications/i/item/who-convened-global-study-of-origins-of-sars-cov-2-china-part.
49. Zhengli Shi, "Reply to Science Magazine," link in Jon Cohen, "Wuhan Coronavirus Hunter Shi Zhengli Speaks Out," *Science*, 2020-07-24, https://www.sciencemag.org/news/2020/07/trump-owes-us-apology-chinese-scientist-center-covid-19-origin-theories-speaks-out; Wen Wang et al., "Coronaviruses in Wild Animals Sampled in and around Wuhan in the Beginning of COVID-19 Emergence," *Virus Evolution*, veac046, 2022-06-04, https://doi.org/10.1093/ve/veac046; "2020春天纪事."

50. Liuyang He and Hui Li, "Failed It or Nailed It: A Historical-Comparative Analysis of Legislating Bushmeat Ban in China," *The Chinese Journal of Comparative Law* 9, no. 2 (2021): 157–177.
51. "国家卫健委高级别专家组就新型冠状病毒肺炎答记者问," 央视新闻客户端, 2020-01-20, http://m.news.cctv.com/2020/01/20/ARTIF4Fl7LEu8TRqIsnde93B200120.shtml; see also "科学家对新冠病毒有了哪些新的认识? 高福院士告诉你," 新华网, 2020-12-30, www.xinhuanet.com/talking/2020-12/30/c_1210954482.htm.
52. CGTN, "Exclusive Interview with Chinese CDC Director Gao Fu."
53. Bob Woodward, *Rage* (New York: Simon & Schuster, 2020), 216.
54. "国家卫健委高级别专家组就新型冠状病毒肺炎答记者问."
55. 许雯, "中疾控独家回应."
56. CGTN, "Exclusive Interview with Chinese CDC Director Gao Fu."
57. "国家卫健委高级别专家组就新型冠状病毒肺炎答记者问."
58. "国家卫健委高级别专家组就新型冠状病毒肺炎答记者问."
59. 许雯, "中疾控独家回应."
60. Ye Qi et al., "Experts' Conservative Judgment and Containment of COVID-19 in Early Outbreak," *Journal of Chinese Governance* 5, no. 2 (2020): 140–159.
61. CGTN, "Exclusive Interview with Chinese CDC Director Gao Fu."
62. On Gao's character, see, 佘惠敏, "中国科学院院士高福: 为人类筑起病毒防火墙," 经济日报, 2016-06-16, http://www.scio.gov.cn/32621/32629/32755/Document/1480478/1480478.htm.
63. CGTN, "Exclusive Interview with Chinese CDC Director Gao Fu."
64. "在一线，疾控勇士与新型冠状病毒赛跑," China-CDC, 2020-02-01, http://www.chinacdc.cn/yw_9324/202002/t20200201_212137.html; I am indebted to a China CDC specialist with experience of dealing with avian influence outbreaks for informative discussions.
65. Chaolin Huang, et al., "Clinical Features of Patients Infected with 2019 Novel Coronavirus in Wuhan, China," *The Lancet* 395, no. 10223 (2020): 497–506.
66. 信娜, "高福."
67. Roy Anderson et al., "Epidemiology, Transmission Dynamics and Control of SARS: The 2002–2003 Epidemic," *Philosophical Transactions of the Royal Society of London. Series B: Biological Sciences* 359, no. 1447 (2004): 1091–1105.
68. 曾光, "流行病学调查在中国 抗疫中的作用和影响," 科普研究 59 (2020): 5–8.
69. 王志虹 et al., "医务人员高暴露人群严重急性呼吸综合征隐性感染与工作强度和工种的相关性研究," 中华结核和呼吸杂志 27, no. 3 (2004): 151–154.
70. "疾控专家专访：武汉肺炎病毒调查进展如何？出院标准是什么?" 央视新闻, 2020-01-14, http://www.nbd.com.cn/articles/2020-01-14/1400410.html; interview with Feng Zijian on China Central Television.
71. Kai Kupferschmidt, "This Biologist Helped Trace SARS to Bats. Now, He's Working to Uncover the Origins of COVID-19," *Science*, 2020-09-30, https://www.science.org/news/2020/09/biologist-helped-trace-sars-bats-now-hes-working-uncover-origins-covid-19; emails obtained by @USRightToKnow, https://usrtk.org/wp-content/uploads/2022/05/UTMB-Shi-Menachery-1.pdf, at 362.
72. Linfa Wang speaking at panel on "Lab Leak or Natural Origin? Scientists Discuss How the #COVID19 Pandemic Began," @ScienceMagazine, 2021-09-30, https://twitter.com/i/broadcasts/1MYGNnZZdknGw.
73. 王广发, "感染新冠肺炎的第一个专家组成员—我的经历," 国讯网, 2021-09-25, https://www.gxrhfz.com/guonei/173872.html.

74. A profile of Zeng Guang in the *China CDC Weekly* lists Zeng as chief epidemiologist for "2000–2019." Peter Hao et al., "Guang Zeng, China CDC's Former Chief Expert of Epidemiology," *China CDC Weekly*, 2020-11-06, 887–888.
75. 曾光, "疫情下完善公共卫生体系的思考," 爱思想, 2020-04-24，https://www.aisixiang.com/data/121012.html.
76. Interview with former colleague of Zeng's.
77. "曾光: 武汉的战役是在敌我界限不清的前提下开始的," 环球人物, 2020-02-11, http://www.hqrw.com.cn/2020/0211/92941.shtml.
78. "流行病学专家曾光: 从事公共卫生40年, 面对疫情我不能袖手旁观!," 西瓜视频, 2020-03-04, video, https://www.ixigua.com/6820331387682292237?id=6800297767441793550.
79. From a Hubei CDC member who was present when Zeng visited with the China CDC team.
80. "卫健委高级别专家组成员: 李文亮、张继先忧国忧民，是可敬的!," 西瓜视频, 2020-03-04, video, https://www.ixigua.com/6820331387682292237?id=6800269418279469579&logTag=399cbd185060d2b22b27.
81. "曾光."
82. "首席流行病专家两次到武汉: 别恐慌, 武汉人不出去就是保护全国," 西瓜视频, 2020-01-22, video, https://www.ixigua.com/6785003304796553741.
83. 彭丹妮, 李想俣, "复盘疫情决策," 中国新闻周刊, 2020-02-27, https://www.sohu.com/a/376165378_220095.
84. 黄思卓, "疾控专家曾光: 我在疫情'风暴中心,'" 南方周末, 2020-12-31, www.infzm.com/contents/198888.

Chapter 8

1. "武汉市卫健委关于不明原因的病毒性肺炎情况通报," 武汉市卫生健康委员会, 2020-01-05, https://wjw.wuhan.gov.cn/gsgg/202004/t20200430_1199589.shtml. Archived at https://zh.wikisource.org/wiki/武汉市卫生健康委员会关于不明原因的病毒性肺炎情况通报.
2. "武汉市卫健委关于不明原因的病毒性肺炎情况通报."
3. "武汉不明原因肺炎，5个你最关心的问题都在这!," 健康湖北, 2020-01-06, https://mp.weixin.qq.com/s/7XNck2ZZSygZ5XR4hh5rsQ.
4. See also comment by a veteran in a Hubei news organization, "我们已知的武汉肺炎的重要消息，都不是武汉官方首发的," 中国数字时代, 2020-01-21, https://chinadigitaltimes.net/chinese/632659.html.
5. Personal interview.
6. "专家解读不明原因的病毒性肺炎最新通报," 武汉市卫生健康委员会, 2020-01-11, http:// https://wjw.wuhan.gov.cn/gsgg/202004/t20200430_1199592.shtml. Archived at https://zh.wikisource.org/wiki/专家解读不明原因的病毒性肺炎最新通报.
7. "新型冠状病毒感染的肺炎疫情知识问答," 武汉市卫生健康委员会, 2020-01-15, https://wjw.wuhan.gov.cn/gsgg/202004/t20200430_1199594.shtml.
8. 中国疾病预防控制中心, "重点传染病和突发公共卫生事件每日情报会商纪要," 2020-01-07.
9. There are three response levels: alert, serious, and emergency. Government of the Hong Kong Special Administrative Region, "Government Launches Preparedness and Response Plan for Novel Infectious Disease of Public Health Significance," Info.gov.hk, 2020-01-04, https://www.info.gov.hk/gia/general/202001/04/P2020010400179.htm.

10. "44 Wuhan-related Cases Detected," News.gov.hk, 2020-01-03, https://www.news.gov.hk/eng/2020/01/20200103/20200103_193832_067.html.
11. 王端, 文思敏, "对话高级别专家组成员袁国勇: 我在武汉看到了什么," 财新网, 2020-03-08, https://china.caixin.com/2020-03-08/101525508.html.
12. The Central Theater Command General Hospital near Wuhan University Zhongnan Hospital also encountered a similar experience, but few details from this military hospital have been released.
13. 王嘉兴, "在钟南山之前，她向附近学校发出疫情警报," 中国青年报客户端, 2020-01-28, https://shareapp.cyol.com/cmsfile/News/202001/28/toutiao320881.html.
14. 吴菁, "党旗所向，白衣为袍，勇当抗疫排头兵—同济医院战疫纪实," 共产党员网, 2020-02-20, https://www.12371.cn/2020/02/20/ARTI1582204911636359.shtml.
15. 唐卫彬 et al., "'与国家同舟, 与人民共济'—新冠肺炎重症救治同济医院战疫直击," 新华网, 2020-02-20, http://www.xinhuanet.com/politics/2020-02/20/c_1125603912.htm.
16. 吴菁, "党旗所向, 白衣为袍, 勇当抗疫排头兵—同济医院战疫纪实"; "李树生: 抗疫急诊冲锋队的定海神针," 同济新闻, 2020–07, https://www.tjh.com.cn/plmnhytf12f3/1/同济新闻/2020/07/抗疫急诊冲锋队的定海神针.pdf; "感染科抗疫先锋队," 同济医院宣传部, 2020-05-11, https://www.tjh.com.cn/contents/585/30445.html; 李朝全, "同济战疫记," 人民网－人民日报, 2020-04-08, http://health.people.com.cn/n1/2020/0408/c14739-31665365.html; "同济时刻," CCTV 央视网, 2020-10-29, video, https://v.cctv.com/2020/10/29/VIDEGz35pUBki6Jhg3y3iy7w201029.shtml.
17. "迎难而上, 引领防控, 负重逆行：湖北省新冠肺炎专家组组长、同济医院呼吸与危重症医学科主任赵建平," 同济新闻, 2020–07, https://www.tjh.com.cn/plmnhytf12f3/1/同济新闻/2020/07/迎难而上%20%20引领防控%20%20%20负重逆行.pdf.
18. 潘俊文, 蓝婧, "武汉红会医院漫长的战争," 红星深度, 2020-03-13, https://new.qq.com/omn/20200313/20200313A0HB6C00.html.
19. 潘俊文, 蓝婧, "武汉红会医院漫长的战争"; 王达, "疫情风暴下，一座医院的坚守: 武汉市红十字会医院抗击新冠肺炎疫情实录," 中国红十字报, 2020-02-28, https://www.redcross.org.cn/html/2020-02/67372.html.
20. 潘俊文, 蓝婧, "武汉红会医院漫长的战争."
21. 雷宇, 王鑫昕, "80后院长的战疫百日记忆," 中国青年报, 2020-04-10, http://www.xinhuanet.com/politics/2020-04/10/c_1125835363.htm.
22. 崔芳, "武汉市红十字会医院: 风暴眼中的生死坚守," 健康报, 2020-03-14, https://www.sohu.com/a/379970400_162422.
23. 杨海, "武汉市中心医院医生: 传染病留给大家反应的时间太短了," 中国青年报-冰点周刊, 2020-03-13, https://terminus2049.github.io/archive/2020/03/13/bing-dian.html.
24. 杨海, "武汉市中心医院医生."
25. Interview with Wuhan Central Hospital doctor in video included in Muyi Xiao et al., "How a Chinese Doctor Who Warned of Covid-19 Spent His Final Days," *New York Times*, 2022-10-06, https://www.nytimes.com/2022/10/06/world/asia/covid-china-doctor-li-wenliang.html.
26. "武汉十七日," CCTV13 央视新闻调查, 2020-02-09, video, https://mp.weixin.qq.com/s?__biz=MjM5MjkxNjU5NA==&mid=2651174469&idx=1&sn=ada2c139b623866109cae5f2291d1c6e.
27. In "武汉十七日," Dr. Du said that the first patients were not from the Huanan Seafood Market and that they had "no exposure history to the Huanan Seafood Market." However, given the circumstances of the interview, it was possible Dr. Du mixed the first patients up with those who came afterward. In April 2020, Both Dr. Du and Dr. Peng Peng said that the

first five or six patients had a history of exposure to the Huanan Seafood Market as vendors and purchasers. 程靖, "很早就在买买买！疫情中，武汉有家不缺防护服的医院," 纵相新闻, 2020-04-16, https://new.qq.com/rain/a/20200416A0VYGW00; 张赫, "武汉市肺科医院院长: 我们从未缺过物资," 健康时报, 2020-04-06, https://new.qq.com/omn/20200406/20200406A0OIZK00.html. I thank Michael Worobey for discussing these reports.

28. 张赫, "武汉市肺科医院院长: 我们从未缺过物资," 健康时报, 2020-04-06, https://new.qq.com/omn/20200406/20200406A0OIZK00.html.
29. Liangjun Chen et al., "RNA Based mNGS Approach Identifies a Novel Human Coronavirus from Two Individual Pneumonia Cases in 2019 Wuhan Outbreak," *Emerging Microbes & Infections* 9, no. 1 (2020): 313–319; on Zhongnan Hospital, I have relied on the extraordinary reporting by 萧辉, 包志明, 高昱, "武汉疫情中的中南医院: 他们打满全场," 财新周刊, no. 14, 2020-04-13, weekly.caixin.com/2020-04-10/101540932.html. This censored report is archived at https://archive.ph/vmPbn.
30. 谢海涛, 张颖钰, "影像医生张笑春的百日抗疫," 中国数字时代, 2021-01-10, https://chinadigitaltimes.net/chinese/661349.html.
31. 萧辉, 包志明, 高昱, "武汉疫情中的中南医院." For a profile of Cheng Zhenshun, see "程真顺：坚守疫情防线 为生命保驾护航," 武汉大学新闻网, 2020-03-12, https://news.whu.edu.cn/info/1002/58245.htm.
32. The SARS test kits were ordered from Guangzhou-based DAAN Gene Co.
33. Quoted in 萧辉, 包志明, 高昱, "武汉疫情中的中南医院."
34. 萧辉, 包志明, 高昱, "武汉疫情中的中南医院."
35. 王珊, "新冠肺炎, 医院的节点," 三联生活周刊, 2020-03-14, https://zhuanlan.zhihu.com/p/113238046.
36. Quoted in 萧辉, 包志明, 高昱, "武汉疫情中的中南医院."
37. 萧辉, 包志明, 高昱, "武汉疫情中的中南医院."
38. 萧辉, 包志明, 高昱, "武汉疫情中的中南医院."
39. 萧辉, 包志明, 高昱, "武汉疫情中的中南医院."
40. "武汉市卫健委关于不明原因的病毒性肺炎情况通报," 2020-01-03, https://wjw.wuhan.gov.cn/gsgg/202004/t20200430_1199588.shtml. Archived at https://zh.wikisource.org/wiki/武汉市卫健委关于不明原因的病毒性肺炎情况通报.
41. 包志明 et al., "武汉中心医院为何医护人员伤亡惨重," 财新网, 2020-03-10, https://china.caixin.com/2020-03-10/101526309.html.
42. "不明原因的病毒性肺炎入排标准."
43. "全国不明原因肺炎病例监测、排查和管理方案," 国家卫生健康委员会办公厅, 2007-08-06, http://www.nhc.gov.cn/bgt/pw10708/200708/4455f46a2f5e4908a8561c079ecbcf0e.shtml.
44. Miguel Delgado-Rodriguez and Javier Llorca, "Bias," *Journal of Epidemiology & Community Health* 58, no. 8 (2004): 635–641.
45. 李想俣, "金银潭副院长黄朝林病愈隔离. 自述被传染和当'试药人'内情," 中国新闻周刊, 2020-02-14, https://mp.weixin.qq.com/s/qpztvhmnkNTtHQZi_e5PNw.
46. 武汉市不明原因的病毒性肺炎应急监测与流行病学调查方案.冠状病毒赛跑," China-CDC, 2020-02-01, http://www.chinacdc.cn/yw_9324/202002/t20200201_212137.html.
47. 许雯, "中疾控独家回应: '人传人'早有推论，保守下结论有原因," 新京报, 2020-01-31, http://www.bjnews.com.cn/news/2020/01/31/682224.html.
48. Moyses Szklo and Javier Nieto, *Epidemiology: Beyond the Basics*, 3rd ed. (Burlington, MA: Jones & Bartlett Learning, 2014), chap. 4.
49. 许雯, "中疾控独家回应."

50. 许雯, “中疾控独家回应.”
51. “武汉市卫生健康委员会关于不明原因的病毒性肺炎情况通报,” 武汉市卫生健康委员会, 2020-01-05, https://wjw.wuhan.gov.cn/gsgg/202004/t20200430_1199589.shtml.
52. 刘志勇, “专访曹彬: 面对新发传染病防控, 没有科研的引导, 就好像走夜路没有路灯,” 健康报, 2020-04-13, https://www.sohu.com/a/387529607_464387.
53. 高昱, “‘华南海鲜市场接触史’罗生门, 武汉市卫健委‘双标’令人迷惑,” 财新网, 2020-01-19, www.caixin.com/2020-02-19/101517544.html.
54. 殷维, “新型冠状病毒疫情处置情况说明,” 2020-02-08, https://mp.weixin.qq.com/s/vBeZKFgCxW_Rnnm04vCRYQ.
55. 杨海, “白皮手册与绿皮手册: 新冠肺炎诊断标准之变,” 中国青年报-冰点周刊, 2020-02-20, https://news.sina.cn/2020-02-20/detail-iimxxstf3065664.d.html.
56. 徐梅, “从发现到封城,武汉一线医护复盘疫情为何爆发,” 南方人物周刊, 2020-02-01, https://static.nfapp.southcn.com/content/202002/01/c3049605.html.
57. 包志明 et al., “武汉中心医院为何医护人员伤亡惨重.”
58. Quoted in 包志明 et al., “武汉中心医院为何医护人员伤亡惨重.”
59. “在一线，疾控勇士与新型冠状病毒赛跑.”
60. 杨海, “武汉早期疫情上报为何一度中断,” 中国青年报-冰点周刊, 2020-03-05, https://mp.weixin.qq.com/s/69pdSrjNH_4qN3RrQ-Yk0Q.
61. 全国传染病与突发公共卫生事件监测日报. The reported information included the sex, age, date of disease onset, and, when available, profession of the patients. The earliest disease-onset date among the 19 patients was December 12, 2019.
62. 杨海, “武汉早期疫情上报为何一度中断.”
63. 杨海, “武汉市中心医院医生.”
64. 杨海, “武汉市中心医院医生.”
65. Quoted in杨楠, 蒯乐昊, 徐梅, “危城勇士: 武汉医疗抗疫一线实录,” 南方人物周刊, 2020-02-27, https://www.nfpeople.com/index.php/article/9880.
66. 杨海, “白皮手册与绿皮手册.”
67. 包志明, 萧辉, 高昱, “武汉火线救人50天现场全记录,” 财新周刊, 2020-02-24, https://weekly.caixin.com/2020-02-22/101518920.html.
68. 张赫, “武汉市肺科医院院长.”
69. 殷维, “新型冠状病毒疫情处置情况说明.”
70. 殷维, “新型冠状病毒疫情处置情况说明.”
71. 殷维, “新型冠状病毒疫情处置情况说明.”
72. 龚菁琦, “发哨子的人,” 人物, 2020-03-10, https://www.weibo.com/ttarticle/p/show?id=2309404480863474679890.
73. 殷维, “新型冠状病毒疫情处置情况说明.”
74. 殷维, “新型冠状病毒疫情处置情况说明.”
75. 殷维, “新型冠状病毒疫情处置情况说明.”
76. 殷维, “新型冠状病毒疫情处置情况说明.”
77. 萧辉, “重症科医生亲述: 我们是怎样抢救危重病人的,” 财经网, 2020-02-05, https://china.caixin.com/2020-02-05/101511802.html.
78. 萧辉, 包志明, 高昱, “武汉疫情中的中南医院.”
79. “黄冈日记: ‘穿防护服戴口罩和护目镜’的人突然来了,” 澎湃新闻, 2020-03-06, https://www.thepaper.cn/newsDetail_forward_6319905.
80. “黄冈抗疫记,” CCTV13-央视新闻调查, 2020-02-24, https://cn.chinadaily.com.cn/a/202002/24/WS5e532638a3107bb6b57a1c4b.html.
81. 萧辉, 包志明, 高昱, “武汉疫情中的中南医院.”

82. 萧辉, 包志明, 高昱, “武汉疫情中的中南医院.”
83. Quoted in 萧辉, 包志明, 高昱, “武汉疫情中的中南医院.”
84. 萧辉, 包志明, 高昱, “武汉疫情中的中南医院.”
85. 高昱, 萧辉, 包志明, “四大ICU主任详解病毒, 来自最前线的防治之策,” 财经周刊, 2020-02-10, https://weekly.caixin.com/2020-02-07/101512870.html.
86. 萧辉, 包志明, 高昱, “武汉疫情中的中南医院.”
87. 萧辉, 包志明, 高昱, “武汉疫情中的中南医院.”
88. Reporter's notes by Xiao Hui (萧辉) of *Caixin* circulated on social media, 2020-04-11. Copy on file.
89. Diane Vaughan, “The Trickle-Down Effect: Policy Decisions, Risky Work,” *California Management Review* 39, no. 2 (1997): 80–102, at 99.
90. “疫情可防可控—武汉市就新型冠状病毒感染的肺炎综合防控工作答记者问,” 新华网, 2020-01-19, www.xinhuanet.com/politics/2020-01/19/c_1125480602.htm.

Chapter 9

1. “专家称武汉不明原因的病毒性肺炎可防可控,” 新华网, 2020-01-11, http://www.xinhuanet.com/local/2020-01/11/c_1125448549.htm. The interview with Wang Guangfa was conducted in the evening of January 10.
2. Jiang Rongmeng was at a meeting in Shanghai and went from Shanghai to Wuhan on January 9. 戴轩, “地坛医院感染二科主任医师蒋荣猛: 转战七个多月‘追疫人’归来,” 新京报, 2020-09-07, http://beijing.qianlong.com/2020/0907/4692290.shtml.
3. 谭畅, “‘建议轻症病人居家隔离’: 对话传染病专家蒋荣猛,” 南方周末, 2020-01-26, https://news.southcn.com/node_64549305f1/fb9873c7f9.shtml; “蒋荣猛,” 百度百科, accessed 2022-03-20, https://baike.baidu.com/item/蒋荣猛/1050718.
4. 俞琴, 黎诗韵, “专访卫健委派武汉第二批专家: 为何没发现人传人?,” 财经E法, 2020-02-26, https://news.caijingmobile.com/article/detail/412839.
5. 张定宇, “我在风暴之眼,” 中央广播电视总台, 武汉! 武汉! *2020*战疫口述实录 (北京: 现代出版社, 2020), 8.
6. “大型纪录片同心战疫,” 新闻频道-央视网, 2020-09-02, episode 1, https://news.cctv.com/2020/09/02/ARTIPf7jQ46IVedUA9VTNjWW200902.shtml.
7. “17例死亡病例病情介绍,” 国家卫生健康委卫生应急办公室, 2020-01-23, http://www.nhc.gov.cn/yjb/s3578/202001/5d19a4f6d3154b9fae328918ed2e3c8a.shtml.
8. 杨楠, 何沛芸, “重组金银潭: 疫情暴风眼的秘密,” 南方周末, 2020-03-05, http://www.infzm.com/contents/178385. Dr. Zhong officially became the captain of the Tongji Hospital First Medical Team to Jinyintan Hospital, though some Tongji medical staff had been at Jinyintan beginning on January 7, 2020.
9. 杨楠, 何沛芸, “重组金银潭.”
10. 杨楠, 何沛芸, “重组金银潭.”
11. 姜天骄, “身先士卒, 忘我战疫—记华中科大同济医院医疗队队长、党支部书记钟强,” 中国经济网, 2020-03-02, https://new.qq.com/omn/20200302/20200302A03LLJ00.html.
12. 杨楠, 何沛芸, “重组金银潭.”
13. 张定宇, “我在风暴之眼,” 11–12.
14. 杨楠, 何沛芸, “重组金银潭.”
15. 田巧萍, “为什么是张定宇,” 长江日报, 2020-02-14, https://www.thepaper.cn/newsDetail_forward_5975974.

16. 国家卫生健康委直属机关党委, "李大川: 始终奔忙在战疫一线," 旗帜网, 2020-03-07, http://dangjian.people.com.cn/n1/2020/0307/c117092-31621766.html.
17. "专家称武汉不明原因的病毒性肺炎可防可控." The interview with Wang Guangfa was conducted in the evening of January 10, 2020.
18. Quoted in 俞琴, 黎诗韵, "专访卫健委派武汉第二批专家."
19. 彭丹妮, 李想俣, "专家复盘：信息报上去了，如何及时转化为防控行动？," 中国新闻周刊, 2020-03-06, https:// https://www.naradafoundation.org/content/6773.
20. 俞琴, 黎诗韵, "专访卫健委派武汉第二批专家."
21. 俞琴, 黎诗韵, "专访卫健委派武汉第二批专家."
22. "新型冠状病毒感染的肺炎疫情知识问答," 武汉市卫生健康委员会, 2020-01-15, https://wjw.wuhan.gov.cn/gsgg/202004/t20200430_1199594.shtml.
23. According to a China CDC source, this table was prepared by Zhou Lei (周蕾), a senior research fellow of the China CDC Health Emergency Response Center.
24. The Novel Coronavirus Pneumonia Emergency Response Epidemiology Team, "The Epidemiological Characteristics of an Outbreak of 2019 Novel Coronavirus Diseases (COVID-19)—China, 2020," *China CDC Weekly* 2, no. X (2020): 1–10; Zheng, Lichun, Xiang Wang, Chongchong Zhou, Qin Liu, Shuang Li, Qin Sun, Mengjia Wang, Qian Zhou, and Wenmei Wang. "Analysis of the Infection Status of Healthcare Workers in Wuhan during the COVID-19 Outbreak: A Cross-Sectional Study," *Clinical Infectious Diseases* 71, no. 16 (2020): 2109–2113.
25. Incidentally, it was on January 12 that Dr. Li Wenliang checked into the Wuhan Central Hospital with the clinical symptoms of novel coronavirus infection.
26. "武汉市15名医务人员确诊为新型冠状病毒感染的肺炎病例," 新华网, 2020-01-21, http://www.xinhuanet.com/politics/2020-01/21/c_1125487270.htm.
27. 田巧萍, "最早上报疫情的她, 怎样发现这种不一样的肺炎?," 长江日报, 2020-02-02, http://wjw.hubei.gov.cn/bmdt/ztzl/fkxxgzbdgrfyyq/fkdt/202002/t20200202_2017829.shtml (byline not listed).
28. 肖欢欢, "'上报疫情第一人'张继先," 广州日报大洋网, 2020-03-08, https://news.dayoo.com/society/202003/08/140000_53178565.htm.
29. 高昱 et al., "现场篇：武汉围城," 财新周刊, 2020-02-03, https://weekly.caixin.com/2020-02-01/101510145_1.html.
30. 王一苇, "一年前的今天：武汉张继先医生看到第一例新冠病人," 知识分子, 2020-12-26, http://www.zhishifenzi.com/depth/character/10623.html.
31. "卫健委高级别专家组成员: 李文亮、张继先忧国忧民, 是可敬的!," 西瓜视频, 2020-03-04, video, https://www.ixigua.com/6820331387682292237?id=6800269418279469579&logTag=399cbd185060d2b22b27.
32. "张继先谈发现疫情: 从1家3口同患病说起, 说人传人时已很麻烦," 梨视频, 2020-03-05, video, https://v.qq.com/x/cover/mzc00200r3dzy7k/v3076z5faf8.html. Video interview with Dr. Zhang Jixian.
33. 王一苇, "一年前的今天."
34. 王一苇, "一年前的今天."
35. 吴岩, 刘志伟, "科学战疫, 循证务实步步为营—记武汉大学中南医院院长王行环," 科技日报, 2020-06-08, http://stdaily.com/index/fangtan/2020-06/08/content_953700.shtml; 萧辉, 包志明, 高昱, "武汉疫情中的中南医院: 他们打满全场," 财经周刊, no. 14, 2020-04-13, weekly.caixin.com/2020-04-10/101540932.html, archived at https://archive.ph/vmPbn.
36. 吴岩, 刘志伟, "科学战疫, 循证务实步步为营."

37. Quoted in 萧辉, 包志明, 高昱, "武汉疫情中的中南医院."
38. "三级综合医院评审标准实施细则 (2011)," 中华人民共和国国家卫生健康委员会, 2011-11-25, www.nhc.gov.cn/wjw/gfxwj/201304/0404f9cd71764ab29b2365e069cfbf2d.shtml.
39. "医院感染管理办法 (2006)," 中央政府门户网站, 2006-07-05, www.gov.cn/flfg/2006-07/25/content_344886.htm.
40. "国家卫生健康委办公厅关于进一步加强医疗机构感染预防与控制工作的通知," 医政医管局, 2019-05-23, http://www.nhc.gov.cn/yzygj/s7659/201905/d831719a5ebf450f991ce47baf944829.shtml； "国家卫生健康委关于南方医科大学顺德医院发生医院感染暴发事件的通知," 医政医管局, 2019-06-18, www.nhc.gov.cn/yzygj/s3594/201906/23e7011c79d449908c234f563cec5992.shtml.
41. "基层医院如何做好院感防控工作," 中国人口报, 2019-07-03, http://wjw.hubei.gov.cn/bmdt/mtjj/mtgz/201910/t20191030_163170.shtml.
42. Jerry Muller, *The Tyranny of Metrics* (Princeton, NJ: Princeton University Press, 2018).
43. 赵孟, 陈鑫, "卫健委专家组成员王广发回应'可防可控,'" 界面新闻, 2020-02-01, https://new.qq.com/omn/20200201/20200201A03EDU00.html.
44. 俞琴, 黎诗韵, "专访卫健委派武汉第二批专家."
45. 王天枀, "华中科技大学同济医学院附属同济医院感染科主任宁琴," 人民政协报, 2020-08-19, http://rmzxb.bzzb.tv/shareart_3311866_5.html.
46. 俞琴 黎诗韵, "专访卫健委派武汉第二批专家."
47. Information from WeChat source, 2020-01-27.
48. "与病毒较量, 经历生死考验," 央视新闻客户端, 2020-02-02, https://china.huanqiu.com/article/9CaKrnKp9qm.
49. 王瑞文, "对话同济医院重症医生陆俊," 新京报, 2020-02-04, https://www.bjnews.com.cn/detail/158082261714403.html.
50. "中国红基会字节跳动医务工作者人道救助基金资助首批医务工作者," 中国红十字基金会, 2020-01-27, https://www.crcf.org.cn/article/19445.
51. 陆俊, "武汉首位新冠重症医生," 环球时报新媒体, 2020-12-08, https://china.huanqiu.com/article/411LyXGPqMF; 王天枀, "华中科技大学同济医学院附属同济医院感染科主任宁琴," 人民政协报, 2020-08-19, http://rmzxb.bzzb.tv/shareart_3311866_5.html; 杨楠, "张霓: 透过护目镜, 护士的眼睛像天上的星星," 南方人物周刊, 2020-09-10, https://www.nfpeople.com/article/10287.
52. 陆俊, "武汉首位新冠重症医生."
53. "迎难而上, 引领防控, 负重逆行: 湖北省新冠肺炎专家组组长、同济医院呼吸与危重症医学科主任赵建平," 同济新闻, 2020–07, www.tjh.com.cn.
54. "迎难而上, 引领防控, 负重逆行."
55. 王瑞文, "对话同济医院重症医生陆俊."
56. 陈红霞, "武汉协和医院门诊办公室主任袁莉: 发热门诊就像战地医院," 21世纪经济报道, 2020-02-18, https://m.21jingji.com/article/20200218/e3112843895dabd0ce57627d9bb01b71.html.
57. "专访武汉协和医院赵洪洋," 神外前沿, 2020-06-24, https://www.sohu.com/a/403808325_130047.
58. 李明子, "'超级传播者': 他转移4次病房, 传染了14名医护人员," 中国新闻周刊, 2020-01-25, https://mp.weixin.qq.com/s/Z8JSBuK_-hEweM_yG9KbBQ; "武汉十七日," CCTV13 央视新闻调查, 2020-02-09, https://mp.weixin.qq.com/s?__biz=MjM5MjkxNjU5NA==&mid=2651174469&idx=1&sn=ada2c139b623866109cae5f2291d1c6e.

59. 童俊, “武汉的伤与痛-对未来心理创伤干预的警示,” 致道中和, 2020-04-12, https://mp.weixin.qq.com/s/qqRTixoNtYnvUtt16nsLbw.
60. 杜玮, “亲历者讲述：武汉市中心医院医护人员被感染始末,” 中国新闻周刊, 2020-02-17, https://mp.weixin.qq.com/s/1zNY2YXy75snzwX3Tg09Cg.
61. 秦珍子, “带着试剂盒跑,” 中国青年报, 2020-02-12, http://zqb.cyol.com/html/2020-02/12/nw.D110000zgqnb_20200212_1-07.htm.
62. “专访武汉协和医院赵洪洋.”
63. “专访武汉协和医院赵洪洋.”
64. 俞琴, 黎诗韵, “专访卫健委派武汉第二批专家.”
65. 杨海, “白皮手册与绿皮手册: 新冠肺炎诊断标准之变,” 冰点周刊: 中国青年报, 2020-02-20，https://news.sina.cn/2020-02-20/detail-iimxxstf3065664.d.html.
66. Quote from a WeChat discussion, 2020-01-27.
67. “目前阶段的关键任务—中国工程院副院长、呼吸与危重症医学专家王辰再谈武汉疫情防控焦点问题,” 新华网, 2020-03-13, http://www.xinhuanet.com/politics/2020-03/13/c_1125708821.htm.

Chapter 10

1. “李克强主持召开国务院全体会议，讨论政府工作报告(征求意见稿),” 中国政府网, 2020-01-14, http://www.gov.cn/guowuyuan/2020-01/14/content_5469057.htm.
2. On the Jiangsu case, see 邱冰清, “国家卫健委确诊江苏首例新型冠状病毒感染的肺炎确诊病例,” 新华网, 2020-01-23, http://www.xinhuanet.com/politics/2020-01/23/c_1125497543.htm.
3. “关于切实加强不明原因肺炎/住院肺炎等呼吸道传染病病例检测的通知,” 江苏省卫生健康委员会, 2019-12-31. Digital copy on file.
4. “北京市卫生健康委员会关于成立北京市突发事件卫生应急专家咨询委员会的通知,” 北京市卫生健康委员会, 2019-02-02, last accessed 2022-02-05, http://wjw.beijing.gov.cn/zwgk_20040/fgwj/wjwfw/201912/t20191219_1301466.html.
5. 赵今朝, 杨睿, “京首例患者就医始末,” 财新网, 2020-02-13，https://china.caixin.com/2020-02-13/101514878.html
6. “北京清华长庚医院战疫满月纪实,” 清华大学附属北京清华长庚医院公众号, 2020-02-17, http://news.39.net/a/200217/7785728.html.
7. 胡宁, 刘世昕, “疫情几起几落, 北京地坛医院打了三场硬仗,” 中国青年报客户端, 2020-08-25, http://news.youth.cn/gn/202008/t20200825_12465879.htm; 王燕, 郑新媚, “北京地坛医院: 抗疫路上, 地坛人74载从未缺席,” 搜狐健康, 2020-03-01, https://www.sohu.com/a/376925081_359980.
8. 赵今朝, 杨睿, “京首例患者就医始末.”
9. “我市新增3例新型冠状病毒感染的肺炎病例.,” 首都健康, 2020-01-20, 06:31, https://www.weibo.com/2417852083/IqovwEeMp.
10. 首都文明办, “吴浩: 接地气儿的基层疫情防控专家,” 中国文明网, http://www.wenming.cn/sbhr_pd/zghrb/jyfx/202009/t20200903_5777128.shtml.
11. For an indication of the WHO's influence in 2003, see Peter Wonacott, “WHO Lifts Last Travel Alert Linked to SARS, for Beijing,” *Wall Street Journal*, 2003-06-24, https://www.wsj.com/articles/SB105644048211588200.

12. Jacky Habib, "This Virus Expert Detected the First Case of COVID-19 outside of China," Global Citizen, 2020-12-23, https://www.globalcitizen.org/en/content/following-the-a-team-Supaporn-Wacharapluesadee/.
13. "Surveillance Case Definitions for Human Infection with Novel Coronavirus (nCoV)," World Health Organization, 2020-01-11, https://apps.who.int/iris/bitstream/handle/10665/330376/WHO-2019-nCoV-Surveillance-v2020.1-eng.pdf.
14. Elizabeth Cheung, "Wuhan Pneumonia: Thailand Confirms First Case of Virus outside China," *South China Morning Post*, 2020-01-13, https://www.scmp.com/news/hong-kong/health-environment/article/3045902/wuhan-pneumonia-thailand-confirms-first-case.
15. World Health Organization, "WHO Statement on Novel Coronavirus in Thailand," 2020-01-13, https://www.who.int/news-room/detail/13-01-2020-who-statement-on-novel-coronavirus-in-thailand.
16. Quoted in Sarah Newey, "WHO Refuses to Rule out Human-to-Human Spread in China's Mystery Coronavirus Outbreak," *Guardian*, 2020-01-14, https://www.telegraph.co.uk/global-health/science-and-disease/refuses-rule-human-to-human-spread-chinas-mystery-virus-outbreak/.
17. Lisa Schnirring, "Report: Thailand's Coronavirus Patient Didn't Visit Outbreak Market," CIDRAP News, 2020-01-14, http://www.cidrap.umn.edu/news-perspective/2020/01/report-thailands-coronavirus-patient-didnt-visit-outbreak-market.
18. "每日情报会商纪要," China CDC, 2020-01-15.
19. "每日情报会商纪要," China CDC, 2020-01-14.
20. 谢玮, "蒋超良的45天," 经济网, 2020-02-14, http://www.ceweekly.cn/2020/0214/285828.shtml.
21. 国务院新闻办公室, "抗击新冠肺炎疫情的中国行动白皮书," 新华社, 2020-06-07, http://www.xinhuanet.com/politics/2020-06/07/c_1126083364.htm. Like Xi Jinping's January 7 "requirements," details of Li Keqiang's January 13 "requirements" have not been made public.
22. 国务院新闻办公室, "抗击新冠肺炎疫情的中国行动白皮书."
23. 国务院新闻办公室, "抗击新冠肺炎疫情的中国行动白皮书."
24. "国家卫生健康委召开全国电视电话会议，部署新型冠状病毒感染肺炎防控工作," 2020-01-14, http://www.nhc.gov.cn/xcs/fkdt/202002/e5e8a132ef8b42d484e6df53d4d110c1.shtml; https://news.sina.com.cn/c/2020-02-27/doc-iimxyqvz6197615.shtml. While this news release carried an official date of January 14, it was posted in late February as the html link with "2020-02" indicates. Sina.com first carried the release on February 27, 2020.
25. "国家卫生健康委召开全国电视电话会议, 部署新型冠状病毒感染肺炎防控工作."
26. "国家卫生健康委召开全国电视电话会议, 部署新型冠状病毒感染肺炎防控工作."
27. "国家卫生健康委召开全国电视电话会议, 部署新型冠状病毒感染肺炎防控工作."
28. An NHC statement of January 19, 2020, referred to a national teleconference in the health system but did not give the date of the meeting.
29. "国家卫生健康委召开全国电视电话会议, 部署新型冠状病毒感染肺炎防控工作."
30. Interview with public health specialists (LF22).
31. See, for example, 王燕, 郑新媚, "北京地坛医院: 抗疫路上, 地坛人74载从未缺席"; "卫健委专家组成员王广发出院了，回答了我们8个问题," 中国青年报-冰点周刊, 2020-02-02, https://mp.weixin.qq.com/s/DWcRVz10zps27VIrml_Khg.
32. 蒋荣猛, "新型冠状病毒肺炎诊疗方案试行第一版至第六版的制修订历程," 中华传染病杂志 38, no. 3 (2020): 129–133.

33. 国家卫生健康委, "国家卫生健康委办公厅关于印发新型冠状病毒感染的肺炎诊疗和防控等方案的通知," 2020-01-15.
34. "国务院新闻办公室2020年1月22日新闻发布会文字实录," 国家卫生健康委员会, 2020-01-22, http://www.nhc.gov.cn/xcs/fkdt/202001/61add0d230e047eaab777d062920d8a8.shtml.
35. "官旭华: 冲锋在传染病防治一线的侦察兵," 湖北e家庭, 2022-07-22, https://m.thepaper.cn/newsDetail_forward_19142402.
36. "武汉机场火车站等地安装红外线测温仪, 加强旅客体温检测工作," 北京日报新媒体, 2020-01-19, https://www.takefoto.cn/viewnews-2023810.html.
37. Ma's January 15 visit was first revealed to the public on January 22 by NHC vice minister Li Bin.
38. "新型冠状病毒感染的肺炎疫情知识问答," 武汉市卫生健康委员会, 2020-01-15, https://wjw.wuhan.gov.cn/gsgg/202004/t20200430_1199594.shtml.
39. "新型冠状病毒感染的肺炎疫情知识问答."
40. "新型冠状病毒肺炎疫情，防控进行时!," 央视网, 20200115, 2020-01-15, https://tv.cctv.com/2020/01/15/VIDEVPaxZBFtDLGUA6mk5PW2200115.shtml.
41. "黄冈抗疫记," CCTV13-央视新闻调查, 2020-02-23, https://mp.weixin.qq.com/s/k48gTZtTevoZBYEL36MxbA. Transcript.
42. Yang Yang et al. "Epidemiological and Clinical Features of the 2019 Novel Coronavirus Outbreak in China," Medrxiv, 2020-02, https://www.medrxiv.org/content/10.1101/2020.02.10.20021675v2.
43. "湖北省卫健委书记被免职事件始末," 网易新闻 政治圈, 2020-02-11, http://www.hxnews.com/news/gn/shxw/202002/11/1858717.shtml.
44. "安评所工会组织全所新春包饺活动," 湖北省疾病预防控制中心, 2020-01-19, http://www.hbcdc.cn/xwdt/gzdt/6657.htm.
45. Personal interview.
46. Jacinta Chen et al., "COVID-19 and Singapore: From Early Response to Circuit Breaker," *Annals, Academy of Medicine, Singapore* 49 (2020): 561–572; Kai Kupferschmidt, "This Biologist Helped Trace SARS to Bats. Now, He's Working to Uncover the Origins of COVID-19," *Science*, 2020-09-30, https://www.science.org/news/2020/09/biologist-helped-trace-sars-bats-now-hes-working-uncover-origins-covid-19.
47. "市文化和旅游局政府购买2020春节文化旅游惠民活动氛围布置服务的公告," 武汉市文化和旅游局, 2020-01-17, http://wlj.wuhan.gov.cn/zwgk_27/zwdt/tzgg/202008/t20200827_1436951.shtml.
48. 陈月芹, "万家宴后的百步亭," 经济观察报, 2020-02-06, http://www.eeo.com.cn/2020/0206/375757.shtml; "封城二十日里的武汉百步亭, 听社区工作者口述," 澎湃新闻, 2020-02-13, https://www.yicai.com/news/100502945.html.
49. "'万家宴'里过小年," 新华网, 2020-01-18, http://www.xinhuanet.com/photo/2020-01/18/c_1125478854.htm.
50. "疫情可防可控—武汉市就新型冠状病毒感染的肺炎综合防控工作答记者问," 新华网, 2020-01-19, www.xinhuanet.com/politics/2020-01/19/c_1125480602.htm.
51. "疫情可防可控—武汉市就新型冠状病毒感染的肺炎综合防控工作答记者问."
52. 孟祥夫, "国家卫生健康委疾病预防控制局: 筑牢坚强屏障 护佑人民健康," 人民网-人民日报, 2021-05-18, http://dangjian.people.com.cn/n1/2021/0518/c117092-32106078.html.
53. 国家卫生健康委直属机关党委, "战疫路上, 他两次逆行," 旗帜网, 2020-03-10, http://www.qizhiwang.org.cn/n1/2020/0310/c431695-31625118.html.

54. 岳琦 et al., “那是最痛苦的回忆: 武汉发热门诊高压60天,” 每日经济新闻, 2020-03-02, http://www.nbd.com.cn/articles/2020-03-02/1413076.html.
55. 国家卫生健康委直属机关党委, “李大川: 始终奔忙在战疫一线,” 旗帜网, 2020-03-07, http://dangjian.people.com.cn/n1/2020/0307/c117092-31621766.html.
56. 俞琴, 黎诗韵, “专访卫健委派武汉第二批专家: 为何没发现人传人?” 财经, 2020-02-26, https://news.caijingmobile.com/article/detail/412839.
57. “民进会员王广发: 在抗击新冠肺炎疫情中奔跑,” 团结网, 2020-07-03, http://www.tuanjiewang.cn/zhuanti/2020-07/03/content_8882261.htm.
58. “卫健委专家组成员王广发出院了, 回答了我们8个问题”; 赵孟, 陈鑫, “卫健委专家组成员王广发回应‘可防可控,’” 界面新闻, 2020-02-01, https://new.qq.com/omn/20200201/20200201A03EDU00.html.
59. “卫健委专家组成员王广发出院了, 回答了我们8个问题.”
60. 王广发, “感染新冠肺炎的第一个专家组成员——我的经历,” 国讯网, 2021-09-25, https://www.gxrhfz.com/guonei/173872.html.
61. “北京大学第一医院医生王广发治愈出院,” 新华网, 2020-01-30, http://www.xinhuanet.com/politics/2020-01/30/c_1125513337.htm.
62. “卫健委专家组成员王广发出院了, 回答了我们8个问题.”
63. An Imperial College team led by Neil Ferguson released the results of their modeling and analysis on January 17, 2020. They estimated that there might be 1,700 cases in Wuhan as of January 12, 2020. This result was picked up by the China CDC monitoring team and summed up in their bulletin for January 19.
64. 高申现, 左丹卉, “李天昊: 职业敏感让我必须跟踪处理,” 深圳晚报, 2020-03-14, https://www.sohu.com/a/380080367_464445 =.
65. 余海蓉, 罗莉琼, “广东第一个发病的家庭是怎么被发现的?” 读特APP-深圳市卫生健康委员会, 2020-02-25, http://www.sz.gov.cn/szzt2010/yqfk2020/szzxd/content/post_6739805.html.
66. Jasper Fuk-Woo Chan et al. “A Familial Cluster of Pneumonia Associated with the 2019 Novel Coronavirus Indicating Person-to-Person Transmission: A Study of a Family Cluster,” *The Lancet* 395, no. 10223 (2020): 514–523.
67. 王端, 文思敏, “对话高级别专家组成员袁国勇: 我在武汉看到了什么,” 财新网, 2020-03-08, https://china.caixin.com/2020-03-08/101525508.html; Chan et al., “Familial Cluster of Pneumonia.”
68. “深圳卫视专访袁国勇: 深圳防控工作真的很严格!,” 深圳卫视深视新闻, 2020-04-06, https://www.sohu.com/a/385953553_626425.
69. 余海蓉, 罗莉琼, “广东第一个发病的家庭是怎么被发现的?”
70. 晶报特别报道组, “深圳为何那么早就发现新冠肺炎人传人?,” 晶报, 2020-04-08, https://www.sznews.com/news/content/2020-04/08/content_23038420.htm.
71. 邹旋 et al., “深圳市新型冠状病毒肺炎应急响应策略和措施效果评价,” 中华流行病学杂志 41, no. 8 (2020): 1225–1230.
72. 余海蓉, 罗莉琼, “广东第一个发病的家庭是怎么被发现的?”
73. 西篱, “抗疫先锋,” 广东文坛, 2020-03-11, http://www.gdzuoxie.com/v/2020/03/12334.html.
74. 余海蓉, 罗莉琼, “广东第一个发病的家庭是怎么被发现的?”
75. 邓惠鸿, “做守护公众健康的忠诚卫士,” 广东省疾病控制中心, 2020-09-24, http://cdcp.gd.gov.cn/ywdt/jkyw/content/post_3447561.html.
76. 晶报特别报道组, “深圳为何那么早就发现新冠肺炎人传人?,” 晶报, 2020-04-08, https://www.sznews.com/news/content/2020-04/08/content_23038420.htm.

77. The Yuen team findings were published on January 24, 2020, as Chan et al., "Familial Cluster of Pneumonia."
78. 王端, 文思敏, "对话高级别专家组成员袁国勇."
79. 郑丽纯, "深圳'人传人'结论是如何得出的," 财新网, 2020-03-01, https://www.caixin.com/2020-03-01/101522551.html.
80. 赵天宇, 朱贺, "国家卫健委专家组袁国勇: '武汉肺炎'尚需确定更准确的病死率," 财经, 2020-01-27, http://m.caijing.com.cn/api/show?contentid=4640435.
81. The China CDC verified the sample for Patient WH, and an NHC expert panel ruled it to be a case of novel coronavirus infection on January 19. 郑丽纯, "深圳'人传人'结论是如何得出的."
82. "As Thailand Notes 2nd nCoV Case, CDC Begins Airport Screening," CIDRAP, 2020-01-17, https://www.cidrap.umn.edu/news-perspective/2020/01/thailand-notes-2nd-ncov-case-cdc-begins-airport-screening.
83. 杨楠, 何沛芸, "重组金银潭：疫情暴风眼的秘密," 南方周末, 2020-03-05, http://www.infzm.com/contents/178385.
84. Personal interview.
85. "新型冠状病毒感染的肺炎诊疗方案(试行第二版)," NHC, 2020-01-18, https://zh.wikisource.org/wiki/新型冠状病毒感染的肺炎诊疗方案（试行第二版）.
86. "面对一场没有硝烟的战疫, 与时间赛跑的科研人员是如何努力'抓到'元凶," CCTV记录, 2021-04-06, video, https://www.youtube.com/watch?v=MkvIo_zsZPE.
87. It also greenlighted the visit of a small WHO team comprised of members of the WHO China Office and the WHO Regional Office for the Western Pacific. Dr. Gauden Galea, the WHO representative in China, was part of this team that visited Wuhan on January 20–21. According to Gauden Galea, the WHO experts were quickly informed during their visit to Wuhan that there were two healthcare worker infections with the novel coronavirus. 萧辉, 包志明, 高昱, "武汉疫情中的中南医院: 他们打满全场," 财经周刊, no. 14, 2020-04-13, weekly.caixin.com/2020-04-10/101540932.html, archived version at https://archive.ph/vmPbn; Tom Cheshire, "Coronavirus: WHO 'Not Invited' to Join China's COVID-19 Investigations," Skynews, 2020-04-30, https://news.sky.com/story/coronavirus-who-not-invited-to-join-chinas-covid-19-investigations-11981193; "WHO Timeline—COVID-19," 2020-04-27, https://www.who.int/news/item/27-04-2020-who-timeline—covid-19.
88. 王端, 文思敏, "对话高级别专家组成员袁国勇."
89. 张丹丹, "73岁李兰娟: 这个险我是一定要冒的," 环球人物, 2020-04-02, https://www.msweekly.com/show.html?id=118124.
90. 高渊, "李兰娟七章: 一位传染病专家的三进武汉," 上观新闻, 2020-11-08, http://baijiahao.baidu.com/s?id=1682758962924572109.
91. "面对一场没有硝烟的战疫, 与时间赛跑的科研人员是如何努力'抓到'元凶."
92. 叶依, 你好, 钟南山 (广州: 广东教育出版社, 2020), 3.
93. "面对一场没有硝烟的战疫, 与时间赛跑的科研人员是如何努力'抓到'元凶."
94. 叶依, 你好, 钟南山, 3.
95. 叶依, 你好, 钟南山, 3.
96. 熊育群, 钟南山: 苍生在上 (广州: 花城出版社, 2020), 4–5.
97. 熊育群, 钟南山, 4–5.
98. 叶依, 你好, 钟南山, 3.
99. Yingdan Lu, Jennifer Pan, and Yiqing Xu, "Public Sentiment on Chinese Social Media during the Emergence of COVID-19," *Journal of Quantitative Description: Digital Media* 1 (2021): 1–47.

Chapter 11

1. “面对一场没有硝烟的战疫, 与时间赛跑的科研人员是如何努力’抓到’元凶,” CCTV记录, 2021-04-06, video, https://www.youtube.com/watch?v=MkvIo_zsZPE.
2. “从香港专家组成员袁国勇了解到深圳的肺炎家庭病例, 引起钟南山的警觉,” 凤凰网视频-问答神州, 2021-04-13, video, https://tech.ifeng.com/c/85P19HlOMFW.
3. “钟南山: 湖北当时的实际情况, 远比公开的要严重,” 健康时报网, 2020-03-19, http://www.jksb.com.cn/html/2020/jjxxgzbd_0319/160807.html.
4. Quoted in 萧辉, 包志明, 高昱, “武汉疫情中的中南医院: 他们打满全场,” 财经周刊, 14, 2020-04-13, weekly.caixin.com/2020-04-10/101540932.html, archived version at https://archive.ph/vmPbn.
5. “杜斌: 最后的坚守,” 央视网, 2020-04-19, video, https://tv.cctv.com/2020/04/19/VIDEbA5FLfiAQEllcqMK5Qxo200419.shtml; 杨楠, 汤禹成, “专访卫健委高级别专家组成员杜斌: 这一切与英雄主义无关,” 南方人物周刊, 2020-03-13, https://www.infzm.com/contents/179126; “曾光: 武汉的战役是在敌我界限不清的前提下开始的,” 环球人物, 2020-02-11, https://www.sohu.com/a/372175280_120118844.
6. “曾光: 疫情发生时专家组去武汉时, 没见到省市主要负责人,” 新京报, 2020-03-25, http://www.bjnews.com.cn/feature/2020/03/25/708524.html.
7. 王端, 文思敏, “对话高级别专家组成员袁国勇: 我在武汉看到了什么,” 财新网, 2020-03-08, https://china.caixin.com/2020-03-08/101525508.html.
8. David Culver and Nectar Gan, “Lack of Immunity Means China Is Vulnerable to Another Wave of Coronavirus, Top Adviser Warns,” CNN, 2020-05-16, https://edition.cnn.com/2020/05/16/asia/zhong-nanshan-coronavirus-intl-hnk/index.html.
9. 王端, 文思敏, “对话高级别专家组成员袁国勇.”
10. “黄冈抗疫记,” CCTV13-央视新闻调查, 2020-02-23, https://mp.weixin.qq.com/s/k48gTZtTevoZBYEL36MxbA.
11. “黄冈抗疫记.”
12. 王端, 文思敏, “对话高级别专家组成员袁国勇”; Culver and Gan, “Lack of Immunity Means China Is Vulnerable.”
13. “一级响应,” 上海广播电视台, 湖北广播电视台, 2021, video, episode 1, https://www.youtube.com/watch?v=mCT2fp7QLlE&t=607s.
14. “国家卫生健康委员会高级别专家组就新型冠状病毒感染的肺炎疫情答记者问,” 2020-01-21, http://www.nhc.gov.cn/xcs/s7847/202001/8d735f0bb50b45af928d9944d16950c8.shtml.
15. 王端, 文思敏, “对话高级别专家组成员袁国勇”; Culver and Gan, “Lack of Immunity Means China Is Vulnerable.”
16. “专访武汉协和医院赵洪洋,” 神外前沿, 2020-06-24, https://www.sohu.com/a/403808325_130047.
17. 胡锡进, “如果钟南山不说, 是不是武汉卫健委会继续隐瞒15名医务被感染?,” 胡锡进微博-凤凰网, 2020-01-21, https://news.ifeng.com/c/7tPeT5QRTsG.
18. 叶依, 你好，钟南山 (广州: 广东教育出版社, 2020), 8.
19. 李兰娟, “如果不封城, 国家的损失就太大了,” 中国卫生杂志, no. 4 (2020): 14–19.
20. 王端, 文思敏, “对话高级别专家组成员袁国勇.”
21. “武汉封城建议者: 向武汉人民致敬，向援助武汉的人致敬,” 凤凰网财经, 2020-05-10, https://finance.ifeng.com/c/7wM0E6Bs8PI.
22. Personal interview.
23. 李兰娟, “如果不封城,国家的损失就太大了.”

24. 西篱, “抗疫先锋,” 广东文坛, 2020-03-11, http://cms.gdzuoxie.com/?c=Article&a=view&id=12334.
25. “环球称: 非典晚报瞒报那样的事在中国不会重演了,” 环球时报, 2020-01-19, https://news.sina.cn/gn/2020-01-20/detail-iihnzhha3580323.d.html.
26. “深圳通报首例肺炎确诊病例情况, 另有8例观察病例隔离治疗,” 新华网, 2020-01-20, http://www.xinhuanet.com/politics/2020-01/20/c_1125486144.htm.
27. 叶依, 你好，钟南山, 8. The State Council Information Office white paper states, “late that night, following careful study and assessment, members of the senior experts’ team [concluded that] human to human transmission of the novel coronavirus has clearly occurred.” 国务院新闻办公室, 抗击新冠肺炎疫情的中国行动, 2020–06, www.gov.cn/zhengce/2020-06/07/content_5517737.htm.
28. 李兰娟, “如果不封城,国家的损失就太大了.”
29. Xi Jinping was Zhejiang governor (October 2002–January 2003) and party secretary (November 2002–March 2007).
30. “一级响应.”
31. 沙雪良, “防控新型冠状病毒，国务院常务会请两位院士建言,” 新京报, 2020-01-21, https://www.bjnews.com.cn/detail/157960330015268.html.
32. 王端, 文思敏, “对话高级别专家组成员袁国勇.”
33. 李兰娟, “如果不封城,国家的损失就太大了.”
34. 王端, 文思敏, “对话高级别专家组成员袁国勇.”
35. Peter Hao et al., “Guang Zeng, China CDC’s Former Chief Expert of Epidemiology,” *China CDC Weekly* 2, no. 45 (2020, November 6): 887–888; Guanfu Fang, Wei Li, and Ying Zhu, “The Shadow of the Epidemic: Long-Term Impacts of Meningitis Exposure on Risk Preference and Behaviors,” *World Development* 157 (2022): 105937; Fan Ka Wai, “Epidemic Cerebrospinal Meningitis during the Cultural Revolution,” *Extrême-Orient Extrême-Occident* no. 37 (2014): 197–232.
36. 曾光, “疫情下完善公共卫生体系的思考,” 爱思想, 2020-04-24, https://www.aisixiang.com/data/121012.html.
37. 高珧, “浙江发现5例武汉来浙发热呼吸道症状患者,” 央视新闻, 2020-01-20, https://weibo.com/2656274875/IqkydFW0z?type=comment#_rnd1633674007213. Citation is to a later and edited version.
38. 李兰娟, “如果不封城, 国家的损失就太大了”; 毛晓琼, 吴晔婷, 王晨, “被新型冠状病毒疫情波及, 浙江是怎样防控的?,” 八点健闻, 2020-01-28, https://zhuanlan.zhihu.com/p/104259366. Dr. Li was in close touch with Zhang Ping, director general of the Zhejiang Provincial Health Commission. A source told me that the NHC leadership was then not happy with Zhejiang releasing the announcement without prior approval by the NHC.
39. The specific timing of this meeting was noted by NHC vice minister Li Bin in “国务院新闻办公室2020年1月22日新闻发布会文字实录,” 国家卫生健康委员会宣传司, 2020-01-22, http://www.nhc.gov.cn/xcs/ptpxw/202001/61add0d230e047eaab777d062920d8a8.shtml.
40. “习近平对新型冠状病毒感染的肺炎疫情作出重要指示,” 新华网, 2020-01-20, http://www.xinhuanet.com/politics/leaders/2020-01/20/c_1125486561.htm.
41. “习近平对新型冠状病毒感染的肺炎疫情作出重要指示.”
42. Personal interview; 杨楠, 汤禹成, “专访卫健委高级别专家组成员杜斌.”
43. Matthew Levy and Joshua Tasoff, “Exponential-Growth Bias and Overconfidence,” *Journal of Economic Psychology* 58 (2017): 1–14; Ritwik Banerjee, Joydeep Bhattacharya, and Priyama Majumdar, “Exponential-Growth Prediction Bias and Compliance with Safety

Measures Related to COVID-19," *Social Science & Medicine* 268 (2021): 113473; Martin Schonger and Daniela Sele, "How to Better Communicate the Exponential Growth of Infectious Diseases," *PLoS One* 15, no. 12 (2020): e0242839.

44. "春节前国务院开的这个常务会,李克强请来钟南山和李兰娟," 中国政府网, 2020-01-21, http://www.gov.cn/premier/2020-01/21/content_5471097.htm.
45. "春节前国务院开的这个常务会,李克强请来钟南山和李兰娟."
46. "一级响应."
47. 叶依,你好，钟南山,9.
48. 何黎 et al.,"李兰娟:昨天建议武汉封城,今天国家行动了," 钱江晚报, 2020-01-23, https://baijiahao.baidu.com/s?id=1656497853691259775.
49. "曾光: 疫情发生时专家组去武汉没见到省市主要领导, 这是遗憾," 健康时报, 2020-03-24, https://www.thepaper.cn/newsDetail_forward_6663300.
50. "疫线疾控人: 6, 使命与担当," 健康报, 2020, https://mp.weixin.qq.com/s/HjMBvIWcZHeSKHhlERAcpw. Video.
51. "中华人民共和国国家卫生健康委员会公告2020年第1号," 2020-01-20, http://www.nhc.gov.cn/jkj/s7916/202001/44a3b8245e8049d2837a4f27529cd386.shtml.
52. "新型冠状病毒感染的肺炎纳入法定传染病管理," 疾病预防控制局, 2020-01-20, http://www.nhc.gov.cn/jkj/s7915/202001/e4e2d5e6f01147e0a8df3f6701d49f33.shtml.
53. "春节前国务院开的这个常务会,李克强请来钟南山和李兰娟."
54. "疫情可防可控——武汉市就新型冠状病毒感染的肺炎综合防控工作答记者问," 新华网, 2020-01-19, www.xinhuanet.com/politics/2020-01/19/c_1125480602.htm.
55. "新型冠状病毒肺炎, 情况如何—白岩松专访国家卫健委高级别专家组组长钟南山," 中国记协网, 2021-10-25, http://www.zgjx.cn/2021-10/25/c_1310257075.htm.
56. Members of the Senior Advisory Panel, except for Du Bin, also met with the press to explain their positions late in the afternoon of January 20. Gao Fu, who had studiously avoided the limelight since the initial outbreak, made his first public comment on the Wuhan situation. However, the edited transcript of this presser event went online after Dr. Zhong's live interview and paled in importance. "国家卫健委高级别专家组就新型冠状病毒肺炎答记者问," 央视新闻客户端, 2020-01-20, http://m.news.cctv.com/2020/01/20/ARTIF4Fl7LEu8TRqIsnde93B200120.shtml.
57. In fact, at the afternoon press event, Zhong had stated that he did not anticipate a major increase in the number of cases during the Lunar New Year. He also did not believe this outbreak would "have as big a social impact and economic damage as SARS did 17 years ago." "国家卫健委高级别专家组就新型冠状病毒肺炎答记者问."
58. "白岩松八问钟南山: 新型冠状病毒肺炎, 情况到底如何?," 央视新闻客户端, 2020-01-21, http://m.news.cctv.com/2020/01/20/ARTIpzG9gFnLXsE7amZvU9MY200120.shtml.
59. "卫健委专家高福院士: 疫区'口罩文化'至关重要," 新京报, 2020-01-24, https://finance.sina.com.cn/china/2020-01-24/doc-iihnzahk6095278.shtml.
60. "春节前国务院开的这个常务会,李克强请来钟南山和李兰娟."
61. "国家卫健委高级别专家组就新型冠状病毒肺炎答记者问."
62. "孙春兰主持召开国务院应对新型冠状病毒感染的肺炎疫情联防联控工作机制会议," 新华社, 2020-01-24, http://www.gov.cn/guowuyuan/2020-01/24/content_5472048.htm.
63. 杨楠,汤禹成,"专访卫健委高级别专家组成员杜斌."
64. "马国强部署武汉市疫情防控工作, 集中一切力量, 坚决遏制疫情蔓延, 湖北日报," 2020-01-23, http://wjw.wuhan.gov.cn/ztzl_28/fk/fkdt/202004/t20200430_1196725.shtml.

65. 郑汝可, “武汉升级防控措施, 成立肺炎疫情防控指挥部,” 新京报, 2020-01-21, http://www.bjnews.com.cn/news/2020/01/21/677247.html.
66. “全力以赴打赢阻击战—专访武汉市市长周先旺,” 新华网, 2020-01-22, http://www.xinhuanet.com/2020-01/22/c_1125495524.htm.
67. “全力以赴打赢阻击战—专访武汉市市长周先旺.”
68. “全力以赴打赢阻击战—专访武汉市市长周先旺.”
69. “武汉今起派送20万张惠民旅游券,” 荆楚网, 2020-01-20, https://news.sina.com.cn/c/2020-01-21/doc-iihnzahk5505095.shtml. A postponement of this activity was announced on January 21, 2020.
70. “1月21日, 2020年湖北省春节团拜会文艺演出在洪山礼堂圆满举办,” 荆楚通讯, 2020-01-23, https://www.163.com/dy/article/F3JLGIII0525DVBA.html.
71. “武汉要求在公共场所佩戴口罩,” 中国新闻网, 2020-01-22, http://www.chinanews.com/gn/2020/01-22/9067622.shtml.
72. 王端, “管轶: 新冠肺炎发展曲线与SARS高度相似,” 财新网, 2020-01-20, https://www.caixin.com/2020-01-20/101506222.html.
73. 王端, 文思敏, “管轶: 去过武汉请自我隔离,” 财新网, 2020-01-23, https://china.caixin.com/2020-01-23/101507672.html.
74. 方毅, 亚泽, 千林, “一个武汉人的隔离33天,” 访他者, 2020-03-11, https://mp.weixin.qq.com/s/J_zVZrcyYT5K-3tocx9ubw.
75. 王端, 文思敏, “管轶: 去过武汉请自我隔离.”
76. “武汉市卫生健康委关于市民关心的几个问题的答复,” 2020-01-23, http://wjw.hubei.gov.cn/bmdt/ztzl/fkxxgzbdgrfyyq/xxfb/202001/t20200123_2014585.shtml.
77. 向凯, “记者凌晨探访武汉发热门诊,” 新京报, 2020-01-22, http://www.bjnews.com.cn/news/2020/01/22/677764.html.
78. 杨楠, 汤禹成, “专访卫健委高级别专家组成员杜斌.”
79. 张定宇, “我在风暴之眼,” 中央广播电视总台, *武汉! 武汉! 2020战疫口述实录* (北京: 现代出版社, 2020), 3–17.
80. 杨楠, 何沛芸, “重组金银潭：疫情暴风眼的秘密,” 南方周末, 2020-03-05, http://www.infzm.com/contents/178385.
81. Robert Anders, “Patient Safety Time for Federally Mandated Registered Nurse to Patient Ratios,” *Nursing Forum* 56, no. 4 (2021), 1038–1043.
82. 张定宇, “我在风暴之眼,” 13.
83. 张定宇, “我在风暴之眼,” 13.
84. 张定宇, “我在风暴之眼,” 13.
85. On the Wuhan Red Cross Society Hospital, see “离华南海鲜市场最近的定点医院 疫情期间经历了什么?,” 央视新闻客户端, 2020-03-28, m.news.cctv.com/2020/03/28/ARTIO3xmwPp9lZ0GCACOL8oe200328.shtml; 杨楠, 蒯乐昊, 徐梅, “危城勇士: 武汉医疗抗疫一线实录,” 南方人物周刊, 2020-02-27, https://www.nfpeople.com/index.php/article/9880.
86. 龚菁琦, “发哨子的人,” 人物, 2020-03-10, https://www.weibo.com/ttarticle/p/show?id=2309404480863474679890.
87. 杨海, “武汉市中心医院医生: 传染病留给大家反应的时间太短了,” 中国青年报-冰点周刊, 2020-03-13, https://terminus2049.github.io/archive/2020/03/13/bing-dian.html.
88. 王达, “疫情风暴下, 一座医院的坚守: 武汉市红十字会医院抗击新冠肺炎疫情实录,” 中国红十字报, 2020-02-28, https://www.redcross.org.cn/html/2020-02/67372.html.
89. 王达, “疫情风暴下, 一座医院的坚守.”

90. "离华南海鲜市场最近的定点医院，疫情期间经历了什么?"; 雷宇，王鑫昕，"80后院长的战疫百日记忆，" 中国青年报，2020-04-10，http://www.xinhuanet.com/politics/2020-04/10/c_1125835363.htm.
91. 王达，"疫情风暴下，一座医院的坚守."
92. Quoted in "离华南海鲜市场最近的定点医院，疫情期间经历了什么?"
93. 萧辉，"封城那一夜，" 2020-01-25, http://xiaohui.blog.caixin.com/archives/220350.
94. Xinhua News Agency, "Xi's Yunnan Tour a Big Push for China's Moderately Prosperous Society," *China Daily*, 2020-01-22, www.chinadaily.com.cn/a/202001/22/WS5e27a6d0a310128217272ace.html.
95. 任志强，"人民的生命被病毒和体制的重病共同伤害，" 中国数字时代，2020-03-12, https://chinadigitaltimes.net/chinese/638127.html.
96. 邓琦 et al., "武汉'封城'背后：确认病毒'人传人'的21天，" 新京报，2020-01-24, http://www.bjnews.com.cn/news/2020/01/24/678679.html.
97. 吴庆才，"专访王广发：'我是怎么被感染的?,'" 中国新闻网，2020-01-23, https://www.chinanews.com.cn/gn/2020/01-23/9068408.shtml.
98. "用活大数据，为疫情防控赢得时间—记交通运输部公路科学研究院高级工程师刘冬梅，" 旗帜网，2020-03-08, http://www.qizhiwang.org.cn/n1/2020/0308/c431695-31621867.html.
99. 新华社记者，"关键时刻的关键抉择—习近平总书记作出关闭离汉通道重大决策综述，" 新华网，2020-09-08, www.xinhuanet.com/politics/leaders/2020-09/08/c_1126464092.htm.
100. "孙春兰在武汉考察新型冠状病毒感染的肺炎疫情防控工作，" 新华社，2020-01-22, http://www.gov.cn/guowuyuan/2020-01/22/content_5471734.htm.
101. 李兰娟，"如果不封城，国家的损失就太大了."
102. "李兰娟：相隔十七年的两次果敢，" 科技日报，2020-06-04, http://www.chinanews.com/gn/2020/06-04/9202771.shtml.
103. 李兰娟，"如果不封城，国家的损失就太大了."
104. 何黎 et al., "李兰娟."
105. World Health Organization, "Statement on the First Meeting of the International Health Regulations (2005) Emergency Committee Regarding the Outbreak of Novel Coronavirus (2019-nCoV)," 2020-01-23, https://www.who.int/news/item/23-01-2020-statement-on-the-meeting-of-the-international-health-regulations-(2005)-emergency-committee-regarding-the-outbreak-of-novel-coronavirus-(2019-ncov).
106. "央视对话武汉市长周先旺实录：封城是艰难决定，疫情太突然，" 澎湃新闻，2020-01-27, https://news.sina.com.cn/c/2020-01-28/doc-iihnzahk6603203.shtml.
107. "央视对话武汉市长周先旺实录."
108. "李兰娟."
109. World Health Organization, "Statement on the First Meeting."
110. 马晓华，"时代的尘埃：一位武汉基层官员眼中的封城之前八小时，" 第一财经，2020-03-15, https://www.yicai.com/news/100548961.html.
111. "2020春天纪事，" CCTV记录，2020-09-08, video, episode 4, https://tv.cctv.com/2020/09/04/VIDA2RwP6u7FU6RPgDzr2wG8200904.shtml.
112. "2020春天纪事."
113. "一级响应."
114. Claire Che et al., "China Sacrifices a Province to Save the World from Coronavirus," Bloomberg News, 2020-02-05, https://www.bloomberg.com/news/articles/2020-02-05/china-sacrifices-a-province-to-save-the-world-from-coronavirus.

115. The Chinese original is 壮士扼腕, 买欣全, "做一名外交战线默默无闻的逆行者," 旗帜网, 2020-02-24, http://www.qizhiwang.org.cn/n1/2020/0224/c431695-31601962.html.
116. "梁军: 塔台上的见证," 央视网-面对面, 2020-04-12, video, https://tv.cctv.com/2020/04/12/VIDEv8K7YgcBP9mGGmOjg0XL200412.shtml.
117. 林志吟, 吴俊捷, 权小星, "多个省市启动一级响应抗击疫情，为何湖北省却不是最快的？第一财经," 2020-01-24, https://www.yicai.com/news/100480475.html.
118. Tibet was the exception, and it activated on January 29. "中国内地31省份全部启动突发公共卫生事件一级响应," 财新网, 2020-01-29, https://china.caixin.com/2020-01-29/101509411.html.
119. 杨楠, 汤禹成, "专访卫健委高级别专家组成员杜斌: 这一切与英雄主义无关," 南方人物周刊, 2020-03-13，https://www.infzm.com/contents/179126.

Chapter 12

1. 陈伟 et al., "我国新型冠状病毒肺炎疫情早期围堵策略概述," 中华预防医学杂志 54, no. 3 (2020): 239–244; "万众一心迎挑战, 众志成城战疫情—全国总动员打响疫情防控阻击战纪实," 新华社, 2020-01-27, http://www.gov.cn/xinwen/2020-01/27/content_5472356.htm.
2. Emily Feng, "Wuhan's Lockdown Memories 1 Year Later: Pride, Anger, Deep Pain," NPR, *All Things Considered*, 2021-01-23, https://www.npr.org/sections/goatsandsoda/2021/01/23/959618838/wuhans-lockdown-memories-one-year-later-pride-anger-deep-pain.
3. Yingdan Lu, Jennifer Pan, and Yiqing Xu, "Public Sentiment on Chinese Social Media during the Emergence of COVID-19," *Journal of Quantitative Description: Digital Media* 1 (2021): 1–47.
4. 上海市卫生健康委员会, 战疫纪事*(上)* (上海: 文汇出版社2020), 139–141; "周新: 首批支援湖北医疗队中最年长的医生, 为了人民, 值得!," 文汇报, 2020-03-02, https://www.sohu.com/a/377150339_120244154; "上海交通大学医学院党委新冠肺炎疫情防控工作优秀共产党员: 陈德昌," 上海交通大学医学院委员会, 2020-03-19, https://www.shsmu.edu.cn/eydj/info/1088/9067.htm.
5. 李强, "抢命金银潭," 中国青年报-冰点周刊, 2020-03-25, https://mp.weixin.qq.com/s/4ej-1OPE47Z2cpy8Z7MbPw.
6. 任志强, "人民的生命被病毒和体制的重病共同伤害," 中国数字时代, 2020-03-12, https://chinadigitaltimes.net/chinese/638127.html.
7. "军队支援地方抗击新冠肺炎疫情新闻发布会," 国新网, 2020-03-02, http://www.scio.gov.cn/xwfbh/xwbfbh/wqfbh/42311/42634/wz42636/Document/1674383/1674383.htm.
8. 崇高使命编写组, 崇高使命: 白衣战士武汉、湖北防疫抗疫纪实 (北京: 新华出版社, 2020), 93–101.
9. Quoted in李春雷, "铁人张定宇," 人民日报, 2020-04-01, 20; 李强, "抢命金银潭."
10. 信娜, "张定宇，生死之外," 财经, 2021-04-12, magazine.caijing.com.cn/20210412/4755047.shtml.
11. "离华南海鲜市场最近的定点医院 疫情期间经历了什么?," 央视新闻客户端, 2020-03-29, http://m.cyol.com/content/2020-03/29/content_18540787.htm.
12. 白剑峰, 李红梅, 申少铁, "把人民生命安全和身体健康放在第一位," 人民日报, 2021-11-02, http://cpc.people.com.cn/n1/2021/1102/c64387-32270959.html.

13. "中共中央政治局常务委员会召开会议, 研究新型冠状病毒感染的肺炎疫情防控工作," 新华网, 2020-01-25, http://www.xinhuanet.com//politics/2020-01/25/c_1125502052.htm.
14. "中共中央印发'关于加强党的领导, 为打赢疫情防控阻击战提供坚强政治保证的通知,'" 新华社, 2020-01-28, http://www.gov.cn/zhengce/2020-01/28/content_5472753.htm; 习近平, "在中央政治局常委会会议研究应对新型冠状病毒肺炎疫情工作时的讲话 (2020-02-03)," 求是, no. 4 (2020), 2020-02-15, http://www.qstheory.cn/dukan/qs/2020-02/15/c_1125572832.htm.
15. "李克强主持召开中央应对新型冠状病毒感染肺炎疫情工作领导小组会议," 新华网, 2020-01-26, https://web.archive.org/web/20200126181054/http://www.xinhuanet.com/politics/2020-01/26/c_1125504004.htm.
16. 江琳, "主题教育, 中央指导组和巡回督导组有啥区别?," 人民日报中央厨房, 2019-10-25, http://politics.people.com.cn/n1/2019/1025/c1001-31420772.html.
17. 付朝欢, "江城今日春已半 丹心一片佑家国—记中央赴湖北指导组成员、国家发展改革委经济运行调节局电力处处长刘琼," 改革网, 2020-04-22, https://www.ndrc.gov.cn/xwdt/ztzl/fkyqfgwzxdzt/djyl/202004/t20200422_1226358.html.
18. David Bandurski, "A New Era of Struggle," China Media Project, 2019-09-19, https://chinamediaproject.org/2019/09/19/a-new-era-of-struggle/.
19. 习近平, "在中央政治局常委会会议研究应对."
20. 杨智杰, "湖北多地宣布'战时管制,' 专家称不应滥用概念," 中国新闻周刊, 2020-02-14, https://mp.weixin.qq.com/s/uoVGSC_N9ByisLSGCA3ptA.
21. 马学玲, "战疫时刻, 习近平不同寻常的八个细节," 中新网微信公众号, 2020-05-20, https://www.chinanews.com.cn/gn/2020/05-20/9190047.shtml.
22. 习近平, "在统筹推进新冠肺炎疫情防控和经济社会发展工作部署会议上的讲话," 新华网, 2020-02-23, http://www.xinhuanet.com/politics/leaders/2020-02/23/c_1125616016.htm.
23. "李克强到湖北武汉考察指导新型冠状病毒感染肺炎疫情防控工作," 中国政府网, 2020-01-27, http://www.gov.cn/guowuyuan/2020-01/27/content_5472525.htm.
24. Sometimes also translated as the Central Steering Team or Central Guiding Group.
25. "李克强到湖北武汉考察指导新型冠状病毒感染肺炎疫情防控工作."
26. 余辉, "2月以来, 国家卫健委主任在武汉都做了什么?," 政知圈, 2020-02-18, https://www.sohu.com/a/373826556_167569.
27. "国务院新闻办就中央赴湖北指导组组织开展疫情防控工作情况举行新闻发布会," 中国网, 2020-02-20, http://www.gov.cn/xinwen/2020-02/20/content_5481420.htm.
28. "战疫27天, 中央指导组金句背后的那些事," 玉渊谭天-新华网, 2020-02-22, http://www.xinhuanet.com/politics/2020-02/22/c_1125612131.htm; 杜茂林, 杨楠, 蒋芷毓, "中央指导组抗疫55天: 小半个国务院入鄂," 南方周末, 2020-03-19, https://www.infzm.com/contents/179549.
29. "中央指导组指导组织湖北疫情防控和医疗救治工作进展—国务院新闻办公室2020年2月28日新闻发布会文字实录," 宣传司, 2020-02-28, http://www.nhc.gov.cn/xcs/s3574/202002/2fb820181d8a41969bca041793c11bcb.shtml.
30. Yingdan Lu, Jennifer Pan, and Yiqing Xu, "Public Sentiment on Chinese Social Media during the Emergence of COVID-19," *Journal of Quantitative Description: Digital Media* 1 (2021): 1–47.
31. "19省份对口支援湖北16市州, 众志成城汇聚决胜之力," 央视新闻客户端, 2020-03-16, http://www.xinhuanet.com/politics/2020-03/16/c_1125718859.htm.

32. "广东战疫力量!," 广州日报客户端, 2020-04-11, https://huacheng.gz-cmc.com/pages/2020/04/11/7429a54e3c024a83936fe93004bdd72f.html.
33. "中央赴湖北指导组成员张宗久表示落实三项举措尽最大可能降低死亡率," 湖北日报, 2020-02-01, https://www.hubei.gov.cn/zhuanti/2020/gzxxgzbd/zy/202002/t20200201_2017115.shtml.
34. "抗疫前线, 张伯礼院士收到了这份特殊的生日礼物," 央视新闻客户端, 2020-03-23, http://www.xinhuanet.com/politics/2020-03/23/c_1125754747.htm.
35. 张伯礼, "中医抗疫的文化自信," 红旗文稿, no. 6 (2021), 2021-03-28, http://www.wenming.cn/ll_pd/whjs/202103/t20210328_5994001.shtml.
36. 杨楠, 汤禹成, "专访卫健委高级别专家组成员杜斌: 这一切与英雄主义无关," 南方人物周刊, 2020-03-13, https://www.infzm.com/contents/179126.
37. Martin Tobin, Franco Laghi, and Amal Jubran, "Why COVID-19 Silent Hypoxemia Is Baffling to Physicians," *American Journal of Respiratory and Critical Care Medicine* 202, no. 3 (2020): 356–360; Evangelia Akoumianaki et al., "Happy or Silent Hypoxia in COVID-19—A Misnomer Born in the Pandemic Era," *Frontiers in Physiology* 12 (2021): 745634. Technically hypoxemia (low blood oxygen level) and hypoxia (low oxygen level in tissues) are different, but they tend to be used interchangeably in clinical research publications.
38. Gentry Wilkerson et al., "Silent Hypoxia: A Harbinger of Clinical Deterioration in Patients with COVID-19," *American Journal of Emergency Medicine* 38, no. 10 (2020): 2243-e5–2243-e6; Ahsab Rahman et al., "Silent Hypoxia in COVID-19: Pathomechanism and Possible Management Strategy," *Molecular Biology Reports* 48, no. 4 (2021): 3863–3869.
39. 牛牛妈, "一位武汉呼吸科医生的口述: 那些和我插肩而过的生命," 海上柳叶刀, 2020-02-07, https://mp.weixin.qq.com/s?__biz=MzU5MTUzMjYzNQ==&mid=2247491480&idx=1&sn=d412b87069a9222f425e08a7c8a97b5e.
40. 田巧萍, "救人医生, 重症病人, 以身试药者黄朝林: 42天用6种身份与病毒较量," 长江日报, 2020-02-09, http://m.cnhubei.com/content/2020-02/09/content_12708093.html.
41. 杨楠, 汤禹成, "专访卫健委高级别专家组成员杜斌."
42. 杨楠, 何沛芸, "重组金银潭：疫情暴风眼的秘密," 南方周末, 2020-03-05，http://www.infzm.com/contents/178385.
43. 萧辉, " 中南医院急诊中心副主任: 这是一场持久战," 财新网, 2020-02-22, https://www.caixin.com/2020-02-22/101519114.html; 王昱倩, "对话中南医院ECMO团队带头人: ECMO应个性化使用," 新京报, 2020-03-04, https://www.sohu.com/a/377667407_114988.
44. 吴靖, "武汉一线医生详解新冠: 对重症病人的损害像'SARS+艾滋病,'" 八点健闻, 2020-03-10, https://mp.weixin.qq.com/s/8ewol1WUOZ_nFYzC-Gv8Ww; Dawei Wang et al., "Clinical Characteristics of 138 Hospitalized Patients with 2019 Novel Coronavirus–Infected Pneumonia in Wuhan, China," *JAMA* 323, no. 11 (2020): 1061–1069.
45. "武汉抗击新型肺炎一线医生、护士自述," 长江日报, 2020-01-26, http://wjw.wuhan.gov.cn/ztzl_28/fk/fkdt/202004/t20200430_1196903.shtml; 杨楠, 蒯乐昊, 徐梅, "危城勇士: 武汉医疗抗疫一线实录," 南方人物周刊, 2020-02-27, https://www.nfpeople.com/index.php/article/9880.
46. 杨楠, 汤禹成, "专访卫健委高级别专家组成员杜斌."
47. 浸月, "氧饱和度骤降、插管时机争议：ICU 新冠患者救治之难," 丁香园, 2020-03-19, https://mp.weixin.qq.com/s/R6yiD983xfZeAJhWwOYE-w; 杨楠, 汤禹成, "专访卫健委高级别专家组成员杜斌"; 李强, "抢命金银潭," 中国青年报-冰点周刊, 2020-03-25, https://mp.weixin.qq.com/s/4ej-1OPE47Z2cpy8Z7MbPw.

48. 凌楚眠, "这是武汉疫线最真实的抢救实况," 海上柳叶刀, 2020-02-18, https://mp.weixin.qq.com/s?__biz=MzU5MTUzMjYzNQ==&mid=2247491472&idx=1&sn=2f978c04aafb172297451aae3bfcbc85.
49. Philippe Rola et al., "Rethinking the Early Intubation Paradigm of COVID-19: Time to Change Gears?," *Clinical and Experimental Emergency Medicine* 7, no. 2 (2020): 78–80.
50. 刘志勇, "生死金银潭," 健康报, 2020-03-09, https://news.sina.cn/gn/2020-03-09/detail-iimxxstf7499522.d.html.
51. A medical team of the Fifth Medical Center of PLA General Hospital in Beijing carried out a biopsy on January 27, 2020; but this was not known in Wuhan immediately. Zhe Xu et al., "Pathological Findings of COVID-19 Associated with Acute Respiratory Distress Syndrome," *The Lancet Respiratory Medicine* 8, no. 4 (2020): 420–422.
52. Xiu-Wu Bian, "Autopsy of COVID-19 Patients in China," *National Science Review* 7, no. 9 (2020): 1414–1418.
53. 丁云, 王诗韵, "'重症八仙'郑瑞强归来, 讲述95天疫线故事," 扬州日报-扬州网, 2020-05-11, http://news.xhby.net/yz/zx/202005/t20200511_6638088.shtml; 国家卫生健康委直属机关党委, "李大川: 始终奔忙在战疫一线," 旗帜网, 2020-03-07, http://dangjian.people.com.cn/n1/2020/0307/c117092-31621766.html; "把'最硬的鳞'留下! 20位专家仍坚守武汉," 新华网, 2020-04-17, http://news.xhby.net/zt/zzccfkyq/zmnxz/202004/t20200417_6607983.shtml; 王卡拉, "杜斌: 不是'逆行出征', 这就是医生的本职工作," 新京报, 2021-09-28, https://www.bjnews.com.cn/detail/163279566414970.html.
54. 杜茂林, 杨楠, 蒋芷毓, "中央指导组抗疫55天: 小半个国务院入鄂."
55. 吴佳佳, "逢疫必上—记北京地坛医院传染病专家蒋荣猛," 经济日报, 2020-03-16, http://news.china.com.cn/2020-03/16/content_75821240.htm.
56. "新型冠状病毒感染的肺炎重症、危重症病例诊疗方案(试行), 医政医管局, 2020-01-23," http://www.nhc.gov.cn/xcs/zhengcwj/202001/9fbefc9a5fe747e98ea5baeedfb68158.shtml. This protocol defines a critical case as a patient with respiratory failure and in need of mechanical ventilation, or had shock, or had other organ failures requiring ICU intensive care.
57. 蒋荣猛, "新型冠状病毒肺炎诊疗方案试行第一版至第六版的制修订历程," 中华传染病杂志 38, no. 3 (2020): 129–133; 马海燕, "20天5个版本诊疗方案, 中国及时总结优化防疫经验," 中国新闻网, 2020-02-05, https://m.chinanews.com/wap/detail/zw/gn/2020/02-05/9080198.shtml.
58. On Zhong Nanshan, see "钟南山战疫60天全记录," 人民日报"微信公众号", 2020-03-26, https://www.12371.cn/2020/03/26/ARTI1585189821141546.shtml.
59. See, especially, Xiaobo Yang et al., "Clinical Course and Outcomes of Critically Ill Patients with SARS-Cov-2 Pneumonia in Wuhan, China: A Single-Centered, Retrospective, Observational Study," *The Lancet Respiratory Medicine* 8, no. 5 (2020): 475–481; Wang et al., "Clinical Characteristics of 138 Hospitalized Patients"; Nanshan Chen et al., "Epidemiological and Clinical Characteristics of 99 Cases of 2019 Novel Coronavirus Pneumonia in Wuhan, China: A Descriptive Study," *The Lancet* 395, no. 10223 (2020): 507–513; Chaomin Wu et al., "Risk Factors Associated with Acute Respiratory Distress Syndrome and Death in Patients with Coronavirus Disease 2019 Pneumonia in Wuhan, China," *JAMA Internal Medicine* 180, no. 7 (2020): 934–943.
60. Jasper Fuk-Woo Chan et al., "A Familial Cluster of Pneumonia Associated with the 2019 Novel Coronavirus Indicating Person-to-Person Transmission: A Study of a Family Cluster," *The Lancet* 395, no. 10223 (2020): 514–523; Peng Wu et al., "Real-Time Tentative Assessment of the Epidemiological Characteristics of Novel Coronavirus

Infections in Wuhan, China, as at 22 January 2020," *Eurosurveillance* 25, no. 3 (2020): 2000044.

61. Qun Li et al., "Early Transmission Dynamics in Wuhan, China, of Novel Coronavirus–Infected Pneumonia," *New England Journal of Medicine* (2020), https://www.nejm.org/doi/full/10.1056/NEJMoa2001316.
62. "武汉新型冠状病毒感染患者救治均由政府买单," 人民日报客户端, 2020-01-21, http://www.bjnews.com.cn/news/2020/01/21/677500.html.
63. 刘璐天, "武汉日记: 风口浪尖," 歌德学院(中国), n.d., https://www.goethe.de/ins/cn/zh/kul/fok/ver/21797734.html.
64. "电波中的抗疫," 湖北省卫生健康委员会, 2021-01-08, http://wjw.hubei.gov.cn/bmdt/ztzl/fkxxgzbdgrfyyq/yxdx/202101/t20210108_3212274.shtml.
65. 张赫, "武汉市肺科医院院长: 我们从未缺过物资," 健康时报, 2020-04-06, https://new.qq.com/omn/20200406/20200406A0OIZK00.html.
66. 田巧萍, "最早上报疫情的她, 怎样发现这种不一样的肺炎?," 长江日报, 2020-02-02, http://wjw.hubei.gov.cn/bmdt/ztzl/fkxxgzbdgrfyyq/fkdt/202002/t20200202_2017829.shtml.
67. The national total was 1,716. 国务院联防联控机制举办的新闻发布会, 2020-02-14, http://www.gov.cn/xinwen/gwylflkjz12/index.htm.
68. 樊巍, 崔萌, 杨诚, "武汉市中心医院医护人员吐真情: 疫情是面照妖镜," 环球时报, 2002-03-17, www.medsci.cn/article/show_article.do?id=2f19190169f7.
69. 钟寅, "300多名维保队员守卫武汉火神山, 雷神山医院," 现代快报, 2020-03-31, http://www.qstheory.cn/zdwz/2020-03/31/c_1125792901.htm.
70. 蒋苡芯, 李屾淼, "那些一直短缺的物资, 都是怎样运进武汉的?," 新周刊, 2020-02-02, https://mp.weixin.qq.com/s/8fAChrvwGiF9whN86pxGcw.
71. "火神山、雷神山医院建设背后的中建科技密码," 中国建设, 2020-02-21, https://www.cscec.com/zgjz_new/xwzx_new/gsyw_new/202002/3020679.html.
72. "分分秒秒跟死神夺命," 中国市场监管报-旗帜网, 2020-02-18, http://www.qizhiwang.org.cn/n1/2020/0218/c431695-31592422.html.
73. "1000万人在线观看直播修医院," 每日经济新闻, 2020-01-28, http://finance.sina.com.cn/wm/2020-01-28/doc-iihnzahk6790806.shtml.
74. See, for example, 徐海涛, "我们不煽情, 我们直接上," 海上柳叶刀, 2020-02-24, https://mp.weixin.qq.com/s/gIctnQ7XlLlLg7UOPa7aDQ.
75. "这些有关雷火神山的记忆, 永不磨灭," 中华儿女报刊社微信公众号, 2020-04-14, https://new.qq.com/rain/a/20210716A0D9GD00.
76. 江月, "除了'雷火', 武汉还有这样一家医院," 三联生活周刊, 2020-03-13, https://mp.weixin.qq.com/s/4IvGptHaIJWPeLH5vtfEDA.
77. 铃雨, "泰康+同济医院, '英雄联盟'携手助力提升公共卫生事件应对能力," 第一财经, 2020-11-12, https://www.yicai.com/news/100834873.html.
78. 孙利, 王锐涛, "记者实地探访湖北省妇幼保健院光谷院区," 央广网, 2020-02-18, https://www.sohu.com/a/374052301_362042; 葛欣, 赖瑜鸿, "湖北省妇幼保健院光谷院区开始全面收治患者," 解放军报, 2020-02-22, https://shareapp.cyol.com/cmsfile/News/202002/22/share336160.html.
79. Transcript of "王辰视频连线'新闻1+1,'" 2020-02-05, https://www.bilibili.com/read/cv4587665; video link at http://www.xinhuanet.com/politics/2020-02/06/c_1125536763.htm.

80. 汤禹成，谭畅，“谁是假阴性新冠肺炎病人，” 南方周末，2020-02-06，https://project-gutenberg.github.io/nCovMemory-Web/post/01b2e63206aa520084a90b32bfaa15a9/.
81. 杜茂林, 杨楠, 蒋芷毓, “中央指导组抗疫55天: 小半个国务院入鄂.”
82. 张旭东，赵文君，方亚东，“关键时期的关键之举—中国工程院副院长、呼吸与危重症医学专家王辰回应武汉疫情防控焦点问题，” 新华网2020-02-05, http://www.xinhuanet.com/politics/2020-02/05/c_1125532030.htm.
83. “战疫27天, 中央指导组金句背后的那些事.”
84. 一人君 (pseudonym)，“周先旺‘消失’的15天，” i看见，2020-03-02 https://mp.weixin.qq.com/s?__biz=MzAwODI5MjU3MQ==&mid=2652174867&idx=1&sn=8e2d36cd112cb1a398ae198c85a76253&chksm.
85. 纪红建，“生命之舱，” 人民日报，2020-03-18, http://www.xinhuanet.com/local/2020-03/18/c_1125727468.htm; 刘璐天, “武汉日记.”
86. “战疫27天, 中央指导组金句背后的那些事.”
87. 中国贸促会直属机关党委, “方舱里的志愿者,” 旗帜网, 2020-02-25, http://www.qizhiwang.org.cn/n1/2020/0225/c431695-31603682.html.
88. Transcript of “王辰视频连线‘新闻1+1.’”
89. 张磊,“被改变的生活，” 健康报，2020-03-10, http://www.nhc.gov.cn/wjw/mtbd/202003/b86ddbc4c5644ae0866eda44eeeffcbd.shtml.
90. X. Wang et al., “Clinical Characteristics of Non-Critically Ill Patients with Novel Coronavirus Infection (COVID-19) in a Fangcang Hospital,” *Clinical Microbiology and Infection* 26, no. 8 (2020): 1063–1068.
91. Quoted in 张磊，“一家方舱医院的创建史，” 健康报，2020-03-10, https://mp.weixin.qq.com/s/5t2fIVrDTRtep-Pxn4QdDA.
92. 刘喜梅，“一个具有‘钉钉子精神’的人，” 人民政协网，2021-03-15, http://www.rmzxb.com.cn/c/2021-03-15/2809190.shtml.
93. 刘喜梅, “一个具有‘钉钉子精神’的人.”
94. 陈玮曦, “武汉重症区六层的日与夜,” 时尚先生, 2020-03-09, https://mp.weixin.qq.com/s/xt7wN0xgvbXe2nlQSeUyoA.
95. 刘远航，黄孝光，李明子，“武汉会战，” 中国新闻周刊，2022-02-17, https://mp.weixin.qq.com/s/4oLP2aEPKYT8qI7l66ZFfw; Yaping Zhong et al., “Experiences of COVID-19 Patients in a Fangcang Shelter Hospital in China during the First Wave of the COVID-19 Pandemic: A Qualitative Descriptive Study,” *BMJ Open* 12, no. 9 (2022): e065799.
96. “新闻办就湖北组织开展疫情防控和医疗救治工作情况举行发布会，” 中国网，2020-02-15, http://www.gov.cn/xinwen/2020-02/15/content_5479126.htm; “方舟共济: 武汉疫情期间6万多张床位是如何变出来的，” 数可视，2020-03-23, https://new.qq.com/omn/20200323/20200323A0542O00.html.
97. Simiao Chen et al., “Fangcang Shelter Hospitals: A Novel Concept for Responding to Public Health Emergencies,” *The Lancet* 395, no. 10232 (2020): 1305–1314.

Chapter 13

1. 李昌禹, “筑牢疫情防控的第一道防线—记抗疫中的社区工作者,” 人民日报, 2020-09-08, http://dangjian.people.com.cn/n1/2020/0908/c117092-31853026.html; 中共民政部党组, “坚决筑牢疫情防控社区防线,” 求是, no. 20 (2020), 2020-10-16, http://www.qstheory.cn/dukan/qs/2020-10/16/c_1126614113.htm; 熊琦, “武汉: 党建引领‘微治理’激活社

区'大动力,'" 新华社, 2021-05-31, http://m.xinhuanet.com/hb/2021-05/31/c_1127515009.htm; "有一种力量, 叫中国网格员," 长安评论, 2020-02-19, https://mp.weixin.qq.com/s/dWFQ6YyXtVl7I8wGe9Gyvw.

2. 易先云, 蔡思, "一首打油诗表达正副书记的豪情壮志: 武汉'小巷总理'身患重症战斗在一线," 中国纪录, 2020-03-14, https://www.sohu.com/a/380008978_99927144; "张践, "武汉一社区临时书记: 腰部疼痛难忍, 有时躺地板上工作," 中国新闻网, 2020-02-09, http://www.xinhuanet.com/2020-02/09/c_1125549840.htm. See also 贺广华 et al., "第一道防线, 守住！武汉疫情防控一线纪实之三," 人民日报, 2020-02-05, http://cpc.people.com.cn/n1/2020/0205/c431601-31571519.html; 王馨娜, "守土有责, 守土尽责: 武汉社区工作者疫情期间工作实录," 社区, no. 6 (2020): 14–16.
3. Alex Jingwei He, Yuda Shi, and Hongdou Liu, "Crisis Governance, Chinese Style: Distinctive Features of China's Response to the Covid-19 Pandemic," *Policy Design and Practice* 3, no. 3 (2020): 242–258; Yujun Wei et al., "COVID-19 Prevention and Control in China: Grid Governance," *Journal of Public Health* 43, no. 1 (March 2021): 76–81; Tianke Zhu, Xigang Zhu, and Jian Jin, "Grid Governance in China under the COVID-19 Outbreak: Changing Neighborhood Governance," *Sustainability* 13, no. 13 (2021): 7089.
4. Fulong Wu, "China's Changing Urban Governance in the Transition towards a More Market-Oriented Economy," *Urban Studies* 39, no. 7 (2002): 1071–1093.
5. Beibei Tang, "Grid Governance in China's Urban Middle-Class Neighborhoods," *China Quarterly* 241 (2020): 43–61.
6. Jean C. Mittelstaedt, "The Grid Management System in Contemporary China," *China Information* 36, no. 1 (2022), 3–22.
7. "'武汉经验'获全国推广! 市域社会治理怎么治、治什么、靠什么？," 澎湃新闻, 2019-12-05, https://www.thepaper.cn/newsDetail_forward_5152222; "中共武汉市委关于实施'红色引擎工程'推动基层治理体系和治理能力现代化的意见 (2017-04-08)," 武汉市住房保障和房屋管理局, 2019-06-04, last accessed 2022-07-04, http://fgj.wuhan.gov.cn/fgdt/ztzl_44/hswy/202001/t20200109_725163.shtml.
8. 金雨蒙, 丁涛, "社区中的'网格英雄,'" 人民网, 2020-02-27, http://www.xinhuanet.com/politics/2020-02/27/c_1125633733.htm.
9. "'武汉经验'获全国推广! 市域社会治理怎么治、治什么、靠什么?"
10. "关于加强和改进城市基层党的建设工作的意见," 新华社, 2019-05-08, www.gov.cn/zhengce/2019-05/08/content_5389836.htm.
11. "陈一新就全国市域社会治理现代化试点工作实施方案作说明时指出以新理念新思路新方式开展试点," 人民法院新闻传媒总社, 2019-12-03, www.court.gov.cn/zixun-xiangqing-205351.html.
12. 吴靖, 王晨, "武汉社区告急: 领导干部亲自搬遗体, 基层防疫压力巨大," 八点健闻, 2020-02-02, https://new.qq.com/rain/a/20200202A0BCAR00.
13. "湖北武汉市武昌区水果湖街：区域化党建引领社区治理创新," 人民网-中国共产党新闻网, 2018-11-01, http://dangjian.people.com.cn/n1/2018/1101/c420318-30375902.html.
14. Marcel at large, "知情者口述: 盛会, 病人, 难以逾越的冬天," 荷戟周戡 2020-03-01，https://mp.weixin.qq.com/s/k0HELMTysMTZyF7ECuDKSA.
15. 刘远航, 黄孝光, 李明子, "武汉会战," 中国新闻周刊, 2022-02-17, https://mp.weixin.qq.com/s/4oLP2aEPKYT8qI7l66ZFfw.
16. "武汉市卫生健康委关于市民关心的几个问题的答复," 武汉市卫生健康委员会, 2020-01-23, http://wjw.hubei.gov.cn/bmdt/ztzl/fkxxgzbdgrfyyq/xxfb/202001/t20200123_2014585.shtml.

17. “武汉部署分级分类筛查：确保无条件收治所有疑似患者,” 长江网, 2020-01-25, https://ie.bjd.com.cn/a/202001/25/AP5e2b9218e4b0745e680ac2de.html.
18. “武汉市卫生健康委关于市民关心的几个问题的答复.”
19. 王姗姗, “陈珺: 一个人折射一段武汉抗疫史,” 中国青年报, 2020-03-24, http://m.cyol.com/yuanchuang/2020-03/24/content_18530971.htm.
20. 温如军, “百步亭在疫情中裸泳,” 中国慈善家, 2020-04-11, https://news.sina.com.cn/s/2020-04-11/doc-iircuyvh7104812.shtml.
21. 叶龙杰, “风雨百步亭,” 健康报, 2020-03-11, www.nhc.gov.cn/xcs/fkdt/202003/60fa2099b8b447b6a8e1f154347fddcf.shtml.
22. The details on Liu and his community are drawn from 叶龙杰, “风雨百步亭.”
23. 叶龙杰, “风雨百步亭.”
24. 房宫一柳 et al., “统计数字之外的人: 他们死于‘普通肺炎’?,” 财经杂志, 2020-02-01, https://mp.weixin.qq.com/s/OQGVZlrJWID9Gn4A_T5u_g. Archived at https://chinadigitaltimes.net/chinese/634014.html.
25. Sharon Chen, Dandan Li, and Claire Che, “Urns in Wuhan Prompt New Questions of Virus's Toll,” Bloomberg News, 2020-03-30, https://www.bloomberg.com/news/articles/2020-03-27/stacks-of-urns-in-wuhan-prompt-new-questions-of-virus-s-toll; Phoebe Zhang and Guo Rui, “Hurried Cremation and Curbed Mourning Rituals in Wuhan Distress Families of Covid-19 victims,” SCMP, 2020-04-03, https://www.scmp.com/news/china/society/article/3078106/hurried-cremation-and-curbed-mourning-rituals-wuhan-distress.
26. 叶龙杰, “风雨百步亭.”
27. Fang Fang, *Wuhan Diary: Dispatches from a Quarantined City*, trans. Michael Berry (New York: Harper, 2020); Thomas Whyke, Joaquin Lopez-Mugica, and Zhen T. Chen, “The Rite of Passage and Digital Mourning in Fang Fang's Wuhan Diary,” *Global Media and China* 6, no. 4 (2021): 443–459; and, more generally, Guobin Yang, *The Wuhan Lockdown* (New York: Columbia University Press, 2022).
28. 陈月芹, “万家宴后的百步亭,” 经济观察报, 2020-02-06, http://www.eeo.com.cn/2020/0206/375757.shtml.
29. Xiaoman Zhao et al., “Online Health Information Seeking Using ‘#COVID-19 Patient Seeking Help’ on Weibo in Wuhan, China,” *Journal of Medical Internet Research* 22, no. 10 (2020): e22910; Lai Wei, Elaine Yao, and Han Zhang, “Authoritarian Responsiveness and Political Attitudes during COVID-19: Evidence from Weibo and a Survey Experiment,” *Chinese Sociological Review* 55, no. 1 (2023): 1–37.
30. 石鸣, “一个武汉志愿者的封城16天,” 一条, 2020-02-07, https://mp.weixin.qq.com/s/mZyzqZbvWNC_zCe5sq45Hw.
31. 陈月芹, “万家宴后的百步亭.”
32. 卫毅 et al., “疫情时期百步亭,” 南方人物周刊, https://www.nfpeople.com/article/9896.
33. 曹政, “武汉封城这一月,” 健康报, 2020-02-20, http://wjw.hubei.gov.cn/bmdt/ztzl/fkxxgzbdgrfyyq/fkdt/202002/t20200220_2142217.shtml.
34. 吴靖, 王晨, “武汉社区告急.”
35. “湖北14名新冠肺炎疫情防控一线牺牲人员被评定为首批烈士,” 新华网, 2020-04-02, http://www.xinhuanet.com/politics/2020-04/02/c_1125806371.htm.
36. “封城二十日里的武汉百步亭, 听社区工作者口述,” 澎湃新闻, 2020-02-13, https://www.chinanews.com.cn/m/sh/2020/02-13/9089208.shtml.
37. Quoted in 卫毅 et al., “疫情时期百步亭.”

38. 陈月芹, "万家宴后的百步亭"; 杜虎, "百步亭居民求援, 超级社区不能为掩旧错犯下新错," 狐度, 2020-02-10, https://m.sohu.com/a/371861602_665455.
39. 卫毅 et al., "疫情时期百步亭."
40. 杜虎, "百步亭居民求援, 超级社区不能为掩旧错犯下新错."
41. 蓝婧, 任江波, 王震华, "曾经举办万家宴的武汉百步亭社区, 如今是这样的," 红星深度, 2020-03-22, https://new.qq.com/omn/20200322/20200322A0FVP200.html.
42. 叶龙杰, "风雨百步亭."
43. 曹政, "武汉封城这一月."
44. "战疫27天, 中央指导组金句背后的那些事," 玉渊谭天-新华网, 2020-02-22, http://www.xinhuanet.com/politics/2020-02/22/c_1125612131.htm; video @央视频, 2020-02-22, https://weibo.com/tv/show/1034:4474874316652558.
45. 杜茂林, 杨楠, 蒋芷毓, "中央指导组抗疫55天: 小半个国务院入鄂," 南方周末, 2020-03-19, https://www.infzm.com/contents/179549.
46. Dr. Wu was also the lead expert advisor on community health for the Beijing Municipal Health Commission.
47. 曹政, "中央赴湖北指导组社区防控基层专家组负责人: 用科学方法, 打好疫情防控人民战争," 健康报, 2020-02-16, https://www.sohu.com/a/373522300_162422.
48. Jinlei Qi et al., "Short- and Medium-Term Impacts of Strict Anti-Contagion Policies on Non-COVID-19 Mortality in China," *Nature Human Behavior* (2021): 1–9.
49. 叶龙杰, "艰难防控路," 健康报, 2020-03-11, http://www.nhc.gov.cn/xcs/fkdt/202003/716dac3668b144199d04ea13a724e520.shtml.
50. 曹政, "武汉封城这一月."
51. 韩飏, "全国政协委员吴浩: 在社区战疫一线履职," 中青在线, 2020-04-22, http://m.cyol.com/yuanchuang/2020-04/22/content_18580072.htm.
52. 曹政, "中央赴湖北指导组社区防控基层专家组负责人."
53. Quoted in 叶龙杰, "艰难防控路."
54. 华凌, "吴浩: 武汉社区防控战场上的'排雷'专家," 科技日报, 2020-05-12, http://digitalpaper.stdaily.com/http_www.kjrb.com/kjrb/html/2020-05/12/content_444622.htm.
55. "武汉全市小区封闭管理, 记者探访社区如何严控流量," 长江日报, 2020-02-12, http://society.people.com.cn/n1/2020/0212/c431577-31583540.html.
56. "下沉社区 战疫有我—省直机关党员下沉社区抗疫先进事迹摘登," 湖北日报, 2020-10-26, https://www.hubei.gov.cn/hbfb/rdgz/202010/t20201026_2974978.shtml.
57. 华 凌, "吴浩."
58. 朱一梵, "吴浩: 51天, 他在武汉带领专家组梳理出1275条问题," 人民网, 2020-05-07, http://politics.people.com.cn/n1/2020/0507/c1001-31699892.html.
59. 郑皓, "来自一线的报道(3)," 中国疾病预防控制中心传染病预防控制所, 2020-03-12, https://www.icdc.cn/plus/view.php?aid=2554; "抓好源头防控、控制增量的社区排查兵," 中国疾病预防控制中心传染病预防控制所, 2020-03-13, https://www.icdc.cn/plus/view.php?aid=2560. Access to these sites was firewalled as of 2023-09-01.
60. For review of Dr. Li's treatment record, see Muyi Xiao et al., "How a Chinese Doctor Who Warned of Covid-19 Spent His Final Days," *New York Times*, 2022-10-06, https://www.nytimes.com/2022/10/06/world/asia/covid-china-doctor-li-wenliang.html.
61. 李慕琰, 杜嘉禧, "'她不用开口, 我们都感同身受': 武汉的九百万种心碎," 南方周末, 2020-02-27, http://www.infzm.com/contents/177848; Jing Xuan Teng, "Death of Chinese

Doctor Fuels Anger, Demands for Change," AFP, 2020-02-07, https://www.macaubusiness.com/death-of-chinese-doctor-fuels-anger-demands-for-change/.

62. Yingdan Lu, Jennifer Pan, and Yiqing Xu, "Public Sentiment on Chinese Social Media during the Emergence of COVID-19, "*Journal of Quantitative Description: Digital Media* 1 (2021): 1–47.
63. 王达, "疫情风暴下, 一座医院的坚守: 武汉市红十字会医院抗击新冠肺炎疫情实录," 中国红十字报, 2020-02-28, https://www.redcross.org.cn/html/2020-02/67372.html. The Wuhan Red Cross Society Hospital issued an official obituary of Dr. Xiao on February 21, 2020. "武汉市红十字会医院医生肖俊因感染新冠肺炎殉职," 中国新闻网, 2020-02-21, http://news.sina.com.cn/o/2020-02-21/doc-iimxyqvz4823953.shtml.
64. "17天内一家4口染病去世, 导演常凯遗书让人泪目," 新华社客户端, 2020-02-17, https://guancha.gmw.cn/2020-02/17/content_33562294.htm; 王润, "78岁乔榛诵读常凯导演绝笔遗书，听众为之动容落泪," 北京日报, 2020-03-12, https://ie.bjd.com.cn/5b165687a010550e5ddc0e6a/contentApp/5b21d73be4b02439500383f1/AP5e69b616e4b05e10384b3fb0.
65. 杨胜慰, "我心中的常凯," 二湘的十一维空间, 2020-05-23, https://mp.weixin.qq.com/s/BictcctU3pDx-NO4gY7ggg.
66. Marcel at large, "知情者口述."
67. Dali Yang, "China's Troubled Quest for Order: Leadership, Organization and the Contradictions of the Stability Maintenance Regime," *Journal of Contemporary China* 26, no. 103 (2017): 35–53.
68. Ran Ran and Yan Jian, "When Transparency Meets Accountability," *China Review* 21, no. 1 (2021): 7–36.
69. 周群峰, 徐天, "湖北换帅: 抗疫迎来大考," 中国新闻周刊, 2020-02-20, https://mp.weixin.qq.com/s/PkQCESwECs8DKFQesj-mgw.
70. 习近平, "在中央政治局常委会会议研究应对新型冠状病毒肺炎疫情工作时的讲话(2020-02-03)," 求是, no. 4 (2020), 2020-02-15，http://www.qstheory.cn/dukan/qs/2020-02/15/c_1125572832.htm.
71. 习近平, "在中央政治局常委会会议研究应对新型冠状病毒肺炎疫情工作时的讲话."
72. This resident used the handle "@野孩子hanniblo" in making the post, which is included in 杜虎, "百步亭居民求援, 超级社区不能为掩旧错犯下新错."
73. "习近平在北京市调研指导新型冠状病毒肺炎疫情防控工作," 新华社, 2020-02-10, www.gov.cn/xinwen/2020-02/10/content_5476997.htm.
74. "习近平在北京市调研指导新型冠状病毒肺炎疫情防控工作."
75. "习近平主持中央政治局常委会会议, 分析新冠肺炎疫情形势研究加强防控工作," 新华社, 2020-02-12, http://www.gov.cn/xinwen/2020-02/12/content_5477883.htm.
76. "武汉全市小区封闭管理, 记者探访社区如何严控流量."
77. "武汉市新冠肺炎疫情防控指挥部明确住宅小区封闭管理主要措施," 武汉市疾病预防控制中心, 2020-02-15, https://www.whcdc.org/view/1840.html; "小区为何要封闭管理? 执行得选样? 居民生活如何保障? 记者探访武汉三镇看执行," 长江日报, 2020-02-16, https://www.hubei.gov.cn/zhuanti/2020/gzxxgzbd/qfqk/202002/t20200216_2038856.shtml.
78. 周群峰, 徐天, "湖北换帅: 抗疫迎来大考."
79. "中央赴湖北指导组: 发起武汉保卫战、湖北保卫战全面总攻," 2020-02-15, 武汉市疾病预防控制中心, https://www.whcdc.org/view/1841.html.
80. "应勇主持召开专题会研究省及武汉市新冠肺炎疫情防控工作," 湖北日报, 2020-02-14, https://www.hubei.gov.cn/zwgk/hbyw/hbywqb/202002/t20200214_2027185.shtml.

81. 周群峰, 徐天, "湖北换帅: 抗疫迎来大考."
82. "陈一新战疫一个月拧紧'水龙头,'" 中央政法委长安剑, 2020-03-09, https://mp.weixin.qq.com/s?__biz=MzI0MjI0Nzc5Mg==&mid=2653919101&idx=1&sn=80db8aa3f9a97172550e99151820a6af.
83. "陈一新：军中无戏言！武汉火速查处225人、火线提拔55人," 中央政法委长安剑-澎湃新闻, 2020-03-18, https://www.thepaper.cn/newsDetail_forward_6566555.
84. 杜茂林, 杨楠, 蒋芷毓, "中央指导组抗疫55天."
85. "湖北省委书记应勇的7天," 政事儿, 2020-02-19, https://www.sohu.com/a/374317972_203783.
86. "武汉市委书记：要集中力量打歼灭战而不是松松垮垮打持久战," 长江日报, 2020-02-16, https://moment.rednet.cn/pc/content/2020/02/16/6731189.html.
87. 卫毅 et al., "疫情时期百步亭."
88. "全市拉网大排查19日交卷! 王忠林: 再发现一例居家确诊病人, 拿区委书记区长是问," 环球网, 2020-02-19, http://www.xinhuanet.com/2020-02/19/c_1125593622.htm.
89. 熊琦, "武汉: 党建引领'微治理'激活社区'大动力,'" 新华社, 2021-05-31, http://m.xinhuanet.com/hb/2021-05/31/c_1127515009.htm.
90. "武汉数万党员干部职工下沉社区, 下沉干部们在忙些啥?" 长江融媒-长江日报, 2020-02-17, https://www.hubei.gov.cn/zhuanti/2020/gzxxgzbd/qfqk/202002/t20200217_2040122.shtml.
91. 王鑫昕 et al., "武汉市开展为期3天的拉网式大排查, '五个百分之百'的决战时刻," 中国青年报, 2020-02-20, http://zqb.cyol.com/html/2020-02/20/nw.D110000zgqnb_20200220_7-01.htm; 韩飚, "全国政协委员吴浩: 在社区战疫一线履职," 中青在线, 2020-04-22, http://m.cyol.com/yuanchuang/2020-04/22/content_18580072.htm.
92. 王鑫昕 et al., "武汉市开展为期3天的拉网式大排查."
93. "拉网大排查3天, 各区交答卷," 长江日报, 2020-02-20, http://3g.wuhan.gov.cn/sy/whyw/202003/t20200316_959791.shtml.
94. 李文峰, "只希望疫情早退, 让网格恢复温暖: 武汉社区网格员的一天," 中央纪委国家监委网站, 2020-02-24, https://www.ccdi.gov.cn/yaowen/202002/t20200224_212087.html.
95. "我市上线'武汉健康码,'" 武汉发布, 2020-02-22, http://www.wuhan.gov.cn/zwgk/tzgg/202003/t20200316_972616.shtml.
96. Qing Miao, Susan Schwarz, and Gary Schwarz, "Responding to COVID-19: Community Volunteerism and Coproduction in China," *World Development* 137 (2021): 105128; "'多闻'的二月," CCTV13 央视新闻调查, 2020-03-01, https://mp.weixin.qq.com/s?__biz=MjM5MjkxNjU5NA==&mid=2651174576&idx=1&sn=e0667391863965bcda8da45ce703eed5.
97. 杨杰, "他们的'证书'是一沓沓接收函," 中国青年报-冰点周刊, 2020-03-28, https://mp.weixin.qq.com/s/s_JpnaPE9AwdzjHIfg2tdA.
98. 王姗姗, "陈珺: 一个人折射一段武汉抗疫史"; 风中葫芦, 武汉封城日记: 一个社区工作者的新冠疫情实录, 博登书屋 (New York: 博登书屋, 2021).
99. Feng Feng was a grid worker for the Huiminyuan Community in Houhu Street of Jiang'an District. 金雨蒙, 丁涛, "社区中的'网格英雄,'" 人民网, 2020-02-27, http://www.xinhuanet.com/politics/2020-02/27/c_1125633733.htm.
100. "武汉一线警务人员的战疫日记," weibo.com, 2020-10-09, https://weibo.com/ttarticle/p/show?id=2309404690309391974991.
101. 王姗姗, "陈珺."

102. Lotus Ruan, Jeffrey Knockel, and Masashi Crete-Nishihata, "Censored Contagion: How Information on the Coronavirus Is Managed on Chinese Social Media," CitizenLab, 2020-03-03, https://citizenlab.ca/2020/03/censored-contagion-how-information-on-the-coronavirus-is-managed-on-chinese-social-media/; 梓鹏, "肺炎疫情: 中国官方正能量宣传引众怒," BBC中文, 2020-02-19, https://www.bbc.com/zhongwen/simp/chinese-news-51555873.
103. Fang, *Wuhan Diary*; Yang, *Wuhan Lockdown*.
104. Liu Jiacheng, "From Social Drama to Political Performance: China's Multi-Front Combat with the COVID-19 Epidemic," *Critical Asian Studies* 52, no. 4 (2020): 473–493.
105. "Video Exposed Cheating Still Exists in Wuhan," *Global Times*, 2020-03-06, https://www.globaltimes.cn/content/1181767.shtml.
106. 风中葫芦, 武汉封城日记: 一个社区工作者的新冠疫情实录 (纽约: 博登书屋, 2021).
107. 王姗姗, "陈珺."
108. 王姗姗, "陈珺."
109. 武汉市新冠肺炎疫情防控指挥部, "关于武汉市新冠肺炎确诊病例数确诊病例死亡数订正情况的通报," 新华社, 2020-04-17, www.gov.cn/xinwen/2020-04/17/content_5503568.htm.
110. Quoted in Emily Feng, "'We No Longer Wish for Much': People of Wuhan Share Stories of Loss and Survival," NPR, 2020-06-26, https://www.npr.org/2020/06/26/882018866/we-no-longer-wish-for-much-people-of-wuhan-share-stories-of-loss-and-survival.
111. Shiyi Cao et al., "Post-Lockdown SARS-Cov-2 Nucleic Acid Screening in Nearly Ten Million Residents of Wuhan, China." *Nature Communications* 11, no. 1 (2020): 1–7.
112. "武汉市无症状感染者及其密切接触者清零," 武汉市卫生健康委员会, 2020-06-16, https://www.wuhan.gov.cn/sy/whyw/202006/t20200617_1380087.shtml.
113. "武汉市无症状感染者及其密切接触者清零."
114. Zhenyu He et al., "Seroprevalence and Humoral Immune Durability of Anti-SARS-Cov-2 Antibodies in Wuhan, China," *The Lancet* 397, no. 10279 (2021): 1075–1084.
115. 中共中央党校(国家行政学院)中共党史教研部, 中国共产党防治重大疾病的历史与经验 (北京: 人民出版社, 2020), 223.

Chapter 14

1. Horst Rittel and Melvin Webber, "Dilemmas in a General Theory of Planning," *Policy Sciences* 4, no. 2 (1973): 155–169.
2. Christopher Ansell, Eva Sørensen, and Jacob Torfing, "The COVID-19 Pandemic as a Game Changer for Public Administration and Leadership? The Need for Robust Governance Responses to Turbulent Problems," *Public Management Review* 23, no. 7 (2021): 949–960; Yibeltal Assefa et al., "Attributes of National Governance for an Effective Response to Public Health Emergencies: Lessons from the Response to the COVID-19 Pandemic," *Journal of Global Health* 12 (2022): 05021.
3. Ilan Alon, Matthew Farrell, and Shaomin Li, "Regime Type and COVID-19 Response," *FIIB Business Review* 9, no. 3 (2020): 152–160; Gabriel Cepaluni, Michael T. Dorsch, and Réka Branyiczki, "Political Regimes and Deaths in the Early Stages of the COVID-19 Pandemic," *Journal of Public Finance and Public Choice* 37, no. 1 (2022): 27–53; Michael Nelson, "The Timing and Aggressiveness of Early Government Response to COVID-19: Political Systems, Societal Culture, and More," *World Development* 146 (2021): 105550; Abiel

Sebhatu et al., "Explaining the Homogeneous Diffusion of COVID-19 Nonpharmaceutical Interventions across Heterogeneous Countries," *Proceedings of the National Academy of Sciences of the United States of America* 117, no. 35 (2020): 21201–21208.

4. Munirul Nabin, Mohammad T. H. Chowdhury, and Sukanto Bhattacharya, "It Matters to Be in Good Hands: The Relationship between Good Governance and Pandemic Spread Inferred from Cross-Country COVID-19 Data," *Humanities and Social Sciences Communications* 8, no. 1 (2021): 1–15.
5. "新型冠状病毒感染的肺炎疫情防控工作新闻发布会第九场," 湖北省人民政府网站, 2020-01-31, http://wjw.hubei.gov.cn/bmdt/dtyw/202001/t20200131_2017018.shtml.
6. Jinghua Gao and Pengfei Zhang, "China's Public Health Policies in Response to COVID-19: From an 'Authoritarian' Perspective," *Frontiers in Public Health* 9 (2021): 756677.
7. Kenneth Lieberthal and David Lampton, eds., *Bureaucracy, Politics, and Decision Making in Post-Mao China* (Berkeley: University of California Press, 1992); Kjeld Erik Brødsgaard, *Chinese Politics as Fragmented Authoritarianism* (New York: Routledge, 2017).
8. Lei Zhou et al., "One Hundred Days of Coronavirus Disease 2019 Prevention and Control in China," *Clinical Infectious Diseases* 72, no. 2 (2021): 332–339; see also 2019-nCoV Outbreak Joint Field Epidemiology Investigation Team and Qun Li, "An Outbreak of NCIP (2019-nCoV) Infection in China—Wuhan, Hubei Province, 2019–2020," *China CDC Weekly* 2, no. 5 (2020): 79–80.
9. 谢玮, "蒋超良的45天：从首批专家组抵达武汉到其被去职," 经济网, 2020-02-14, http://www.ceweekly.cn/2020/0214/285828.shtml.
10. Irving Janis and Leon Mann, *Decision Making: A Psychological Analysis of Conflict, Choice, and Commitment* (New York: Free Press, 1977); T. K. Das and Bing-Sheng Teng, "Cognitive Biases and Strategic Decision Processes: An Integrative Perspective," *Journal of Management Studies* 36, no. 6 (1999): 757–778.
11. 韩挺, "武汉时间：从专家组抵达到封城的谜之20天," 经济观察报, 2020-02-07, http://www.eeo.com.cn/2020/0207/375826.shtml.
12. 沈岿, "传染病防控信息发布的法律检讨," 爱思想, 2020-02-13, https://www.aisixiang.com/data/120144.html.
13. 杨海, "武汉早期疫情上报为何一度中断," 中国青年报-冰点周刊, 2020-03-05 https://mp.weixin.qq.com/s/69pdSrjNH_4qN3RrQ-Yk0Q.
14. "疫情可防可控—武汉市就新型冠状病毒感染的肺炎综合防控工作答记者问," 新华网, 2020-01-19, www.xinhuanet.com/politics/2020-01/19/c_1125480602.htm.
15. "疫情可防可控."
16. "疫情可防可控."
17. "国家卫生健康委积极开展新型冠状病毒感染的肺炎疫情防控工作," 卫生应急办公室, 2020-01-09, http://www.nhc.gov.cn/yjb/s7860/202001/de5f07afe8054af3ab2a25a61d19ac70.shtml.
18. "央视新闻面对面: 董倩专访武汉市长," 央视新闻, 2020-01-27, https://w.yangshipin.cn/video?type=0&vid=k000016zn3l. Video.
19. "央视新闻面对面."
20. "央视新闻面对面."
21. Elizabeth W. Morrison and Frances J. Milliken, "Organizational Silence: A Barrier to Change and Development in a Pluralistic World," *Academy of Management Review* 25, no. 4 (2000): 706–725.

22. For transmission in Wenzhou, see Wenning Li et al., "An Evaluation of COVID-19 Transmission Control in Wenzhou Using a Modified SEIR Model," *Epidemiology & Infection* 149 (2021): e2.
23. Kathy Leung et al., "First-Wave COVID-19 Transmissibility and Severity in China outside Hubei after Control Measures, and Second-Wave Scenario Planning: A Modelling Impact Assessment," *The Lancet* 395, no. 10233 (2020): 1382–1393.
24. 黄丽娜 et al., "全民战疫, 广东出击," 羊城晚报, 2020-02-05, https://m.thepaper.cn/newsDetail_forward_5827758.
25. Charles Perrow, *Normal Accidents: Living with High-Risk Technologies* (New York: Basic Books, 1984); Michael Watkins and Max Bazerman, "Predictable Surprises: The Disasters You Should Have Seen Coming," *Harvard Business Review* 81, no. 3 (2003): 72–85.
26. Paul Nutt, "Types of Organizational Decision Processes," *Administrative Science Quarterly* (1984): 414–450; Michaéla Schippers and Diana C. Rus, "Optimizing Decision-Making Processes in Times of COVID-19: Using Reflexivity to Counteract Information-Processing Failures," *Frontiers in Psychology* 12 (2021): 650525.
27. Scott Halpern, Robert Truog, and Franklin Miller, "Cognitive Bias and Public Health Policy during the COVID-19 Pandemic," *JAMA* 324, no. 4 (2020): 337–338.
28. "2020年1月26日新闻发布会文字实录," 国家卫生健康委员会, 2020-01-26, http://www.nhc.gov.cn/wjw/xwdt/202001/12ec9062d5d041f38e210e8b69b6d7ef.shtml.
29. "2020年1月26日新闻发布会文字实录."
30. "科学家对新冠病毒有了哪些新的认识? 高福院士告诉你," 新华网, 2020-12-30, www.xinhuanet.com/talking/2020-12/30/c_1210954482.htm.
31. 萧辉, 包志明, 高昱, "武汉疫情中的中南医院: 他们打满全场," 财经周刊, 14, 2020-04-13, weekly.caixin.com/2020-04-10/101540932.html; archived at https://archive.ph/vmPbn.
32. 中共中央党史和文献研究院编, 习近平关于全面从严治党论述摘编 (北京: 中央文献出版社, 2021), 153.
33. Albert Camus, *The Plague*, trans. Stuart Gilbert (New York: Modern Library, 1948), 230.
34. World Health Organization, "Naming the Coronavirus Disease (COVID-19) and the Virus That Causes It," n.d., https://www.who.int/emergencies/diseases/novel-coronavirus-2019/technical-guidance/naming-the-coronavirus-disease-(covid-2019)-and-the-virus-that-causes-it.
35. Shibo Jiang et al., "A Distinct Name Is Needed for the New Coronavirus," *The Lancet* 395, no. 10228 (2020): 949; Guizhen Wu, Jianwei Wang, and Jianqing Xu, "Voice from China: Nomenclature of the Novel Coronavirus and Related Diseases," *Chinese Medical Journal* 133, no. 09 (2020): 1012–1014.
36. World Health Organization, "Naming the Coronavirus Disease."
37. "突发急性传染病预防控制战略 (2007)," 国家卫生健康委员会, 2007-07-05, http://www.nhc.gov.cn/zwgk/wtwj/201304/5d2e5a8f7b6a4ec8951d6a1454512e43.shtml.
38. World Health Organization, "Surveillance Case Definitions for Human Infection with Novel Coronavirus (nCoV)," 2020-01-11, https://apps.who.int/iris/handle/10665/330376.
39. At least one China CDC senior official blamed the NHC leadership for squandering the opportunity gained at the end of December 2019.
40. Angran Li et al., "Human Mobility Restrictions and Inter-Provincial Migration during the COVID-19 Crisis in China," *Chinese Sociological Review* 53, no. 1 (2021): 87–113; Suoyi Tan et al., "Mobility in China, 2020: A Tale of Four Phases," *National Science Review* 8, no. 11 (2021): nwab148; Xiaoming Zhang, Weijie Luo, and Jingci Zhu, "Top-Down and

Bottom-Up Lockdown: Evidence from COVID-19 Prevention and Control in China," *Journal of Chinese Political Science* 26, no. 1 (2021): 189–211; Pengyu Zhu and Yuqing Guo, "The Role of High-Speed Rail and Air Travel in the Spread of COVID-19 in China," *Travel Medicine and Infectious Disease* 42 (2021): 102097.

41. Xu-Sheng Zhang et al., "Transmission Dynamics and Control Measures of COVID-19 Outbreak in China: A Modelling Study," *Scientific Reports* 11, no. 1 (2021): 1–12; 王思聪 et al., "基于人口流动数据研究武汉"封城"对中国2019冠状病毒病疫情态势的影响," 浙江大学学报 (医学版) 50, no. 1 (2021): 61–67.
42. Matteo Chinazzi et al., "The Effect of Travel Restrictions on the Spread of the 2019 Novel Coronavirus (COVID-19) Outbreak," *Science* 368, no. 6489 (2020): 395–400.
43. Zifeng Yang et al., "Modified SEIR and AI Prediction of the Epidemics Trend of COVID-19 in China under Public Health Interventions," *Journal of Thoracic Disease* 12, no. 3 (2020): 165–174.
44. Zhang et al., "Transmission Dynamics and Control Measures."
45. Based on data analytics, there was a total of about 9,600 visitors to the Huanan Seafood Market in the month of December 2019. 张丹丹, "73岁李兰娟: 这个险我是一定要冒的," 环球人物, 2020-04-02, https://www.msweekly.com/show.html?id=118124 .
46. "武汉市卫健委关于当前我市肺炎疫情的情况通报," 武汉市卫生健康委员会, 2019-12-31, https://wjw.wuhan.gov.cn/gsgg/202004/t20200430_1199576.shtml.
47. Yingdan Lu, Jennifer Pan, and Yiqing Xu, "Public Sentiment on Chinese Social Media during the Emergence of COVID-19, "*Journal of Quantitative Description: Digital Media* 1 (2021): 1–47.

Appendix 2

1. "传中风入院'神隐'42天, 湖北省长王晓东露面," 2020-11-04, https://www.zaobao.com.sg/realtime/china/story20201104-1098225.
2. 蒋子文, "王艳玲任湖北省人大常委会党组书记·马国强任副书记," 澎湃新闻, 2023-01-18, https://www.thepaper.cn/newsDetail_forward_21601713.

Index

For the benefit of digital users, indexed terms that span two pages (e.g., 52–53) may, on occasion, appear on only one of those pages.

Tables and figures are indicated by *t* and *f* following the page number